STRINGS ATTACHED

AIDS and the Rise of Transnational Connections in Africa

PROCEEDINGS OF THE BRITISH ACADEMY • 194

STRINGS ATTACHED

AIDS and the Rise of Transnational Connections in Africa

Edited by
NADINE BECKMANN,
ALESSANDRO GUSMAN
AND
CATRINE SHROFF

Published for THE BRITISH ACADEMY
by OXFORD UNIVERSITY PRESS

Oxford University Press, Great Clarendon Street, Oxford OX2 6DP

First edition published in 2014

British Library Cataloguing in Publication Data
Data available

Library of Congress Cataloging in Publication Data
Data available

Typeset by Keystroke, Station Road, Codsall, Wolverhampton

Printed in Great Britain by

TJ International, Padstow, Cornwall

ISBN 978–0–19–726568–0

ISSN 0068–1202

FSC
www.fsc.org
MIX
Paper from responsible sources
FSC® C013056

Contents

Preface and Acknowledgements

This book is the result of the conference *Sexuality, AIDS and Religion: Transnational Dynamics in Africa*, which was held at Oxford University in September 2011. The Fertility and Reproduction Studies Group (FRSG) at the University of Oxford, and the Religion, Aids and Social Transformation in Africa research network (RASTA) co-hosted the event. Our heartfelt thanks go to the John Fell Fund, the Institute of Social and Cultural Anthropology, the African Studies Centre and St Antony's College at the University of Oxford for providing the necessary funds to bring together scholars and practitioners working on HIV/AIDS and religion in sub-Saharan Africa, the region of the world hardest hit by the global AIDS pandemic.

While much has been written about religions' and religious institutions' roles in the unfolding of HIV/AIDS epidemics in different parts of the world, little attention has been paid to the ways in which transnational relations influence the interrelations between religion, sexuality and AIDS in Africa. Most religious institutions and faith-based organisations work together with partners inside, as well as outside, the continent, but although these relations are known to be crucial for the flows of ideas and resources in relation to HIV/AIDS, there is very limited knowledge on the transnational dynamics of views on sexuality in relation to HIV/AIDS and religion in Africa. The conference explored these themes through a number of exciting panels, analysing the negotiation of policies within transnational faith-based organisations and the roles of diaspora in transnational collaboration, issues of technology and transnational family planning, the role of sexual networks and the value of sex, homosexuality and transgressive sexualities, and the creation of transnational moralities through HIV programmes.

We were fortunate to have an excellent range of speakers, including some of the pioneers in the field of AIDS research, a number of younger academics from various European, North American and southern African countries, many of whom presented data fresh from the field, and activists and practitioners working in the UK and on the African continent. We thank Professor Terence Ranger, Professor Brooke Grundfest Schoepf, Professor Robert Thornton, Professor Suzette Heald, and Reverend Ijeoma Ajibade for inspirational keynote presentations and for their valuable contributions to the discussions.

A major theme emerging from the conference papers and debates was the diversification of transnational approaches to fighting HIV/AIDS in Africa, and an apparent trend towards conservatism within global agendas in the field. For a long time, religion has been regarded as an obstacle to the successful implementation of HIV/AIDS intervention programmes, especially in the realm of prevention. However, numerous presentations showed that we can no longer equate religion with conservative approaches, or transnational dynamics with largely promoting more liberal agendas. We thank our discussants Professor Elisabeth Hsu, Professor Rijk van Dijk, Professor Hansjörg Dilger, Dr Ben Jones, Dr Marian Burchardt and Dr Ruth Prince for raising important questions on these themes.

Professor Rijk van Dijk has been an indispensable colleague in our struggle to understand the transnational dynamics of AIDS and religion in Africa. Thank you for teaming up with us in the introductory chapter and for taking the discussions one step further in the epilogue.

Our special thanks to all the participants, who made this work such an exciting and rewarding endeavour, and to the reviewers for their productive comments on the manuscript.

Nadine Beckmann, Alessandro Gusman and Catrine Shroff
September 2013

Contributors

Reverend Ijeoma Ajibade is a Church of England priest, ministering at St Philip's Church, Earls Court and at Southwark Cathedral in London. Alongside ministry she has worked in the UK public sector for twenty-three years. Her work on HIV has involved seeking to mobilise the church to address HIV through its ministry and mission. In 2009 she developed a training course for clergy in the diocese of Southwark which looks at the issue of HIV from theological and ethical perspectives. Ijeoma has also been involved in governance for UK-based sexual health organisations including the Naz Project London, where she was vice-chair, and the African Health Policy Network, where she was secretary to the board.

Brenda Bartelink is finalising her PhD thesis on religion, HIV/AIDS and sexuality in transnational development relations at the University of Groningen, the Netherlands. Since June 2012, she has worked at the Knowledge Centre on Religion and Development to facilitate and stimulate reflections on religion by Dutch development NGOs. She holds an MA in the Academic Study of Religion and a BA in Nursing.

Nadine Beckmann is a lecturer in social anthropology at the University of Roehampton. She holds a PhD from the University of Oxford (2008), where she was a postdoctoral researcher and deputy director of the Fertility and Reproduction Studies Group before joining Roehampton in 2012. Her research focuses on HIV/AIDS and Islam, the management of sexuality and reproduction, bio-politics, and notions of morality and uncertainty in Zanzibar.

Anaïs Bertrand-Dansereau is a sociologist with an interest in gender, health and youth in postcolonial contexts. She holds a PhD (2013) from the Graduate Institute of International and Development Studies (IHEID), in Geneva, and a master's (2010) from UQÀM, in Canada. Her research focuses on the lives of young people in Malawi, understood through both discourses of HIV prevention and the narratives of their own experiences of love, relationships and intimacy. She is now a post-doctoral researcher at the Centre on Population Dynamics, at McGill University.

Astrid Bochow is a research fellow at the Max Planck Institute for Social Anthropology Halle/Saale (since 2010). She was previously a researcher and PhD candidate at the University of Bayreuth (2004 to 2009) and a postdoctoral researcher at the Freie Universität Berlin (2009). She publishes on reproduction, sexuality,

Christianity and HIV/AIDS, and has authored a monograph entitled 'Intimacy and Sexuality before Marriage in Kumasi, Ghana' (in German). In 2012 she was a Visiting Scholar at Oxford University, and she was granted a junior fellowship at the University of Constance in 2012–13.

Lindsay Ehrisman is a graduate student of African History and Gender at San Francisco State University. Her research explores the ways in which historical epistemologies inform contemporary normative sexual identities in Uganda.

Alessandro Gusman (PhD, 2008) is a postdoctoral researcher in anthropology at the University of Turin. Since 2004 he has been a member of the Italian Ethnological Mission in Equatorial Africa. His research focuses on the social and political impact of Pentecostal churches in Uganda, and on the link between religion and the HIV/AIDS epidemic in the country. Since 2005 he has also conducted research in Italy, in the field of the anthropology of death and in medical anthropology, with a particular focus on funeral rites among migrant communities, and on palliative care. He is the author of a book, *Antropologia dell'olfatto* (2004), and of several articles which have appeared in national and international books and journals.

Erik Meinema is a recent graduate of the Research Master Religion and Culture at the University of Groningen. During his studies, he did fieldwork on religion, sexuality and youth in Kenya and Uganda, and youth peace-building initiatives in Ambon, Indonesia.

Alexandra Müller is a postdoctoral research fellow in the School of Public Health and Family Medicine at the University of Cape Town (South Africa). She holds a PhD in Medical Sociology from the University of Göttingen (Germany), and is a qualified physician. She identifies as a queer, white, anti-racist, feminist scholar, and her work focuses on health rights for sexual minorities, medical education and critical whiteness.

Isak Niehaus is a lecturer in social anthropology at Brunel University in London. He has done extensive research on issues such as witchcraft, politics and masculinity in South African rural areas. He is the author of *Witchcraft, Power and Politics: Exploring the Occult in the South African Lowveld* (with Eliazaar Mohlala and Kally Shokane, 2001), *Magic* (with Fraser McNeill, 2010) and *Witchcraft and a Life in the New South Africa* (2013).

Christine Obbo is a Ugandan social cultural anthropologist who has done extensive research in both rural and urban areas on issues of gender and social change. This focus inevitably led to work on HIV/AIDS, highlighting rights and responsibility. Her writing examines how Christianity and economic development exacerbate local ideologies that frame and perpetuate social and economic gender inequalities. She was a professor at Wheaton College and Wayne State University, in addition to brief visits to other institutions; and has been a consultant for international organisations on identifying unwitting constraints of development policies, and recommending participatory research strategies that promote the success of food poverty and HIV/AIDS projects.

Amy S. Patterson is Professor of Politics at the University of the South, Tennessee. She is author of *The Politics of AIDS in Africa* (2006) and *The Church and AIDS in Africa: The Politics of Ambiguity* (2011). She was a Fulbright scholar in Zambia in 2011. She teaches courses on African politics, global health governance, and political development.

Louise Mubanda Rasmussen is Assistant Professor in International Development Studies at Roskilde University, Denmark. Between 2006 and 2009 she researched various HIV/AIDS interventions in Uganda with an emphasis on Catholic organisations. She obtained her PhD in African Studies from the University of Copenhagen in 2011 on the basis of a thesis titled 'From dying with dignity to living with rules: AIDS treatment and "holistic care" in Catholic organisations in Uganda'. She is currently working on a research project on the local experiences with celebrity-driven development projects in Malawi.

Joanna Sadgrove is a specialist on religion, sexuality and cross-cultural encounter. Her early work focused on Uganda; more recently she has worked on southern Africa, India and the Caribbean. She has published on homosexuality in Uganda and the Anglican Communion, sexual behaviour and religious belonging, and religious identities and cross-cultural change. She currently works as a researcher for the United Society (formerly USPG) and as a consultant for the Anglican Communion-affiliated *Continuing Indaba* project.

Brooke Grundfest Schoepf is an economic and medical anthropologist (PhD Columbia University, 1969). Following fieldwork in England, France and the US, she began research and teaching in Zaire (now Democratic Republic of Congo) in 1974. With African colleagues in Kinshasa in 1985, Schoepf began to study popular representations of AIDS. The *Projet CONNAISSIDA* (knowledge of AIDS) used an approach linking political economy with culture and agency to demonstrate the role of gender relations, poverty and global inequality in driving the epidemic, and experimented with community-based empowerment methods for HIV prevention. From 1991, she drafted AIDS prevention policy strategies as a consultant to UNICEF, UNDP, WHO, and UNAIDS. Schoepf has worked in fourteen countries in Africa.

Catrine Shroff (formerly Christiansen), PhD, is a social anthropologist with extensive research experience on the intersection of religion, health, and development. She has published on religion in development aid, church development, youth and social becoming, and the social impact of HIV/AIDS in Uganda. She is vice-chair of the research network on Religion, AIDS and Social Transformation in Africa (RASTA). She lives in Kenya where she works as a researcher and a consultant.

Jonas Svensson is Associate Professor in the Study of Religion, with a PhD in Islamic Studies. He is currently Senior Lecturer at Linnaeus University, Sweden. Mainly specialising in contemporary Muslim religious discourses on issues such as gender and human rights, he has also done fieldwork on Islamic religious education in Kisumu, Kenya. His chapter in this volume is part of a project on contemporary Muslim theological thinking on HIV/AIDS and Islam financed by Riksbankens Jubileumsfond.

Jack Ume Tocco is Visiting Assistant Professor of Anthropology at Rutgers University. He holds a 2013 PhD in anthropology and a master's in public health from the University of Michigan. His research on HIV/AIDS and Islam focuses on prophetic and biomedical treatment modalities, kinship and sexuality, and masculinities in Northern Nigeria. He has conducted research as a consultant for several international organizations in Nigeria.

Rijk van Dijk is an anthropologist and senior researcher at the African Studies Centre at the University of Leiden. He is an expert on Pentecostalism, globalisation and transnationalism, migration, youth and healing, in Malawi, Ghana and Botswana. He is the author of *Young Malawian Puritans* (1993) and has co-edited seven other books including *The Quest for Fruition through Ngoma* (with Ria Reis and Marja Spierenburg, 2000) and *Situating Globality: African Agency in the Appropriation of Global Culture* (with Wim van Binsbergen, 2004). His current research deals with religious, in particular Pentecostal, engagement with the domains of sexuality and HIV/AIDS in Botswana. He is also chair of the research network on Religion, AIDS, and Social Transformation in Africa (RASTA), and editor-in-chief of the journal *African Diaspora: A Journal of Transnational Africa in a Global World*, which has been published by Brill since 2008.

1

Introduction

Strings Attached: AIDS and the Rise of Transnational Connections in Africa

NADINE BECKMANN, ALESSANDRO GUSMAN,
CATRINE SHROFF AND RIJK VAN DIJK

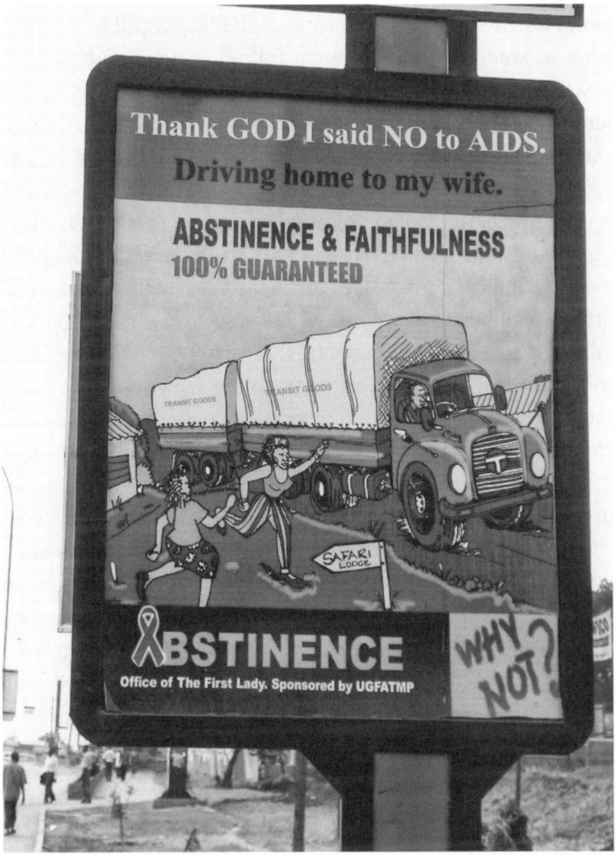

Uganda poster, 2005

Proceedings of the British Academy **194**, *1–27*. © The British Academy 2014.

Transnational dynamics in the AIDS pandemic in Africa

DURING THE LAST TWENTY-FIVE YEARS, AIDS has profoundly impacted the African continent, not only at the epidemiological level, but also in the social, political and economic realm. Not least, it has changed the way people look at sexuality. In this process, HIV prevention campaigns placed sex at the centre of the AIDS pandemic, and early risk group categorisations, combined with the voices of religious leaders and local networks of rumour and gossip, lent the pandemic strong moral connotations at global as well as at local levels. Hence, popular understandings of the disease and risk of infection frequently refer to an interpretative grid that draws on a religious moral framework. In many parts of Africa (and the world at large) AIDS is represented as 'God's punishment' for social corruption and moral decay. This is particularly true in the increasingly popular Pentecostal churches, but a similar approach is also present among mainstream Christians and in various Muslim discourses.

AIDS has not left the religious landscape unaffected. Similar to earlier pandemics in Africa, such as smallpox and the great influenza pandemic of 1918, religious innovation – which does not by definition preclude but which may very well include the strengthening of conservative demands – has been part of the response to the crisis brought about by a disease threatening the collapse of societies. According to the historical literature on the connections between religious renewal and disease in Africa, epidemics trigger movements of prophetic innovation within African religious traditions, Christianity and Islam (Ranger 1992). In Nigeria, for example, the Aladura prophetic healing churches arose out of the memory of a quarter of a million people who died during the influenza pandemic in 1918, and it was in the context of epidemics and upheaval that a movement of popular Islam arose on the East African coast and Islam spread for the first time from the coast to the societies in the interior (Ranger 1992). Concurrent with the rapid emergence and persistence of AIDS, leading to millions of deaths and leaving an even larger number of children orphaned, Christian and Muslim renewal movements, 'characterised by their demand for exclusive commitment and for a fundamentally restructured everyday life, often focusing on mundane practices' (Becker and Geissler 2009: 6), have spread across Africa.

Besides contributing to the emergence of new, radical religious movements, AIDS has presented an opportunity for many religious organisations to take a more prominent role in the public sphere (Gusman 2009; Christiansen[1] 2009; Prince *et al.* 2009). Religious institutions, such as churches and mosques, and faith-based development organisations, such as World Vision, have been active in promoting sexual education and HIV prevention programmes and are at the forefront of providing for the sick. However, these organisations have been criticised for increasing the stigmatisation of people living with the disease and for promoting

[1] Christiansen was the maiden name of Catrine Shroff, one of the co-authors.

ineffective ways of prevention, for example through over-emphasising abstinence and faithfulness while condemning condom use. In other words, religious groups and institutions have been playing a crucial role in the moralisation of the disease and in the setting of public and private moral agendas concerning sexuality, the body and relationships.

These processes are shaped by local particularities, but also take place within a context of extensive transnational interrelationships. How precisely these religious groups and institutions are placed in a modern world of global exchanges and local interactions is the focus of this book. Many religious bodies are profoundly interconnected with similar bodies elsewhere, outside of their local context and even outside the continent. The proliferation of programmes in the fight against AIDS, as well as the moral agendas that have come to be part of it, have been developed in exchange with, and are heavily supported by, organisations and institutions that have their headquarters in other parts of the world, especially in the West. While many of the religious and AIDS-based groups in Africa have been actively pursuing transnational connections with overseas organisations, or, vice versa, have become the target, or perhaps even the product, of these transnational relations, these connections are never devoid of underlying, scripted, hidden, or rather explicit moral codes or agendas for social action. In other words, *there are strings attached.* While scholars have pointed to the important roles religion plays in the moralisation of sexuality throughout the African continent, the roles of transnational connections in shaping this interaction with HIV/AIDS have remained largely unexplored. Most religious institutions and faith-based organisations work together with partners in and outside the continent, but although these connections are known to be crucial for the flows of ideas and resources in relation to HIV/AIDS, there is very limited knowledge of the transnational dynamics of views on sexuality in relation to HIV/AIDS and religion in Africa.

Against this background, this book is concerned with the ways in which transnational connections influence the interrelations between religion, sexuality, and AIDS in Africa. More specifically, it explores the relationship between transnationalism and the forceful introduction of specific moral agendas in the local scene, cultivating the common reference to a religious moral framework for understandings of the pandemic in Africa.

We regard this powerful religious framework as often enacting a conservative moral agenda promoting hetero-normativity, faithfulness and non-marital abstinence and conservative family values, which appears in stark juxtaposition with liberal 'safe-sex' approaches often found in the West. Arguing that matters of sexual morality have been at the centre of conservative political agendas and a central concern in religious and transnational public health interventions, we thus highlight the links between conservatism and a dominant trajectory in the flows of (religious) transnational resources, ideas, attitudes and expertise. We find this linkage deeply problematic since it seems to corroborate stereotyped ideas of what religion is doing in the context of AIDS and sexuality, while ignoring counter-movements among both Christian and Muslim communities and organisations aiming to move away from that conservatism and find new ways of approaching the moral dilemmas posed by HIV/AIDS. Moreover, this linkage raises the question of what exactly conservatism is in an African context, since we cannot a priori assume that our Western categories of conservatism and progressiveness correspond with African perceptions. The different perceptions and local uses of the categories 'liberal' and 'conservative' have been well described for example in studies on Pentecostalism in Africa, as Pentecostalism seems to pursue the rise of the modern, individual believer whose subjectivity enacts anti-traditional, anti-cultural stances that seem very critical of the position of the otherwise conservative views of elderly authority or the conservative mainline Christianity. This is known as the Pentecostal 'break with the past' (Meyer 1998; van Dijk 1998), which seems to promote a more liberal attitude of the individual, but which should not be mistaken for its otherwise highly conservative agenda when it comes to gender-roles, and the disciplining of sexuality and of relationships.

Not all transnational connections in the domain of religion, AIDS and sexuality are necessarily conservative in their socio-political meaning and effects; there are counter-movements to the permeating conservative agenda that vie for more liberal openings in public debates and (governmental) policies. This creates a triangle of transnationalism, conservatism and liberalism within the domain of AIDS and sexuality in Africa. Homosexuality is an excellent example of a 'double loop' where transnational advocacy networks try to contest conservatism by arguing for the universality of a human right to sexual freedom and liberalism, and explicitly reject Christian public morality, at the same time as Christian (especially) transnational alliances work towards enhancing Christian public morality and government policies that criminalise homosexual practices. It is from an analytical starting point in a triangle consisting of transnational connections, conservative moral agendas, and various forms of contestation that this book contributes to the fields of AIDS, religion, sexuality, and transnationalism in Africa.

Transnational relations and conservative agendas

In AIDS research, especially in various parts of Africa, the so-called global-health perspective has become dominant in the past years (Smith and Whiteside 2010; Holden 2003). Through this perspective attention has been drawn to the processes of the circulation, distribution and engagement with a range of AIDS-related biomedical interventions, pharmaceuticals, policies and flows of resources in which international donors play a substantial part. In particular, this perspective analyses how knowledge and technologies that are globally produced in the world of biomedical treatment, prevention and care interact with and encroach upon local medical practices. It investigates interdependencies as well as the power relations and moralities that govern these relationships, unequal as they largely are since local medical providers, institutions or cultural arrangements usually lack the means to produce this global engagement on their own terms.

Whereas in the study of AIDS, devoting attention to local-global relations is pertinent and it has become clear that many of the international players, institutions, agendas and policies have been impacting on local realities in Africa, the precise nature of the linkages and connections across borders and an international field of relations has not been well understood. This can be explored from the perspective of transnational studies. The interrelations and interdependencies between local bodies, individuals, groups, institutions and their counterparts elsewhere are part of a field of transnational relations in which these connections manifest themselves *directly* in the life-worlds of AIDS patients and their caretakers. In many cases AIDS groups maintain a set of international links that are of direct importance for their operation, their resources, their notions of behavioural change policies, and their links with the structures of (political) power in their respective societies. We are introducing a transnational perspective in this field and argue for the analytical distinction between a global perspective on AIDS and a transnational perspective on AIDS. There are many reasons to propose this.

First of all, we must keep in mind that the HIV/AIDS pandemic and its interventions are not exclusively nationally contained or globally shaped, but effectively transnational. A transnational perspective on AIDS draws attention to the crossing of nation-state borders and boundaries. As such it recognises the need to acknowledge that AIDS – as a disease and as a phenomenon of producing specific interventions, policies, discourses, practices and disciplines – is not contained by individual nation-states. While states are based on the control of territory and their people, the relationship between people, culture and place is highly intersected in the context of AIDS (Ferguson and Gupta 1997). AIDS does not stop at the border, and many aspects of the spread of the disease as well as efforts to curb it seem to undercut the control of the state over a particular territory and its people. This does not make the experience of the disease on the part of the nation-state in any particular sense 'global', as it relates more directly to the limitations of the state's (biomedical) institutions of control in curtailing the flow of the disease, its control over the people who cross borders and are involved in its spread, or over the organisations, movements and groups that are forging links across distances.

Secondly, a transnational perspective draws attention to those institutions and organisations that aim to transform subjectivities and create a new or different sense of belonging; a belonging to wider communities, to wider frames of identification with changing notions of citizenship. In a profound way the transnational perspective is a critical perspective, as it points at those configurations of identity formation that nation-states do not control, or that even oppose, contest or reject a society's established forms of power, citizenship or cultural identity. This perspective has been studied particularly in the context of sociological enquiries of social movements whereby attention was drawn to the rise of so-called transnational advocacy networks (TANs). Examples of these can be found in such organisations as Greenpeace, Amnesty International, Human Rights Watch, Survival International, or the Treatment Action Campaign (TAC). As Nguyen (2009) shows in his work on 'therapeutic citizenship', AIDS has provided a space for people to form communities and share identities on the basis of a common plight and a common agenda across national and cultural divides. Through the modern media and means of communication these processes of shaping one's identity in conjunction with those of likeminded people in an entirely different part of the world have not only become extremely powerful – for instance in the way these processes of forming patient-interest and support bodies impact governmental policies – but have become significant in penetrating relatively marginalised places in Africa. One of the most well-known examples of this form of transnational advocacy network that managed to create an internal power-base within African societies can be found in AIDS self-help and support groups (such as TASO originating in Uganda) and in the South African Treatment Action Campaign, vying for the introduction of free antiretroviral medicines for a community of sufferers. The kind of identity formation emerging within social movements that cross-cut borders and boundaries in itself does not say much about the social-political nature of the critical agenda that might be pursued; in other words this transnational advocacy can contain both 'conservative' and 'progressive' moral notions in its agenda.

A third dimension that renders a transnational perspective on AIDS relevant is to gain a better understanding of the internal dynamics of an international body, organisation or institution. Based on an understanding of organisations as sites of heterogeneity and contradictions rather than static systems of rationalism and unity (Kassimir 2001; Wright 1994; March and Olsen 1989), the internal dynamics of organisations can be conceptualised as 'politics' in the sense of power struggles for the fixation of meaning, decision-making, and resource allocation, or for constituting social interactions in certain ways (Laclau and Mouffe 1985). Thus all actors involved in the establishment, maintenance or contestation of the policy and practices in an organisational context engage in 'politics' (Mosse 2005; Hilhorst 2003). An (AIDS) organisation may have its headquarters in the West and an office in Africa, thereby forging an internal transnational connection between the two along which people, ideas, policies and resources may flow. This internal transnational dynamic shows institutional autonomy (March and Olsen 1989) and demonstrates how relative autonomy arises in ways of operation at different sites of a transnational organisation (DiMaggio and Powel 1983). The latter is particularly relevant in development aid where a 'long chain of organisation' connects various types of organisations operating at different levels and in different contexts (Mosse 2005; Ferguson 1990).

This raises questions as to how organisations formulate policies on sexuality; who is involved in the process, and who has the power to make the decisions?

Considering the transnational flows of ideas and resources, predominantly from the West, but increasingly also from other parts of the world, such as the Arab countries, to Africa and vice versa, what is the room for manoeuvre for staff in African contexts to reconcile the organisational policy on sexuality with their own views or local circumstances? How do changing practices on the ground – for example Baptist pastors who decide to encourage the use of condoms because they observe that abstinence does not work – feed into policy revisions at the level of the headquarters of a transnational body? In other words, what characterises the flows of ideas from the local to the global in terms of altering organisational policy? Do the kinds of negotiations differ between religious organisations, such as churches, and religious development organisations, such as Muslim Aid or Christian Aid?

One of the most important fields of research on this point has been the study of the transnational dynamics of religious organisations in Africa and beyond. How exactly are international connections, linkages and flows engaged, by whom and for what reasons? In Africa, religion is a domain where linkages with bodies and institutions in other parts of the world have been considered crucial for institution-building, access to resources (both material and immaterial), the circulation of people and leadership, and the negotiation of moral notions and agendas. These concrete transnational linkages may mean a great deal for the positioning of its internal leadership, the ways in which external resources are attracted to particular initiatives within its local work and the ways in which leaders feel they are related to wider frameworks of identity and action.

Fourthly, a transnational perspective is particularly related to notions of mobility; one line of transnational study is focusing on the rise of so-called 'transnational social fields' (Glick Schiller 2005a, 2005b; Caglar 2006). This line of investigation analyses migration and the ways in which migrants forge intricate international networks through which both 'home' and their location elsewhere remain connected in one sphere of social interaction and exchange. It signals the loss of sharp cultural and geographical divides: the ability to make use of all the modern means of transport and communication means that migrants do not simply leave one cultural domain and face the difficulty of establishing and integrating in another cultural domain. In the domain of AIDS in Africa this aspect of transnational research on the rise and formation of transnational social fields has become particularly relevant in understanding the effect of mobility and the structural implications for AIDS care, treatment and prevention. While migration and mobility may have been causative factors in the spread of AIDS (truck-drivers, sex workers, migrant relationships, transnational marriages, and the like), the same factors also had effects on how AIDS patients were treated and cared for at home; the rendering available of resources, medicines, knowledge, and so forth.

Yet, in addition to migration and the creation of transnational social fields, mobility must also be understood in terms of the flows of ideas, knowledge, images and techniques along similar lines. For example the rise of images of AIDS celebrities that entered the public profiling of AIDS organisations in the West (usually in the service of fundraising campaigns) can be analysed as the result of social fields that link localities and institutions intimately in different parts of the world. Biomedical and social techniques (such as the introduction of the condom, counselling and behavioural change campaigns, or antiretroviral treatment) similarly travel along transnational paths, interconnecting a community of clients, users, experts and professionals along similar notions. In one sense these trajectories thereby create corridors for the introduction of liberal notions on sexuality, the body and relationships that are particularly supported by the rise of the modern media; young people in Africa share views about the adoption of liberal ideas and techniques with their counterparts in other parts of the world through the use of the internet, Facebook, mobile phones and so forth. Yet while this global world of exchange has opened up, in the context of this book we note the remarkable capacity of transnational linkages also to introduce rather opposing views about sexuality, the body and relationships; views that in particular exchange ideas on discipline, bodily control and the containment of sexuality within rigid moral and doctrinal lines. While many African societies have been marked by high 'expectations of modernity', as Ferguson (1999) called it, the transnational connections that many groups and institutions in Africa engaged in were and are often not pursuing a liberal modernist view of the person and of society. In many cases, transnational organisations such as PEPFAR, World Vision and a range of other faith-based organisations active in Africa do have great difficulty with advocating a liberalist modernity in Africa that would promote sexuality as the free right of every sexually active person, sexuality as a domain of pleasure and play, or the right of women to have full control over their reproductive capacities and hence their bodies. While Africa increasingly became part of a global modernity in terms of the ways in which modern means of communication, education and development became part of everyday life and the creation of modern subjectivities, the transnational connections were and are not evidently and automatically part of that process, nor do they declare themselves a priori to be congruent with a modernist agenda.

Transnational powers and local agency: trajectories of a conservative agenda

One of the main themes emerging from the essays composing the present volume is the existence of significant gaps between 'top-down' policies and practices 'on the ground'; between the intentions of international donors funding HIV/AIDS prevention and care programmes and the obtained results; and between the 'official', public face of this prevention, and the practised, private, interventions observed in the work of those involved in such programmes in religious organisations (i.e. the discrepancy reported in this volume by Louise Mubanda Rasmussen between AIDS prevention education and HIV counselling in a Catholic organisation in Uganda; or the colliding viewpoints and negotiations between donors and local faith-based organisations (FBOs) highlighted in Brenda Bartelink and Erik Meinema's analysis).

So, on the one hand, one can observe the presence of powerful transnational forces directing the development of HIV prevention programmes through the injection of large amounts of money and the design of universal, blueprint approaches to HIV interventions implemented across the globe; on the other hand, ethnographic research evidences the presence of a certain room for manoeuvre at the local level, where the universal, often oversimplifying messages contained in international policies are re-elaborated and negotiated to fit with local contexts. Health professionals, 'volunteers' and employees of the local organisations are often able to overcome the rules and the restrictions contained in the policies designed far from the place where they operate, and this is at least in part due to the loose nature these rules have because of their universality. The level of heterogeneity observed in local religious actors' responses to AIDS thus not only reflects diversities among different religious affiliations, but also highlights the adaptation of international programmes to local realities (see Patterson, Chapter 6, this volume).

These considerations raise essential questions about the interactions between global and local levels, concerning, on the one hand, how and to what extent transnational powers are able to direct religious responses and to shape local moral worlds in accordance with the 'transnational morality' pushed by the conservative agenda, and conveyed amongst other ways through HIV/AIDS programmes; and, on the other, how and to what extent local religious, political and social actors' agency is able to create forms of resistance, negotiation and sometimes even subversion of these global-local flows.

The importance of understanding how the macro-level political economies affect socio-cultural dynamics at the micro-level, including the social response to epidemics, was clear from the beginning of the AIDS epidemic (Schoepf 1988). Paul Farmer was one of the first to illustrate with ethnographic richness the fact that local moralities and sexualities need to be understood in connection with the global system, his focus being especially on the constraining historical and economic processes and forces that limit people's agency (Farmer 1999). In his analysis, suffering is the result of 'structural violence', the incorporation of global forces largely overcoming the individual's possibilities of acting reflexively to decide for his/her own life. While Farmer is right in arguing that structural forces often limit individuals' agency at the local level, the claim that structural forces practically pre-define individual destinies is not substantiated in most of the cases discussed in this volume. However, his call for a 'geographically broad' analysis in order to understand the local dynamics has been pivotal to at least partially refocusing AIDS prevention in terms of structural conditions instead of 'individual risk behaviour'.

A different perspective has been recently elaborated, which starts from James Ferguson's proposal to situate grassroots analysis within the new, transnational 'power topographies' that have emerged in the contemporary situation (Ferguson 2006). Ferguson's concept of power topographies is not only thought-provoking, but also very relevant to the topic we are investigating: according to Ferguson, the increased interest for 'civil society' which anthropologists and political scientists have been showing since the 1990s rests upon the assumption of the existence of a 'vertical topography of power' in which the local, national and global levels are analytically subdivided, and where, following the Hegelian dialectic scheme, civil society stays as a medium term between the state and the family. Starting from this view, the state in Africa has been increasingly considered as an obstacle to 'development', and civil society as a local, dynamic space suffocated by the presence of often despotic states; thus, empowering the intermediate level would result in a limitation of the power of the state, and provide new routes to democratisation and individuals' participation in society and politics. Ferguson's critique of this perspective focuses on the fact that this scheme gives the African state a much bigger power than it has in reality, forgetting that the dominant forces in the continent have usually been external forces, eroding the sovereignty of the state: colonial governments and missions in the past, transnational organisations and institutions such as the World Bank and the International Monetary Fund today. Indeed, according to Ferguson, the view that opposes state and civil society is misleading in that it hinders an accurate understanding of the work of governance which transnational actors exercise in the African continent. Moreover, it often naively assumes a 'civil society' that is largely composed of 'local' organisations; but, as Ferguson notes, most of the organisations that operate in Africa today, including churches and FBOs, cannot be described as 'national' or 'local', but are on the contrary 'transnational' in their nature, or at least maintain important transnational connections. Thus, these organisations do not easily fit in the vertical topography of 'state – civil society – individuals', but are 'integral parts of a new transnational apparatus of governmentality' (Ferguson 2006: 103); they are not below the state, but operate at a horizontal level with it, and in the same space.

Ferguson's arguments resonate with the idea of 'extraversion' proposed by Jean-François Bayart, in which dependence may become a 'mode of action' (2000); in both perspectives, the marginalisation of Africa in the contemporary world does not mean that there are no ties between the African continent and the rest of the world, but rather that these connections assume the nature of ties of dependence, from which an African elite benefits. Thus, patron–client networks, that have been common in African politics for a long time, extend to the relationships among donors and local organisations in the context of AIDS governance (Swidler 2007, 2009); dependence becomes a strategy to connect to the world and to attract funds from external donors, a way of maintaining a form of agency within an unequal relation, both in the political and in the religious sphere (Maxwell 2000). The need, and desire, for transnational connections in order to establish and to enlarge a religious congregation, or to start a programme in a faith-based organisation, clearly contrasts with the asserted 'independence' of many churches (mainly Pentecostal), and creates specific religious forms of extraversion, with many of the emerging local congregations largely depending on external connections for their existence (Englund 2003). In this way, as Erica Bornstein (2002) has pointed out, development becomes more NGO-driven than state-driven, as these organisations receive funds directly from international sources. This is especially true in exceptional situations of crisis, as in the case of Zimbabwe in the late 1990s analysed by Bornstein, but more and more also in 'normal' conditions, with churches and FBOs changing their focus and planning their interventions according to the availability of international funds for specific programmes (Patterson 2011; Christiansen 2010).

These considerations are clearly also valid with regard to HIV/AIDS policies: although World Health Organization (WHO) and UNAIDS policy statements advocate bottom-up, 'community-based' approaches, most of the programmes are still rather top-down in terms of the messages that are passed on and the underlying frameworks on which the programmes are based. The call for projects that are more responsive to local communities still largely has to be transformed into concrete interventions: as money comes from elsewhere, so the purse is still held elsewhere (Heald 2003). The adoption of this 'NGO-model' for AIDS policies shows to what extent they are bound to neoliberal politics aiming at reducing state control and at empowering organisations with transnational connections. These same forces are at work in the realm of religious dynamics on the African continent. Recently, James Pfeiffer has drawn attention to parallels between Pentecostal expansion and the spread of HIV/AIDS in Mozambique. Pfeiffer's aim is not to suggest that Pentecostalism might be responsible for the growth in HIV prevalence, but rather that 'Pentecostalism and HIV have travelled along similar vectors and have been propelled by the same recent socio-economic and political transformations' (Pfeiffer 2011: 164), pushed by the World Bank and the IMF. After the adoption of a structural adjustment project (SAP), Mozambique's gross domestic product (GDP) began to grow rapidly at the end of the 1990s, but with a significant increase in social inequalities and economic vulnerability. In the same period, the country experienced a growth in HIV rates, and a rapid expansion of Pentecostal churches.

The case of Mozambique shows that the assumption of transnationalism equalling liberal values is unsustainable, as transnational forces frequently push for a conservative agenda. The most well-known example of external funding of AIDS prevention programmes with specific conservative goals is PEPFAR (the US President's Emergency Plan for AIDS Relief). This plan, approved by the US Congress in 2003, has been the major fund for the treatment and prevention of

HIV/AIDS. According to the plan, 55 per cent of the total sum goes to treatment, and 20 per cent to prevention; yet, here prevention is mainly conceived in terms of abstinence-only and fidelity programmes, resulting in an increasing emphasis on 'morality' and 'sin' as a part of sex education and HIV prevention (Susser 2009).

The Ugandan case is emblematic in this respect: this country has been considered as a model in the struggle against AIDS due to the results obtained, with a fall in the incidence from 18 per cent in 1992 to 6.1 per cent in 2001. However, since the injection of PEPFAR funds in 2004, Uganda's HIV/AIDS prevention programmes began to place an almost exclusive emphasis on the 'Abstain' and 'Be Faithful' components of the 'ABC' strategy, leaving the 'C' (Use Condoms) out (Epstein 2007). Here, as elsewhere in the continent, a number of religious leaders and FBOs have been quick to embrace this shift in prevention strategies, with their claim for 'sexual probity' as the main instrument to fight AIDS, especially promoting abstinence-only programmes among young Ugandans (Gusman 2009). During the last decades, Pentecostal churches have been growing fast in the religious arena throughout the continent, with their aggressive approach calling to transform local societies, and ultimately the whole world. In this view, morality, and especially sexual morality for young people, has been viewed as the fundamental basis for change, placing a strong emphasis on behavioural change. Sexuality has thus become a central focus in the competition to occupy the religious space: as had already been the case in the past with other diseases, especially sexually transmitted infections, public health measures have been used as instruments of social and sexual control (de Waal 2003). In this context, AIDS is instrumentalised as a means to push for an exclusively heterosexual and – in Christian arenas – monogamist model of sexual relationships, and in the Muslim world, to emphasise the destructive force of sex outside of marriage, and the need to combine marital faithfulness and premarital HIV tests to ensure that all polygamous partners would be HIV-free (Beckmann 2010).

The availability of funds directed specifically to abstinence as a prevention strategy has provided a significant incentive for an increasing moralisation of sexuality and AIDS, and religious leaders and organisations were able to align their moral views with restrictions on prevention programmes. Once again, agency seems to be a quality restricted only to an elite (religious or political) able to enter the transnational networks in a position of dependence, to attract funds and to improve their position. Apart from this restricted group of people, Africans are often depicted by media as victims of global processes, unable to overcome the constraining structures that are present in their everyday lives, as these structures are located mostly at a transnational level, and thus even more difficult to address. Yet, some of the cases reported in this volume show that it is not possible to understand structures without considering actors, and vice versa (van Dijk *et al.* 2007) and that it is in dialectical relations that agency emerges, though sometimes with heavy limitations. Without considering this space for agency, 'structures' might appear strict and rigid (even more than they are), and it would be difficult to explain the heterogeneity of religious responses to the epidemics, the ways people respond to policies coming from external sources, for example by refusing to test (see Niehaus, Chapter 9, this volume), or to understand the public/private face of HIV prevention. A room for manoeuvre is still present even in the presence of powerful transnational forces, or perhaps precisely because of their transnational nature. These forces seem to provide a framework in which local actors are able to act reflexively to navigate within, if not to transform the structure. Although religious discourses and faith-based programmes have frequently framed HIV infection as a moral issue, aiming to direct people's actions into socially acceptable forms of behaviour, there is a discrepancy between these discourses and teachings, and the way people put them into practice in their everyday lives. With a look at the grassroots level, it becomes evident that what people say is not necessarily what they do, especially in such a contested sphere as sexuality, where hiding a 'wrong' behaviour may be necessary in order to 'keep up appearances' (Sadgrove 2007).

What we learn from this is that the trajectory of a conservative agenda *vis-à-vis* modernist views of the body, sexuality and relationships is not an uncontested one. While transnational conservative agendas have power, because of the ways in which they are backed by external resources, flows of people, educational material, awareness-raising campaigns and the like, they cannot deny the fact that sexuality in Africa has been changing dramatically since colonial times. Modern views of sexuality have emerged on the continent, in part provoked by the introduction of Western biomedicine itself. The ways in which, as Foucault and Giddens indicated for Western societies, a separation between sexuality and reproduction has emerged precisely because of the introduction of biomedical technologies of contraception, has been meaningful on the African continent, as well. Through transnational trajectories of biomedical relations (the circulation and flow of medical staff, resources, technologies and so forth) a channelling of modernist interventions in the domains of sexuality and reproduction became possible in Africa, too (see Vaughan 2007 [1991] on the early colonial medical experiences of this). Therefore, by looking at the significance of transnational relations in Africa through the lens of sexuality we are discovering that these relations never are 'neutral' in the kind of agendas they propose; in the variety of transnational relations and in the variety of how they propose a 'modern sexuality' a variety of moral strings are attached. How has a modern sexuality emerged in Africa?

A brief history of approaches to sexuality and AIDS in Africa

The generalised nature of HIV epidemics in many sub-Saharan African countries, where HIV is transmitted largely via heterosexual contacts within the broad, 'normal' population, has revived old debates around sexuality on the African continent. Historians have highlighted the long and fraught relationship between the missions, the colonial governments, and the 'natives' sexuality'. Colonial records abound with descriptions of sexual practices, beliefs, and values which problematised 'African sexuality' as excessive, dirty, and diseased. The medical discourse on Africa, Vaughan (2007 [1991]: 19) points out, was highly sexualised and promoted a pathologised view of African sexuality in which Africans came to represent sexual instinct and a 'genital potency beyond all moralities and prohibitions' (Fanon 1986 [1952]: 177). There were two main variations on this theme: for some, African sexuality was 'primitive' and uncontrolled, steeped in exotic customs and traditions, and represented the dangers of the 'dark continent'. Others regarded African sexuality as 'innocent' – an expression of the view that Africans' minds were child-like – and saw the danger rather in the degeneration of this innocent sexuality through the rapid social and economic changes brought about under colonialism and Christianisation (Vaughan 2007 [1991]: 129).

The continuity of these tropes becomes visible in debates around HIV/AIDS, particularly in the early years of the pandemic. Historical analyses of colonial explanations of venereal disease epidemics in the early twentieth century show striking similarities with epidemiologists' and social scientists' more recent explanations of why Africa was hit so hard by HIV/AIDS. Both drew on the arguments of primitiveness and excess, and a racialised, flawed modernisation, describing the epidemics as symptoms of an imperfect adjustment to modern conditions, including labour migration, rapid urbanisation, and the breaking apart of traditional hierarchies and structures of authority, resulting in a lack of control over sexuality, unstable marriage unions, and widespread 'promiscuity' and 'prostitution' (cf. Vaughan 2007 [1991]: 132ff.; Pigg and Adams 2005: 31).

In early studies of HIV/AIDS in Africa sweeping statements were made about Africans' sexual practices. Scanning the existing ethnographic literature for data on sexual morality, a new model of a distinctly 'African sexuality' was postulated, mainly inspired by the demographers Caldwell, Caldwell and Quiggin's hypothesis of a 'distinct and internally coherent African system embracing sexuality, marriage, and much else' (1989: 187). Although very diverse accounts of sexual practice in Africa exist for example in the anthropological literature, an image of a homogeneous, essentialised and rigid kind of 'African sexuality' was proposed which was in turn understood as exotic, highly permissive and promiscuous, imprisoned in tribal taboos and prohibitions, or as exclusively focusing on reproduction. The model portrayed Africans as deviant and immoral and posed 'culture' as an obstacle to the successful implementation of behaviour change.

According to Caldwell *et al.*, lineage organisation and ancestor worship form the characteristic criteria of African societies, placing much importance on fertility and reproduction, which consequently led to fairly permissive sexual attitudes and extensive sexual networking. Their claim that 'Africans neither placed aspects of sexual behaviour at the centre of their moral and social systems nor sanctified chastity' (Caldwell *et al.* 1989: 194) highlights the persistent racism and stigmatisation of Africans in scientific research, and was criticised harshly by anthropologists who pointed to methodological problems (e.g. Le Blanc *et al.* 1991; Ahlberg 1994) on the one hand, and to the racist interpretation of the available data on the other (Bibeau and Pedersen 2002). Heald, for example, highlights the preoccupation of many East African societies with the monitoring of sexuality, so that the controls surrounding sex, and the self-control that one must exercise with regard to it, epitomise social and moral behaviour: 'Coitus is fraught with danger, circumscribed by taboo and subject to restrictions unknown in the West' (1995: 492).

While the 'African sexuality' hypothesis has been discarded, interest in identifying patterns of sexual practice which can account for the rapid spread of HIV in parts of sub-Saharan Africa continues. Recent studies have focused on multiple concurrent sexual partnerships (MCPs), which play an important role in the creation of sexual networks in which HIV can flow freely and spread rapidly. HIV can spread efficiently through populations in which MCPs are common and it increases everyone's risk, including persons who are monogamous (Halperin and Epstein 2007). If someone in such a sexual network becomes infected with HIV, it increases the risk of HIV spreading to everyone in the network. The presence of MCPs, which are claimed to be widespread in Africa (Mah and Halperin 2010),[2] thus raises questions about the extent to which individual behaviour change can influence the course of an HIV epidemic.

For three decades individual sexual behaviour has been portrayed as the main driver of the pandemic in sub-Saharan Africa, the world's most severely affected region. Recent studies, however (e.g. Thornton 2008), have started to challenge this narrow focus and highlight the importance of analysing the shape of sexual networks to understand the way HIV (and other sexually transmitted diseases) spread throughout a population. What are the factors that influence the shape of the sexual network in a specific location? How does religious discourse and practice affect attitudes towards and patterns of intimacy, sexual relationships, ideas of love, and reproductive goals and practices? What influence do transnational flows of ideas, values and people have on the ways these concepts and practices may change? Sexual networks are intimately linked to mobility; one may only think of the main 'risk groups' – long-distance truck-drivers and prostitutes catering to their needs – identified as vectors of infection in the early days of the African AIDS crisis (cf. Obbo 1993). Transnational connections add another dimension to the role of mobility and create new links between existing sexual networks. At the same time, HIV intervention programmes designed by global stakeholders and transnational

[2] The data are not conclusive, however, and this claim has been contested (cf. Wellings *et al.* 2006).

advocacy networks influence and – perhaps to a lesser extent – are influenced by the local shaping of the disease. These processes are accompanied by flows of money to an unprecedented extent. The roles which political, economic and religious considerations play at the local, national and global levels are therefore essential in understanding the ways in which sexual networks are shaped.

MCPs have recently become a key focus of HIV programmes in eastern and southern Africa, but debate continues over the precise role of MCPs in the African epidemics, and over different forms of interventions. One group of scientists and public health experts (e.g. Helen Epstein, Halperin, UNAIDS) starts from individual sexual behaviour and seeks to define 'improved behaviour-change interventions'. They suggest a 'shift in social norms emerging from a deeper appreciation of the importance of avoidance and addressing concurrency, not only for those whose behaviour is "risky" according to conventional standards, but also for those whose behaviour is not considered risky, such as monogamous women' (Halperin and Epstein 2007), and thus rely on the old ABC approach focusing on individual sexual behaviour. One example is the One Love campaign.

Other researchers (including Mark Lurie, Robert Thornton, and some Southern organisations, such as SAfAIDS) argue that we first need to understand the underlying reasons for having multiple concurrent partnerships. They envisage interventions in improving individuals' risk perception and thereby increasing condom use. In their view, it is vital to acknowledge the existence of sexual networks. Drawing attention to social, economic and gender forces, they address the question of why people have multiple sexual partners and analyse the links sexual activity has to the pursuit of influence, control and power. According to Thornton, any individual behaviour-change intervention, including partner reduction, has little impact given the important effect of the inter-connectivity of the sexual network. It is therefore, he argues, not so much about the number of sexual contacts (multiple concurrency) or the time over which they occur (long-term concurrency) but rather 'the frequency with which they *change*, and the fact that this strategy entails maintaining several relationships at the same time, moving between them according to specific social and economic needs and social rules' (Thornton 2009: 7).

Transnational ideas and sexual practice

The above-mentioned view towards culture in attempts to explain the spread of HIV in Africa is of course nothing new: frequently faced with major epidemics, colonial administrations regarded Africans as reservoirs of disease. With a wider shift in colonial discourse from an emphasis on racial difference towards a 'liberal' cultural relativist position in the 1930s, colonial public health discourse started to focus on cultural practices as the cause of Africans' susceptibility to disease (and no longer emphasised living conditions and environmental factors) (Vaughan 2007 [1991]: 46). Sexuality took centre stage in these discussions on culture and disease, and Vaughan demonstrates how sexual practices, values, and beliefs have been at the heart of the civilising mission in Africa, as well as a focal point for colonial domination through the fight against disease.

While the medical discourse on Africa was very deeply concerned with sexuality, initially, the colonial gaze focused on African men, who had been in closer contact with social transformations, those modernising forces, which were held to corrupt their 'primitive minds'. African women, by contrast, were regarded as repositories of 'tradition' and order in the midst of rapid economic and social change. Vaughan argues that it was mainly when women resisted this role (e.g. by becoming migrant workers themselves) that they became 'the object of a particularly heightened concern over social disintegration' (2007 [1991]: 22), a concern which found evidence in the medical literature in falling birth rates, infertility and sexually transmitted diseases (STDs), which were analysed in terms of female immorality.

In missionary medical discourse, however, African women had always been a central focus: it was precisely their perceived role as repositories of tradition which served to identify African women with all that was seen to be dark and evil in African cultures and practices, exemplified by their roles as midwives, and as central figures in initiation and fertility rituals and other traditional religious practices. In missionaries' eyes, these had to be broken to pave the way for Christianity. Medical missions approached this concern with a focus on maternal and child health, expressed in terms of 'liberating' women from what was regarded as subjugation, but simultaneously exalting women's reproductive roles and 'domesticity' (Vaughan 2007 [1991]: 23). In the missionary medical discourse, body and soul were referred to as indivisible. The diseases of Africa, Vaughan points out, stood for larger spiritual ills, for the sickness of their souls. Mission medicine thus used the powerful tool of biomedicine for social control, but allied it to a moral and religious discourse (ibid.: 73).

Sexual practices have often been the focus of efforts to reform and modernise the nation, and contemporary sexual education and reproductive health interventions can be analysed with reference to colonial programmes 'to intervene in health by way of sexual regulation, medico-legal mechanisms to control venereal disease, missionary projects focussing on the moral reform of the native through sexual and reproductive practices and nationalist efforts to ensure a robust population' (Pigg and Adams 2005: 12f.). Today's efforts at sexual reform and intervention are still linked both to advancing ideas of what it means to be modern, and to larger national projects of development. Health, social reform and population control projects are spaces in which sexuality is negotiated, where target populations (such as men having sex with men (MSM), or commercial sex workers (CSW)) are generated, and where sexual practices are discouraged, promoted, named, and reframed (ibid.: 11). In such bio-political projects, the most intimate decisions on sexual practice are made into questions of life and death, and thus questions of national interest. In this sense, humanitarian projects aimed at preventing death are prime examples of a new, distinctly modern kind of 'government at a distance', which draw on epidemiological technologies of data collection and frameworks for risk reduction that enable authorities to act upon the conduct of persons (Rose 2007: 16).

What concept of sexuality is being promoted through sexual education and public health campaigns? While the early development programmes had targeted fertility, in the era of AIDS sex has become the target of interventions, and sexuality has become scripted through the imperative of disease intervention. This represents a significant shift in how sex is framed: as a set of sexual practices, identities and risk, tightly interwoven with science (Pigg and Adams 2005: 19). Stacey Leigh Pigg in turn argues that HIV prevention programmes, just like programmes on reproductive health, family planning, or STD control, 'are based on and promulgate a particular set of ideas about the sexual and reproductive body' which are fundamentally informed by the sexual sciences (2005: 40). This biologised notion of sex, with its focus on reproductive organs and genitalia, on hormones and menstrual cycles, on ovulation and fertilisation, and on the spread and replication of viruses via the bloodstream and mucous membranes, has come to dominate sexual education programmes worldwide, internationalised by a set of institutional networks that largely work within a Western, secular frame of thinking. The sexual sciences thus increasingly standardise and define a baseline of normality, and make other ways of knowing and having a sexual body merely local and cultural 'beliefs', to be replaced by biological 'facts' (ibid.: 58).

Sex education ostensibly aims at providing people with a knowledge base from which they can make informed decisions, thus improving both their autonomy and their health. However, Pigg reminds us that in many countries there are few other arenas outside the globally devised public health education programmes around HIV/AIDS or family planning where this specific kind of scientific knowledge about the sexual and reproductive body would be encountered. In a scientific view of sexuality, where individuals are called upon to 'break the silence' and talk boldly and frankly about sex in the name of reducing risk, ensuring health, and ultimately saving lives, biological facts are 'endowed with a magical ability to change people's consciousness. Calling on them is construed as a socially neutral act, a way of stepping outside of moral debate and even cultural particularism itself' (Pigg 2005: 61).

Yet, while such scientific knowledge about sex is presented as neutral and objective, it is deeply embedded in moral discourses around what kinds of sexuality are normal (e.g. masturbation, oral sex, consensual and voluntary sex between adults, 'safer' sex) or permissive (e.g. homosexual relationships, anal sex), and thus contributes to the creation of modern sexual normativities which are defined in opposition to 'deviant' and pathologised practices. These sexual morals are based on sexual health insights on medically 'risky' sex and human rights discourses around individual free choice and mutual consent that may not always fully overlap with local knowledge and attitudes to what constitutes morally permissible, healthy or normal sexuality. We must keep in mind that the particular concept of sex which is promoted in globally devised sex education programmes is a product of social and scientific processes in nineteenth-century Europe and North America which led to the emergence of the concept of personal life, individuality, and self-development, and the development of sex as a personal behaviour and an act of self-expression. This excision of sexuality as 'sex' from its entanglement in moral social relationships, the focus on the body parts, practices and behaviours, often does not easily resonate with local lived realities (ibid.: 40–1, 50).

What happens when such a concept of sex divorced from its social and moral embeddedness is promoted through funding streams and aggressive 'marketing'? And how is this negotiated by religious institutions and FBOs that increasingly are roped in to implement health and sexual risk awareness programmes? Several essays in this volume address these questions, reminding us that global and local discourses on sex have not only been shaped by scientific, biological views; sexual issues have also been at the heart of religious moral discourses, which act as a powerful counterbalancing force against scientific 'objective' and 'neutral' information on sex. While religious discourses do draw on medical, biological concepts of sex and disease (cf. missionary medicine's use of biomedical authority, or the teaching of biological basics in some FBOs' sex education programmes), they fill a gap by presenting a moral approach to sexuality in which religious norms and moral values – as opposed to health risk and Western human rights – define the baseline of normality. Thus providing another powerful source of authority on sex, Christian and Muslim religious ethics provide a counter-discourse to the medical focus on 'saving lives': while striving for health is often regarded as a spiritual imperative and divine blessing, the matter of ultimate importance is the saving of souls.

In this light, the push for 'progressive', 'liberal' agendas in the realm of sexuality and sexual and reproductive health can easily backfire, especially in countries that have a history of colonialism. The local interpretation of open talk about sex and condom promotion as the real cause of HIV/AIDS in several African societies (cf. Heald 2003 for Botswana; Beckmann 2009 for Zanzibar) is a case in point.

Transnational identities and homosexuality

A current and striking example of widespread resistance against liberal agendas is the outrage triggered by British prime minister David Cameron's demand that British aid be conditional upon the decriminalisation and respect for the human rights of sexual minorities (*Guardian*, 30 October 2011). The international gay movement creates a narrative of progress that contrasts pre-modern 'closeted' homosexualities with a modern sexual and political subject. Pigg and Adams (2005: 36) argue that these distinctions offer both possibilities and limitations for 'gay' people outside of Euro-America (see for example Cohen 2005). Sexual minority rights worldwide have experienced a backlash in recent years, and African countries have been particularly condemning of homosexual practices. A wave of anti-gay legislation and persecution of homosexuals has swept across the continent, alongside reaffirmation that 'such practices' were entirely 'un-African'. In this context, Cameron's claim came as an affront, widely debated in African newspapers, web blogs and social networking sites around the world. It had not been forgotten that England had the earliest anti-sodomy laws in Europe (instituted in 1533) and had exported these to its colonies, and only rather recently (in 1967 for England and Wales, and as late as 1992 in the Isle of Man) had decided to withdraw the legislation. Even in South Africa, which has one of the most progressive legislations on sexual minority rights whose protection is written into the post-apartheid constitution, calls have become louder to rewrite the constitution in favour of more conservative values. These recent debates demonstrate once more that sexuality is a sensitive topic, not only in African societies. As many of the essays in this volume show, it is surely far from resolved in Western faith communities, too. The recent scandal around child abuse in the Catholic Church and the way it has been handled – with secrecy and reluctance to allow full disclosure and the prosecution of perpetrators by state authorities – is but one example highlighting the uneasy relationship between sexuality (especially in what is regarded as its 'deviant' forms) and religious institutions.

Framing global HIV prevention and sexual health education campaigns in a rights-based rhetoric, programmes are usually required to promote an empowerment approach which emphasises the importance of 'coming out', standing up for one's rights, and claiming an 'HIV-positive', 'sex worker', or 'gay' identity. The emphasis on disclosure is also justified through medical reasoning: disclosure is regarded as an essential step towards a healthy life with HIV, a life as a responsible, treatment-adherent citizen-patient. However, ethnographic evidence points out that this may actually be counter-productive and harmful to both the health and lives of individuals who claim a stigmatised identity, and thus contradict the harm reduction approach that is also promoted by many organisations. In Muslim contexts, for example, transparency is regarded as problematic and private matters are kept hidden from prying eyes; illicit affairs are managed through secrecy in order to protect the wider social network's honour and reputation. While homosexual relationships are often tolerated as long as they are kept secret, coming out and assuming a 'gay identity' is usually strongly condemned and frequently leads to violence and social isolation. Similarly, women involved in transactional sexual relationships often would not identify as sex workers, because there is nothing to gain: they would have to endure societal condemnation and potentially prosecution. Instead, framing their activities as 'having boyfriends' allows these women to keep a positive self-image, guard their respectability, and appear as caring mothers who look after their families by seeking a male provider. In this context one could argue that secrecy and concealment are forms of harm reduction, since keeping it secret – even if it is an open secret – opens up routes for agency and negotiation.

Yet, globally designed blueprint approaches to HIV/AIDS prevention and treatment tend to ignore these complex entanglements and subtle meanings and press for the medicalisation of sexuality, the 'empowerment' of women, men and youth as rational, free, and individual actors, and disclosure and 'coming out'. The renewed focus by donors and public health planners on most-at-risk persons (MARPs) in the fight against HIV/AIDS poses a particular dilemma for people living with HIV/AIDS (PLHA). After decades of PLHAs' struggles against stigma and discrimination, and efforts to re-build a 'normal' life and portray themselves as moral persons, the international focus on MARPs has started to force them to accept people who are considered undesirable, immoral, and deviant into their midst – i.e. sex workers, men having sex with men, and intravenous drug users – and to support them. In some cases this has been easily achieved and community organising around AIDS has opened up spaces for homosociality (cf. Nguyen 2005). In many other places, however, this has not only resulted in bitterness among those PLHAs that consider themselves 'normal' and moral persons, and nevertheless suddenly find themselves neglected by the new donor agendas, but also increased fears of having their reputation as a group damaged by embracing such 'undesirable' members. In contexts where associating oneself with the 'wrong' persons inspires rumours and gossip and leaves a bad reputation on everybody involved, such support groups may feel that their endeavours to reconstruct their respectability in the eyes of the public are endangered. The strategy of identifying and naming MARPs, and singling them out for targeted programmes, can, and does, therefore easily lead to discrimination and hostility within the very groups that are often considered to be the last resort for support for already marginalised people.

Outline of the book

The book consists of four sections, which highlight different issues of the transnationalism of the AIDS pandemic in Africa. Combining a range of disciplinary approaches, the volume traces continuities with the past, showing how contemporary dynamics have antecedents in the colonial era; it looks at current developments, providing a nuanced, yet broad analysis of the role religious and political, local and international forces play in creating competing and sometimes conflicting agendas for AIDS and sexuality; and it attempts an outlook into the future of such agendas.

The first section, 'Transnational Relations and Conservative Agendas', looks at how transnational relations have brought conservative models and agendas to the continent, often in conjunction with neoliberal economic approaches. Christine Obbo provides a historical background to the volume, shedding light on approaches to AIDS in the early years of the pandemic. Drawing on her empirical data from Uganda, she traces the development of Uganda's sexual networks by analysing the socio-political changes and the transformations in sexual and moral models starting from the colonial era, when missions and colonial governments imported and sought to impose monogamy, with the effect of producing 'informal polygamy'. She shows how this story of externally imposed models continues with PEPFAR; based on Obbo's experience not only as a scholar, but as a consultant for UNAIDS, her analysis highlights the simplistic nature of the 'ABC' approach to HIV prevention, criticising the lack of attention to central factors such as gender relations and economic vulnerability.

After Obbo's retrospective, Brooke Schoepf's chapter offers an analysis of contemporary developments and provides a prognosis for the future. Drawing on decades of experience as a researcher and high-level consultant since the beginning of the AIDS pandemic, Schoepf analyses how American HIV/AIDS politics have been shifting during the Obama administration, and discusses the future of PEPFAR. She explores how transnational relations, and especially transoceanic relations between the USA and Africa, have fuelled poverty and inequality in the continent, thus creating space for the spread of the epidemic. PEPFAR here is considered as an example of political pressures from the USA shaping the agenda of HIV prevention and education in Africa and introducing ideas that then rapidly circulate around the continent.

With Ajibade's and Sadgrove's chapters the section shifts to the grassroots level, where responses, contestation and negotiations of these external discourses take place. From her perspective as an Anglican priest in the UK, Ijeoma Ajibade offers a view from within a religious organisation: how it responds to the epidemic, and negotiates the different positions on morality and sexuality. Her contribution offers a vivid account of the impact transnational dynamics have on the everyday lives of the people assisted by the organisation she works with, showing also that models seldom fit with people's experience. In the final chapter of this section, Joanna Sadgrove explores the competition of alternative views of love, intimacy and sexuality taking place in Uganda; religious models promoted especially by evangelicals are highly influential here, but find a counterpart in moral registers proposed by human rights networks and secular non-governmental organisations (NGOs). Young Ugandans are thus positioned amidst competing moral discourses of sexuality and selfhood, and negotiate this puzzled moral arena often by oscillating opportunistically between different models.

The second section on 'Transnational Power and Local Agency' opens with Amy Patterson's analysis of the disjuncture between top-down, homogeneous prevention messages, and the actual practices taking place at the local level, with a focus on Zambia. Starting from a reflection on extraversion and resistance in the context of AIDS policies, the chapter discerns five major reasons for the gap between programmes and practice. Louise Rasmussen brings the focus back to Uganda in her analysis of Catholic organisations. She shows how the official prohibition of condom use is negotiated in the everyday practice of people working in these organisations. In particular, Rasmussen's chapter highlights a contrast between HIV prevention education and HIV counselling, and thus between the public and the private spheres of interventions. Brenda Bartelink and Erik Meinema's contribution also points to a gap between ideals and practices by investigating the negotiation taking place around AIDS prevention strategies between Dutch FBOs and their Ugandan partner organisations in the Christian Educaids network. Contradictions are most visible in debates on abstinence and condom use; however, the strong moral positions taken by Ugandan actors in the network are often combined with pragmatic approaches to sex education in practice. Finally, Isak Niehaus provides an alternative point of view on the reasons why people locally may oppose international HIV policies. Drawing on extensive fieldwork in the Bushbuckridge municipality in South Africa, Niehaus shows that resistance to testing, especially in the rural areas, is only partially explained by the presence of stigmatisation of HIV-positive people, and needs to be connected to the idea that words are understood to have agency in causing disease, and that talking about HIV has the power to kill.

The third section, 'Transnational Ideas and Local Discourses about Sexuality', opens with Anaïs Bertrand-Danserau's study of HIV prevention programmes with young people in Malawi; she focuses on the existence of a strict moral hierarchy between 'good sex' and 'bad sex', based not only on transnationally conveyed ideas, but also on local ideas of sexuality. Her case study is an example of how secular approaches to sex have led to paralysis and may even be harmful in terms of HIV intervention, while more sex-positive messages come from unexpected sources, i.e. the churches and FBOs she studied. The chapter illustrates once more the theological and political negotiations that take place as religious organisations grapple with moral imperatives, real-life situations, donor demands and young people's needs. With Jonas Svensson's chapter, the volume moves to Islamic discourses and provides an example of resistance to the promotion of conservative values. It explores the South African organisation Positive Muslims' development of a 'theology of compassion' as an alternative to the dominant 'Islamic view' on sexuality, AIDS and prevention in the face of the dramatic reality of the epidemic. The chapter contests the widespread idea of a monolithic Islam and analyses the personal and ideological relationships between Positive Muslims and the transnational movement of Progressive Islam. Astrid Bochow's contribution analyses the stories of several women belonging to the emerging cosmopolitan elites in Botswana to provide an understanding of how ideas about fertility changed due to the AIDS epidemic. If in the past fertility was equal to prosperity, the author argues, in the current situation socio-economic transformations and the fear of HIV/AIDS advance the notion of a need to 'control' reproduction, so that having children, in these women's view, is becoming more of a personal decision, and not a social obligation.

The fourth and final section of the volume, 'Transnational Identities and Homosexuality', deals with the very sensitive topic of homosexuality, which has been heavily debated in recent years. Lindsay Ehrisman provides a historical perspective on homophobia in Uganda, which she shows to be a historical product connected to the action of missionaries during the colonial era, rather than a recent phenomenon. Silence around same-sex sexuality, the author argues, was already present in missionary archives, as well as the myth of a 'traditional' Ugandan sexuality, with homosexuality considered as something imported by foreigners. Alexandra Müller's contribution looks at contemporary Uganda, with a discussion of the proposed introduction of the death penalty for HIV-positive homosexuals who infect a partner, and then goes on to analyse three sets of transnational dynamics (the human rights approach to HIV prevention; US domestic and global policies on AIDS; and evangelical organisations' aggressive attitude in prevention) and their respective impact on national policies in Africa. The chapter examines the interconnection of funding priorities and moral ideologies, and the consequent invisibility of homosexuals in HIV policies. Finally, Jack Ume Tocco brings our attention to another form of silence: in the north of Nigeria, where *sharia* is the official law, transmission of HIV via male–male sexual contacts is silenced; as a result, there has been a complete lack of initiatives to prevent this form of transmission. Tocco's chapter shows that this silence has failed to appreciate social and epidemiological implications, as homosexuals are often integrated into larger sexual networks via heterosexual relationships.

References

Ahlberg, B.M. 1994. 'Is there a distinct African sexuality? A critical response to Caldwell', *Africa* 64(2): 220–42.

Bayart, J.-F. 2000. 'Africa in the world: a history of extraversion', *African Affairs* 99: 217–67.

Becker, F. and P.W. Geissler. 2009. 'Introduction: searching for pathways in a landscape of death: religion and AIDS in Africa', in F. Becker and P.W. Geissler (eds), *Aids and Religious Practice in Africa*. Leiden: Brill, 1–29.

Beckmann, N. 2009. 'AIDS and the power of God: narratives of decline and coping strategies in Zanzibar', in F. Becker and P.W. Geissler (eds), *AIDS and Religious Practice in Africa*. Leiden: Brill, 119–54.

Beckmann, N. 2010. 'Pleasure and danger: Muslim views on sex and gender in Zanzibar', *Culture, Health and Sexuality* 12: 619–32.

Bibeau, G. and D. Pedersen. 2002. 'A return to scientific racism in medical social sciences: the case of sexuality and the AIDS epidemic in Africa', in M. Nichter and M. Lock (eds), *New Horizons in Medical Anthropology: Essays in Honour of Charles Leslie*. New York: Routledge, 141–71.

Bornstein, Erica. 2002. 'Developing faith: theologies of economic development in Zimbabwe', *Journal of Religion in Africa* 32: 4–31.

Caglar, A. 2006. 'Hometown associations and grassroots transnationalism', *Global Networks* 6(1): 1–22.

Caldwell, J., P. Caldwell and P. Quiggin. 1989. 'The social context of AIDS in sub-Saharan Africa', *Population and Development Review* 15(2): 185–234.

Christiansen, C. 2009. 'The new wives of Christ: paradoxes and potentials in the remaking of widow lives in Uganda', in F. Becker and P.W. Geissler (eds), *AIDS and Religious Practice in Africa*. Leiden: Brill, 85–118.

Christiansen, C. 2010. 'Development by churches, development of churches: institutional trajectories in rural Uganda'. Unpublished PhD thesis, University of Copenhagen.

Cohen, L. 2005. 'The Kothi wars: AIDS cosmopolitanism and the morality of classification', in V. Adams and S.L. Pigg (eds), *Sex in Development: Science, Sexuality, and Morality in Global Perspective*. Durham, NC: Duke University Press, 269–304.

de Waal, Alex. 2003. 'A disaster with no name: the HIV/AIDS pandemic and the limits of governance', in G. Ellison, M. Parker and C. Campbell (eds), *Learning from HIV and AIDS*. Cambridge: Cambridge University Press.

DiMaggio, P.J. and W.W. Powel. 1983. 'The iron cage revisited: institutional isomorphism and collective rationality in organizational fields', *American Sociological Review* 48(2): 147–60.

Englund, H. 2003. 'Christian independency and global membership: Pentecostal extraversion in Malawi', *Journal of Religion in Africa* 33: 83–111.

Epstein, H. 2007. *The Invisible Cure: Africa, the West and the Fight against AIDS*. New York: Farrar, Straus and Giroux.

Fanon, F. 1986 [1952]. *Black Skin, White Masks*. London: Pluto Press.

Farmer, P. 1999. *Infections and Inequalities: The Modern Plagues*. Berkeley: University of California Press.

Ferguson, J. 1990. *The Anti-Politics Machine: 'Development', Depoliticization and Bureaucratic Power in Lesotho*. Cambridge: Cambridge University Press.

Ferguson, J. 1999. *Expectations of Modernity: Myths and Meanings of Urban Life on the Zambian Copperbelt*. Berkeley: University of California Press.

Ferguson, J. 2006. *Global Shadows: Africa in the Neoliberal World Order*. Durham, NC: Duke University Press.

Ferguson, J. and A. Gupta. 1997. *Culture, Power, Place: Explorations in Critical Anthropology*. Durham, NC: Duke University Press.

Glick Schiller, N. 2005a. 'Transnational social fields and imperialism: bringing a theory of power to transnational studies', *Anthropological Theory* 5(4): 439–61.

Glick Schiller, N. 2005b. 'Transnationality', in D. Nugent and J. Vincent (eds), *A Companion to the Anthropology of Politics*. Malden, MA: Blackwell, 448–67.

Guardian, 30 October 2011. 'Countries that ban homosexuality risk losing aid, warns David Cameron'. http://www.guardian.co.uk/politics/2011/oct/30/ban-homosexuality-lose-aid-cameron (accessed 28 January 2012).

Gusman, A. 2009. 'HIV/AIDS, Pentecostal churches, and the 'Joseph Generation' in Uganda', *Africa Today* 55: 67–86.

Halperin, D.T. and H. Epstein. 2007. 'Why is HIV prevalence so severe in southern Africa? The role of multiple concurrent partnerships and lack of male circumcision: implications for AIDS prevention', *Southern African Journal of HIV Medicine* 8(1): 19–25.

Heald, S. 1995. 'The power of sex: some reflections on the Caldwells' 'African Sexuality' thesis', *Africa* 65(4): 489–505.

Heald, S. 2003. 'An absence of anthropology: critical reflections on anthropology and AIDS policy and practice in Africa', in G. Ellison, M. Parker and C. Campbell (eds), *Learning from HIV and AIDS*. Cambridge: Cambridge University Press.

Hilhorst, D. 2003. *The Real World of NGOs, Discourses, Diversity and Development*. London: Zed Books.

Holden, S. 2003. 'AIDS as a development issue', in *AIDS on the Agenda: Adapting Development and Humanitarian Programmes to Meet the Challenges of HIV/AIDS*. Oxfam.

Kassimir, R. 2001. 'Producing local politics: governance, representation, and non-state organizations in Africa', in T.M. Callaghy, R. Kassimir and R. Latham (eds), *Intervention and Transnationalism in Africa: Global-Local Networks of Power*. Cambridge: Cambridge University Press, 93–114.

Laclau, E. and C. Mouffe. 1985. *Hegemony and Socialist Strategy: Towards a Radical Democratic Politics*. New York: New Left Books.

Le Blanc, M.-N., D. Meintel and V. Piché. 1991. 'The African sexual system: comment on Caldwell et al.', *Population and Development Review* 17(3): 497–505.

Mah, T. and D. Halperin. 2010. 'The evidence for the role of concurrent partnerships in Africa's HIV epidemics: a response to Lurie and Rosenthal', *AIDS and Behaviour* 14: 25–8.

March, J.G. and J.P. Olsen. 1989. *Rediscovering Institutions: The Organizational Basis of Politics*. New York: Free Press.

Maxwell, D. 2000. '"Catch the cockerel before dawn": Pentecostalism and politics in post-colonial Zimbabwe', *Africa* 70: 249–77.

Meyer, B. 1998. 'Make a complete break with the past: Time and modernity in Ghanaian Pentecostalist discourse', in R.P. Werbner (ed.), *Memory and the Postcolony*. London: Zed Books, 182–208.

Mosse, D. 2005. *Cultivating Development: The Ethnography of Policy and Practice*. London: Pluto Press.

Nguyen, V.-K. 2005. 'Uses and pleasures: sexual modernity, HIV/AIDS, and confessional technologies in a West African metropolis', in V. Adams and S.L. Pigg (eds), *Sex in Development: Science, Sexuality, and Morality in Global Perspective*. Durham, NC: Duke University Press, 245–68.

Nguyen, V.-K. 2009. 'Government-by-exception: enrolment and experimentality in mass HIV treatment programmes in Africa', *Social Theory and Health* 7: 196–222.

Obbo, C. 1993. 'HIV transmission through social and geographic networks in Uganda', *Social Science and Medicine* 36: 949–55.

Patterson, A. 2011. *The Church and AIDS in Africa: The Politics of Ambiguity*. Boulder, CO: First Forum Press.

Pfeiffer, J. 2011. 'Pentecostalism and AIDS treatment in Mozambique: creating new approaches to HIV prevention through anti-retroviral therapy', *Global Public Health* 6: 163–73.

Pigg, S.L. 2005. 'Globalizing the facts of life', in V. Adams and S.L. Pigg (eds), *Sex in Development: Science, Sexuality, and Morality in Global Perspective.* Durham, NC: Duke University Press, 39–66.

Pigg, S.L. and V. Adams. 2005. 'Introduction: the moral object of sex', in V. Adams and S.L. Pigg (eds), *Sex in Development: Science, Sexuality, and Morality in Global Perspective.* Durham, NC: Duke University Press, 1–38.

Prince, R., P. Denis and R. Van Dijk. 2009. 'Introduction to special issue – Engaging Christianities: negotiating HIV/AIDS, health, and social relations in East and southern Africa', *Africa Today* 56(1): v–xvii.

Ranger, T. 1992. 'Plagues of beasts and men; prophetic responses to epidemic in eastern and southern Africa', in T. Ranger and P. Slack (eds), *Epidemics and Ideas: Essays on the Historical Perception of Pestilence.* Cambridge: Cambridge University Press, 241–68.

Rose, N. 2007. *The Politics of Life Itself: Biomedicine, Power, and Subjectivity in the Twenty-First Century.* Princeton, NJ: Princeton University Press.

Sadgrove, J. 2007. '"Keeping up appearances": sex and religion amongst university students in Uganda', *Journal of Religion in Africa* 37: 116–44.

Schoepf, B. 1988. 'Women, AIDS, and economic crisis in Central Africa', *Canadian Journal of African Studies* 22(3): 625–44.

Smith, J.H. and A. Whiteside. 2010. 'The history of AIDS exceptionalism', *Journal of the International AIDS Society* 13: 47. http://www.jiasociety.org/content/13/1/47.

Susser, I. 2009. *AIDS, Sex, and Culture.* Oxford: Blackwell.

Swidler, A. 2007. 'Syncretism and subversion in AIDS governance: how locals cope with global demands', in N. Poku, A. Whiteside and B. Sandkjaer (eds), *Aids and Governance.* Aldershot: Ashgate, 145–63.

Swidler, A. 2009. 'Dialectics of patronage: logics of accountability at the African AIDS-NGO interface', in S. Heydemann and D.C. Hammack (eds), *Philanthropic Projections: Sending Institutional Logics Abroad.* Bloomington: Indiana University Press, 192–222.

Thornton, R. 2008. *Unimagined Community: Sex, Networks and AIDS in Uganda and South Africa.* Berkeley: University of California Press.

Thornton, R. 2009. 'Sexual networks and social capital: multiple and concurrent sexual partnerships as a rational response to unstable social networks', *African Journal of AIDS Research* 8(4): 1–9.

van Dijk, R. 1998. 'Pentecostalism, cultural memory and the state: contested representations of time in postcolonial Malawi', in R. Werbner (ed.), *Memory and the Postcolony: African Anthropology and the Critique of Power.* London: Zed Books, 155–81.

van Dijk, R., M. de Bruijn and J.-B. Gewald. 2007. 'Social and historical trajectories of agency in Africa: an introduction', in M. de Bruijn, R. van Dijk and J.-B. Gewald (eds), *Strength Beyond Structure: Social and Historical Trajectories of Agency in Africa.* Leiden: Brill, 1–16.

Vaughan, M. 2007 [1991]. *Curing Their Ills: Colonial Power and African Illness.* Stanford, CA: Stanford University Press.

Wellings, K., M. Collumbien, E. Slaymaker, *et al.* 2006. 'Sexual behaviour in context: a global perspective', *The Lancet* 368: 1706–28.

Wright, S. 1994. *Anthropology of Organizations.* London: Routledge.

Part 1

TRANSNATIONAL RELATIONS AND CONSERVATIVE AGENDAS

2

Sponsored Sexuality, Aids and Tough Choices

CHRISTINE OBBO

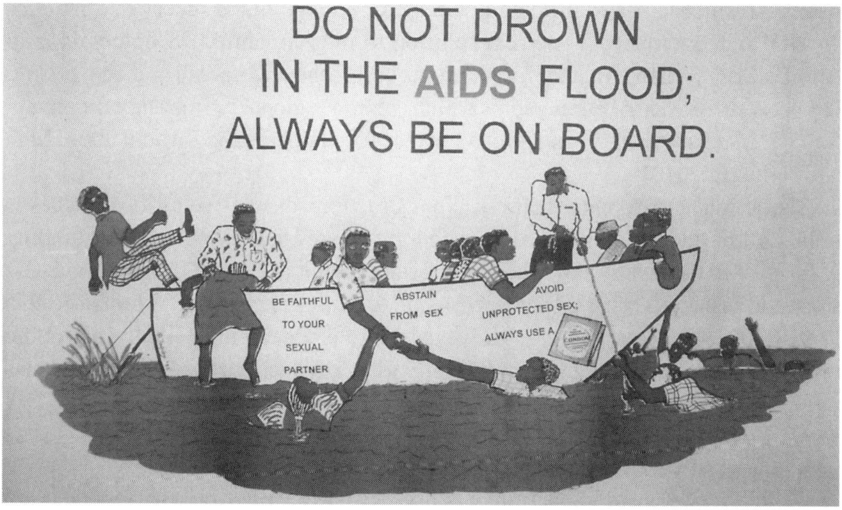
DO NOT DROWN
IN THE AIDS FLOOD;
ALWAYS BE ON BOARD.
BE FAITHFUL
TO YOUR
SEXUAL
PARTNER
ABSTAIN
FROM SEX
AVOID
UNPROTECTED SEX;
ALWAYS USE A

Uganda poster, 1995

THE DOMINANT ZEITGEIST IN AFRICA during the past four decades of the AIDS epidemic has been cultural-religious fundamentalism. A UNAIDS (2005) extensive consultative survey presenting three possible 2025 scenarios on AIDS in Africa identified these tendencies together with poverty, underdevelopment and marginalisation in a globalising world as AIDS deepened entrapments that would demand tough policy choices. AIDS control agendas in countries with varying economic, educational and social potential are dictated by conservative tendencies nurtured by foreign funding and advice.

Every generation of Africans has faced tough choices negotiating around foreign-imposed religious values on sexuality. This is an account of the unbroken

Proceedings of the British Academy **194**, *31–41*.

saga of top-down paradigms promoting monogamy and fidelity since colonial contact; and how social, political and economic hardships make people vulnerable to the dictates of rescuers. AIDS is now a matter of life and death fuelled by the intractable problems of ignorance, poverty and disease. This has set a perfect stage for the foreign macro-managing of response choices by promoting paradigms and practice that silence Ugandans long involved in designing diverse HIV prevention approaches which acknowledge that the sexually active who fall short of the ideals of chastity before and fidelity after marriage should be encouraged to seek the public health option of condom use. This promotes HIV self-protection and responsibility for the safety of others from infection. The current neo-colonial Christian anti-sex-condom crusade ignores gender inequality, poverty and power as the structural drives of the epidemic (Schoepf 2001) and discusses abstinence, fidelity and sexual networks without historical or cultural context.[1]

Fidelity (Epstein 2004) emerged as the coalescence model for expounding the ABC (Abstinence, Be faithful and perhaps Condoms) brand theory and practice on HIV risk avoidance.[2] The real solution to the African AIDS epidemic is to enforce ABC with the 'fidelity fix' through curbing the widespread practice of long-term concurrent sexual partnerships which create a regional 'virtual superhighway' for HIV in Africa (Morris and Kretzchmar 1997; Halperin and Epstein 2004; Mah and Halperin 2010).

The primacy of foreign theoretical constructions dismissive of local voices is important to understanding the anti-condom debates that inform current funding policies. ABC sponsors and scholar advocates laud it as core to Uganda's success story and insist it is what Africa needs and 'African leaders want' (Human Rights Watch 2005; Fogelberg 2005). However, there is a deafening silence about the economic incentives that buttress the support of key local advocate actors (Rawls 2012).

Sex and marriage choices during colonialism

'Too much' African sex emerged as a policy issue at the turn of the twentieth century with the advent of British colonialism. Accordingly, legislation and church sermons discouraged practices such as beer drinking, celebratory and ritual dances, and polygamous marriages. The same practices were identified as engendering the spread of HIV in the 1990s WHO surveys on cultural and behavioural practices.

[1] I have been involved in anthropological AIDS research since 1989. My involvement is particularly focused on Action Research to empower youth and women with skills to negotiate safer sex and to challenge men into harnessing their social and cultural privileges to take responsibility for curbing the epidemic.

[2] The global impact of the American Ivy League universities-generated brand marketing theorising (Applbaum 2004) has rationalised ABC, the motor for the evangelical morality-driven PEPFAR.

Colonial missionaries promoted nuclear families. Polygamous men demonstrated their true conversion to Christianity by choosing one wife for a monogamous 'ring' marriage licensed by church ceremonies, in response to the offered incentives of education, chieftainship and landownership. But the mentality that men are forced to have one wife by poverty persisted. Thus while monogamy was the legally enforced practice for modern families, men maintained women in long-term relationships outside marriage. Thus in a parallel universe monogamy and modernised polygamy flourished under the radar of foreigners' gaze. This practice continues in a climate undermining condom use but promoting abstinence and fidelity (Parikh 2007; Carpenter *et al.* 1999).

Under both customary and statutory laws, men could divorce women for infidelity, but women were not accorded the same rights. A woman demanding statutory divorce on grounds of cruelty or infidelity was required to demonstrate that the husband was mad. Needless to say divorces initiated by women were rare. The common recourse for women was desertion.

Ugandan men as the dominant cultural authorities had always had vested interests in promoting chastity for young people and fidelity for women in marriage (Southall 1960). Bride wealth transferred control over the sexual, productive and reproductive rights of a woman from her father and brothers to her husband. The value of the bride wealth depended upon the virginity of a woman on the eve of the wedding. A father's sister (actual or appointed female relative), the chief adviser to the bride, was responsible for ascertaining this. In many groups, the last bride wealth 'gift', coded with names querying whether the woman was still a virgin, was brought at dawn on the wedding day. While in some societies the rights the husband acquired were earmarked by specific payments, in others the rights were revealed by the fines demanded to redress transgressions. For example, fornication and impregnating a girl were fined as transgressions against virginity and childbearing value respectively. If a woman deserted her husband or was divorced for laziness, barrenness or adultery, the husband had a right to demand the return of the bride wealth as compensation for his loss of the woman's wealth-generating services of economic labour and producing heirs. In gender-cultural prescriptions women are central to food production; to nurturing the physical, psychological and social needs of the family; and to providing a man with sexual gratification and offspring. Many proverbs underscore this by emphasising that unmarried men cannot be homeowners even when they own their residential houses.

In some societies, if a woman died, a sister replaced her as compensation for the husband's loss. Likewise, if a man died, his male relatives inherited his widow who continued to perform the services that were exchanged for bride wealth. In societies where bride wealth was low, women deserted their husbands and worked to repay the bride wealth if their male relatives were unable or refused to do so. Deserting women and widows who did not remarry set themselves up as independent homeowners. With time they formed a socially accepted named category.

Modernisation and religion

The rapid extensive social, political and economic changes that occurred in the 1960s were characterised as consequences of modernisation: another name for prosperity. But as poverty persisted, religious organisations offered relief while entrenching their power.

Economic prosperity from the export of coffee and cotton cash crops enabled parents to educate their children; unmarried women bought land and supported themselves growing food and cash crops, or migrated to urban areas to exploit new income-generating activities catering to the surging urban population. The production of alcoholic drinks and the associated sexual liaisons characterised the low-income areas while modern hotels and nightclubs catered for the leisure activities of the new elites and aspirant poorly educated young people.

In the late 1960s, the Family Planning campaign to space out children in marriage was launched, promoting both birth control pills and condoms. Doctors concerned about rates of abortions and STD infections among university students encouraged condom use as central to the health promotion strategy for males. Unfaithful elite Christian men used condoms to avoid the marital awkwardness of possible 'outside' children. Condoms unintentionally captured the local men's imagination as something to use with women of questionable morals and presumed sexual disease vectors.

Since the early 1960s the dates of political independence from the metropolitan colonisers have been annual celebrations in most African countries. The reins of power were taken up by the first Western-schooled generation of leaders who assumed control over foreign development aid grants and loans that were enthusiastically promoted by accompanying advisers and managers (Timberlake 1986). Despite the different possible development trajectories suggested by existing education and national wealth, leaders in each country mismanaged the money, using it for their personal aggrandisement and expanding their personal power through nepotism and cronyism. This led to the erosion of political institutions and civil society rights. The combination of economic mismanagement, political disenfranchisement and the top-down economic policies resulted in the 'under-development' phenomenon characterised by economic and moral impoverishment at personal, community and national levels. Rural poverty drove people to cities with no jobs and infrastructure to support them. The wealth disparity between rich and poor, rural and urban, gave rise to programmes funded by NGOs with the declared mission of redressing poverty by integrating all into the development enterprise.

By the 1980s, the World Bank and the International Monetary Fund advisers and managers had imposed debt collection policies called Structural Adjustment Programmes (SAP) as conditions for further funding (Jauch 1999). Fiscal reforms to increase efficiency required balancing national budgets, in particular by reducing expenditure through trimming public sector jobs. The centrepiece of SAP was the opening up of the local market to foreign competition through the privatisation of public enterprises and land reforms.

The Uganda narrative begins with the power struggles over controlling development wealth, which culminated in the lost decade of the 1970s. The 1971 military *coup d'état* led not only to the disintegration of the economy and social services, but to a reign of terror which destroyed the judiciary, political parties and the press; and anarchy which threatened lives and property with destruction. There was a revival of many traditional practices that had been partly eclipsed by the modernisation impulses of the 1960s. These included neighbourliness in times of need, divination cures and social control notions of 'good women'.

SAP in Uganda (Jauch 1999; Naiman and Watkins 1999) led to a 40 per cent growth in GDP, which temporarily made it a heavily indebted poor country (HIPC) success story. The main beneficiaries of fast privatisation, and trade liberalisation involving the progressive reduction of export taxation on cash crops, were the enterprises of elites and foreigners. SAP policies were macro in scope and far removed from the reality of who gets access to the means of production, who controls surplus produce and profits, and who is able to respond to the added incentives to produce. Women were dominant among the majority of small-scale farmers receiving poor remuneration because they had limited property rights. The small private sector was unable to cope with the unemployment rates resulting from the retrenchment of about 350,000 public service employees. Women bore the brunt of SAP policies because of their gender responsibilities for the welfare of families. Commoditising education and health services under the 'cost sharing' schemes increased hardship for the poor, who struggled to find hospital and school fees.

In the early 1990s, the Jubilee 2000 coalition campaign, demanding debt relief for the poorest countries by the millennium, was the culmination of many NGOs' campaigns against extensive SAP-induced poverty. In 1997, Uganda was the first country to get the debt relief nod, but a delay of one year left it still servicing the SAP debt. Despite receiving $650 million multilateral debt relief, Uganda was forced back to the status of HIPC with an unsustainable debt-servicing burden by 1999 because the projected earnings from trade export revenues had failed to materialise.

The breakdown of social services in the 1970s and the general impoverishment drove people to seek refuge in religion. Traditional healers and independent churches that had been suppressed during colonial times had surreptitiously expanded during the 1960s. After political independence in 1962, Anglicanism had continued its colonial status as part and parcel of the dominant political framework, and Catholicism continued its successful rural penetration. But since the Anglican and Catholic churches were plagued by the same social disintegration symptoms of corruption, personal rivalry and ethnic conflict, independent churches blossomed as they embarked on the task of mending the social and moral fibre. By the 1980s, the gravity of the moral decay was widely acknowledged. Foreign religious NGOs whose overt agenda was to combat poverty and win souls for God became increasingly focused on moral rehabilitation. I attended many brainstorming sessions on strategies for moral rehabilitation but the most memorable one involved an outlandish proposal to install a television in every village for providing all-day religious broadcasts. Lack of rural electrification put a stop to the idea. The focus of evangelical and Pentecostal missionaries was economic assistance to schools, where ambitious young men were encouraged to preach the gospel, with the possibility of overseas training and, when successful, being rewarded with church ownership.

The days of AIDS

At this critical juncture Uganda was hit by an epidemic of a unique wasting illness, '*slimu*' (AIDS). In the mid-1980s, the earliest deaths were reported in the fishing village of Kasensero, a Lake Victoria landing point in Rakai District, which was the highway of a flourishing but dangerous smuggling trade between Uganda, Kenya and Tanzania. Survival depended on protective sexual and business networks. AIDS was initially blamed on witchcraft and cultural transgressions. Suspected culprits included rejected women and cheated business partners. However, AIDS proved incurable, responding neither to traditional nor biomedical remedies. As AIDS was spread predominantly through sexual activity, cultural explanations turned their attention to women's non-observance of reproductive taboos on abortion. Abortion was polluting and required ritual cleansing. Unsuspecting men allegedly acquired HIV through sexual congress with uncleansed women, especially in urban areas lacking cultural controls. The message emanating from the Christian pulpit was that it was punishment from God for sexual indulgences.

By 1986 Uganda and African sex were rocketed into the international glare through medical reports and mass media, following the identification of AIDS as a fatal sexually transmitted disease. Uganda was overrun by WHO AIDS Global Initiative public health experts and in 1987 WHO sponsored the first AIDS Control Programme. People became well informed about the disease and how to prevent it, but translating this into knowledge for survival revived the debate on sexuality. Condoms were promoted as the appropriate public health technology to curb the epidemic. The condom distribution campaign initially targeted prostitutes and their obvious clients, long-distance truck-drivers. Free condoms were made available in the city health clinics. Educated mothers who suspected their adolescent sons of being sexually active encouraged them to get condoms, and sneaked condoms into their travelling husbands' luggage. These women were roundly condemned from the pulpits and by the press.

Urban condom legends about increased sexual activity became widespread. Condoms were condemned as offensive and a threat to communal moral sensibilities, by corrupting the youth, and endangering lives. The litter of carelessly disposed condoms around churches and mosques was offensive, and was dangerous to playing children, who suffocated, mistaking them for balloons, and to small livestock which choked on them when grazing. The most ubiquitous urban legend staple in pulpits went as follows:

> In one boarding school the headmaster distributed several condoms to each teenage boy after morning school assembly. Towards the end of the day there was a stream of boys knocking on his door, each saying: 'They are finished, I need more!'

The moral of the story was that condom distribution in schools was corrupting the youth and distracting them from schooling. The Ministry of Education was forced to dump thousands of much needed books for primary schools. The beautifully illustrated books, a donation by the French Danielle Mitterrand Foundation, featured a mango addressing the subject of sexual development and how to avoid the ubiquitous AIDS disease.

The AIDS Control Programme (ACP) in collaboration with the African Medical Research Foundation mounted a socially playful but conceptually aggressive campaign message 'zero grazing' to target the youth and married men. People understood the need to tether animals to restrict their feeding radius space in order to stop them from damaging crops and endangering communal goodwill. For humans, 'zero grazing' restrictions translated into assuming responsibility to spouses through faithfulness or preparedness to use condoms with partners. The AIDS prevention picture at the turn of the century was a mosaic.

The infection rates among women were double those of men because they depended upon the goodwill of men for condom protection. Their relatively weak economic and social position eroded their power to refuse sex which was seen as a requirement for procreation and a marital obligation. Older men continued resisting condom use, philandering, and preferring younger women for partners. Such men were openly vocal in their resistance to condoms as not natural sex.

But the men and women willing to use condoms faced the difficult hurdle of 'exceptionalism' posed by beauty or emotional closeness. Sex workers did not insist on condom use with special boyfriends. Several elite men independently confessed to routinely 'not leaving home without a condom' but frequently failing to use them when overwhelmed with beauty. A telling case is that of a senior ACP official who, after conducting a community workshop on the necessity of proper and consistent condom use in avoiding contagion, propositioned and grappled one of the female volunteers. When she challenged him on why he seemed not to need condom protection, he asserted that he knew she was HIV-free because she was young and beautiful. Her cackle as she walked away attracted our attention to his hypocrisy.

Young people were responding to information as knowledge for empowerment. They were learning new skills for negotiating sexual autonomy with their peers on a wide range of issues, including condom use when necessary. Nurses in clinics distributing free condoms reported a trend in youth consultations about sexually transmitted diseases and HIV testing when picking up condoms.

Foreign funding had peaked in the early 1990s, with over 600 AIDS-related programmes, including community-based drama groups, sexually transmitted disease control clinics, and orphan care. Most community-based projects largely focused on knowledge for survival by promoting condom acceptability through orientations courting the approval of religious and other conservative leaders. Traditional Muslim and Christian women were very active in condom promotion because they knew that most of them were being infected by husbands on whose goodwill to use condoms they depended. They wanted to save their children from certain death.

Prompted by the need to evaluate the success of projects for continued funding, WHO, as the leader in the war on AIDS and sponsor of the ACP campaigns, schematised the general picture of what was happening in Uganda as Abstinence, Be faithful and Condom use (ABC).

The United States through its aid agency USAID was from the beginning of the epidemic the largest funder of AIDS prevention programmes. An official boasted to me in 1991, 'We are doing it all.' In 1992 Uganda benefited further when Zaire was relegated to the status of international pariah by funding agencies as punishment for its President's corruption. Following a model that had been successfully developed in Zaire, USAID sponsored private companies to promote condom social marketing, which encouraged people to pay a small fee for condoms. But mostly USAID donated condoms for free distribution in government clinics. The local joke was that the embassy leaned over like the tower of Pisa in Italy from the weight of condoms. The urban youth who had witnessed the horrors of AIDS illness and deaths were scared into embracing condoms as the common-sense preventive measure. But the driving catalyst for their positive response was the availability of free condoms, and the opening of clinics for free confidential HIV testing and counselling.

A paper at the 1995 International Conference on AIDS and STDs in Africa, held in Kampala, reported a drop in HIV prevalence rates from the 18 per cent peak in 1992 among urban youths and mothers attending antenatal clinics. UNAIDS, newly formed to coordinate the AIDS prevention efforts of several UN organisations, joined in the self-congratulatory collective sigh of relief by researchers. With UNAIDS' acknowledgement of Uganda's success story status (1999), many organisations vied to share the credit. Religious groups aggressively claimed that their abstinence and fidelity formula had effectively stemmed the epidemic. Their position was strengthened in 2003.

By 1999 evangelical Christians had made extensive inroads in Africa. During the 1990s in America, chastity-until-marriage pledges, violent anti-abortion campaigns and the condemnation of condoms as promoting promiscuity and homosexuality had crystallised into benchmarks of cultural wars between religious-social conservatives and civil libertarians. These proxy wars were stealthily imported through their sponsored satellite churches in Africa. In Uganda, ambitious locals were encouraged to preach, and they were awarded scholarships to theological colleges. Trained pastors went on carefully guided tours of America that exposed them to the opulent lives of 'prosperity gospel' televangelists who promised material, financial, physical and spiritual success to believers. On their return pastors were encouraged by their American advisers, preachers and fundraisers to groom the power elite in the same way they had been groomed, with prayer and prospects of monetary rewards (see Rawls 2012).

In 2003, conservative religious sponsors of a new American AIDS funding proposal, the President's Emergency Plan For AIDS Relief (PEPFAR), invited targeted Ugandans to give testimonials. Prominent witnesses were Pastor Martin Ssempa, then a protégé of Rick Warren, pastor of the American Saddleback Church; and Janet Museveni, wife of the President and Ssempa's millennium eve born-again convert. Their verbal narratives, supported by handwritten notes distributed to congressmen, attributed the 'Uganda success story' entirely to abstinence (Bryton 2009). There was no mention of the aggressive condom educational campaign of the 1980s and the 1990s which had reduced the rate of HIV infection from 30 per cent in the 1980s to 6.4 per cent in the mid-1990s. In reward, Uganda was among the first countries to receive funding from PEPFAR. Foreign academic advisers (Hogel 2002), evangelical church leaders and political elites revised the AIDS control narrative and endorsed caveats against funding family planning, abortion and condoms. Sex education in and out of school and condom use became marginalised to the point of obscurity. In 2004, the existing successful American-funded condom-promoting AIDS prevention was dismantled when the government stopped the distribution of free condoms in clinics, and later imposed a tax on them. The new policy emphasis was on antiretroviral treatment. Sex education in schools was discouraged. Virginity-until-marriage pledges borrowed by advocates from the United States reinvented the wedding-morning virginity expectations. Young people are awarded cards and buttons, which they exchange for a ceremonial lantern on their wedding morning. Billboards promoting 'condomising' for survival were replaced by abstinence-pledging young people, and irresponsible women straying from the path of fidelity were ridiculed.

In this changed climate, those seeking PEPFAR funding capitulated. Project designers became skilled in self-censoring their experiential grassroots knowledge in favour of condom marginalisation. Concerns over rising infection rates because abstinence was not being practised were drowned by the din of revisionist scholars promoting ABC and blaming condom funders for creating a false sense of security for Africans (Green 2003).

Concluding remarks

Uganda has received $1.7 billion from PEPFAR to fight AIDS, and drugs spent on the prevention of mother-to-child transmission are saving babies. However, the anti-condom education and the anti-abortion policies are moral punishment strings that collectively deprive sexually active people of protection against STDs and deny women access to reproductive health services.

The general preference for the behavioural-change sexual paradigm in 'scientific' and social-cultural discourses buttresses the PEPFAR sponsorship of sexual morality in Africa. In true 'hidden persuaders' (Packard 1957) style, the co-opted locals echo the din emanating from foreigners about the appropriateness and authenticity of ABC as the endogenous cultural formulation. However, AIDS is high politics and when ideology drives the dissemination of information, survival knowledge is compromised.

Current HIV/AIDS prevalence is reported at 7.3 per cent, an increase from 6.4 per cent in 2005. HIV is spreading most not among sex workers or youth, but among married people. Infection rates are higher in women (8.3 per cent) than in men (6.4 per cent), with one in ten women in their thirties infected, compared to one in ten men in their forties (New Vision 2012; *New York Times* 2012). Health experts want a return to the strong government leadership and effective public education campaigns that contributed to the reduction in infection rates during the 1990s and earned Uganda acclaim and vast amounts of money. Furthermore, they urge that reports of emerging resistant HIV strains locally are the result of increased risky behaviour. Fear of HIV has been eroded by perceptions that antiretroviral drugs are managing and even curing AIDS (Tenywa 2008); and increasing claims of religious miracle cures. Health experts demand a new aggressive campaign reinstating the public health message of safer sex with condoms on equal footing with chastity and fidelity depicted in the 1995 poster.

The discourse pushing solely the 'partner reduction' solution presents Africans with false dilemmas. The 'abstain or die' anti-condom policy is a tough Hobson's choice relegating the 1990s Uganda success story to the 'back to the future' narrative.

References

Applbaum, K. 2004. *The Marketing Era: From Professional Practice to Global Provisioning*. New York: Routledge.

Bryton, E. 2009. 'The truth about Rick Warren and AIDS in Africa. Dispatches from the cultural wars: thoughts from the interface of science and religion'. http://scienceblogs.com/dispatches/2009/01/09/the-truth-about-rick-warren-an/.

Carpenter, L., A. Kamali, A. Ruberantwari, S.S. Malamba and J.A. Whitworth. 1999. 'Rates of HIV-transmission within marriage', *AIDS* 13(9): 1083-9.003.

Epstein, H. 2004. 'The fidelity fix', *New York Times*, 13 June.
Fogelberg, K. 2005. 'Not as easy as "ABC"; Uganda's approach to HIV and implications for the PEPFAR', *Michigan Journal of Public Affairs* 2.
Green, E.C. 2003. *Rethinking AIDS Prevention: Learning from Successes in Developing Countries*. New York: Praeger.
Halperin, D.T. and H. Epstein. 2004. 'Concurrent sexual partnerships help to explain Africa's high HIV prevalence: implications for prevention', *Lancet* 364(9428): 4–6.
Hogel, J.A. (ed.) 2002. *What Happened in Uganda? Declining HIV Prevalence, Behavior Change and National Response*. US Agency for International Development.
Human Rights Watch. 2005. 'U.S.-funded "abstinence-only" programs are jeopardizing Uganda's successful fight against HIV'.
Jauch, H. 1999. *Structural Adjustment Programmes: Their Origin and International Experiences*. Namibia: Labour Resource and Research Institute.
Mah, T.L. and D.T. Halperin. 2010. 'Concurrent sexual partnership and HIV epidemics in Africa: evidence to move forward', *AIDS Behaviour* 14(1): 11–16.
Morris, M. and A. Kretzchmar. 1997. 'Concurrent partnership and the spread of HIV', *AIDS* 11(5): 641–8.
Naiman, R. and N. Watkins. 1999. *A Survey of the Impacts of IMF Structural Adjustment in Africa: Growth, Social Spending, and Debt Relief*. Centre for Economic Research, Dakar-Codesria.
New Vision. 2012. 'Uganda medics attack religious leaders over HIV/AIDS', 5 July.
New York Times. 2012. 'Uganda', 2 August.
Packard, V. 1957. *The Hidden Persuaders*. New York: David McKay.
Parikh, S.A. 2007. 'The political economy of marriage and HIV: the ABC approach, "safe" infidelity and managing moral risk in Uganda', *American Journal of Public Health* 97(7): 1198–208.
Rawls, K. 2012. 'How deep is the Republican Christian Right's connection to the anti-gay bills sweeping Sub-Saharan Africa?', *AlterNet*, 6 February.
Schoepf, B.G. 2001. 'International AIDS research in anthropology: taking a critical perspective on the crisis', *Annual Review of Anthropology* 30: 335–61.
Southall, A. 1960. 'On chastity in Africa', *Uganda Journal* 24(2): 207–16.
Tenywa, G. (and Agencies). 2008. 'Uganda: stick to condom use', *All Africa News*, 10 February.
Timberlake, L. 1986. *Africa in Crisis*. London: Earthscan.
UNAIDS. 1999. *Uganda: Best Practice Collection*. Geneva: UNAIDS.
UNAIDS. 2005. *AIDS in Africa Three Scenarios to 2025*. Geneva: UNAIDS.

3

Hands across the Sea: Religion, Politics, Gender and Sex, in the US and Africa

BROOKE GRUNDFEST SCHOEPF

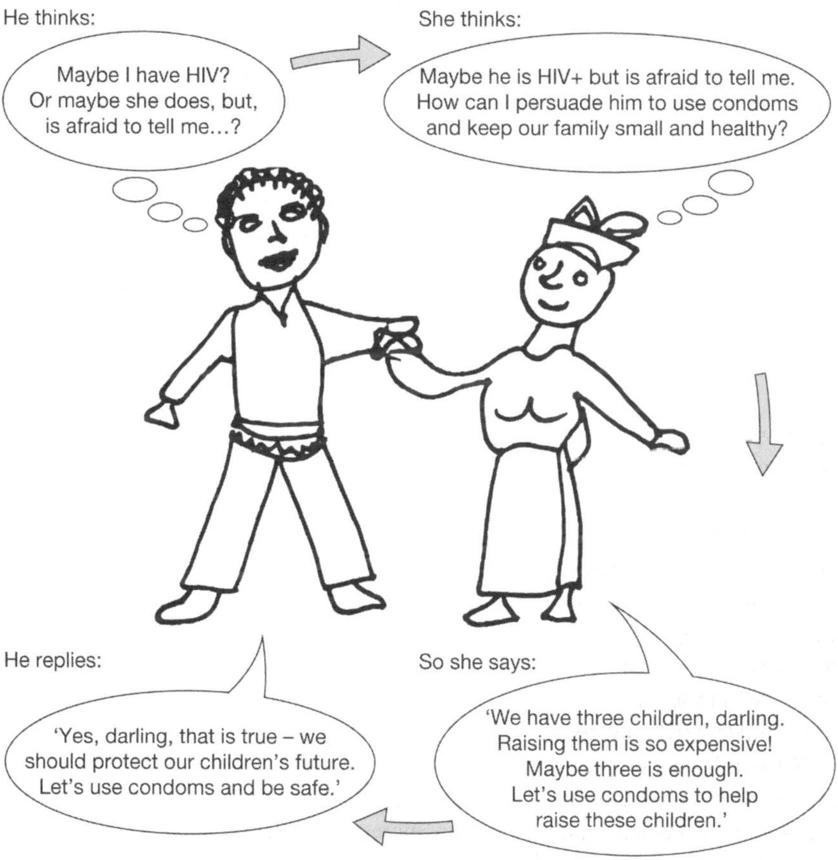

Dialogue of a couple afraid to disclose HIV status

Proceedings of the British Academy **194**, *43–67*.

Introduction

AIDS, LIKE MANY OTHER EPIDEMICS, is socially produced. Societal responses to AIDS in Africa, including disease control policies, from the outset have been propelled by cultural politics forged in the history of relations between Africa and the West (Schoepf 1991). Sexually transmitted and subject to discursive elaboration, 'AIDS brings to the fore in public discourse ideological representations that support and reproduce already constituted gender, colour, class and national hierarchies' (Schoepf 1992: 260). It was clear from the outset that 'structural violence', including poverty, and gender inequality rendered women particularly vulnerable to infection (Schoepf *et al.* 1988).

As the most important civil society institutions in many African countries today, churches act in a complex changing social field. In the context of HIV/AIDS, researchers have looked especially to the effects of Catholic, evangelical and fundamentalist Christian religious leaders' stress on pre-marital abstinence and marital fidelity as ways to prevent infection. The influence of charismatic pastors grew markedly with deepening poverty in the 1980s and 1990s. Their conservative moralist strictures against comprehensive science-based sex education and condom use, as well as their sometimes stigmatising views of sufferers, have left many people, especially girls, women, and men who have sex with men, disarmed and vulnerable to HIV infection, unable to use condoms and fearful to test or to seek treatment. These practices constitute violations of the human rights to health, to bodily integrity and to life itself. In this chapter, I show that many African religious leaders' rejection of public health advice resonates with and, indeed, has emanated from and been supported by the ultra-conservative Christian 'religious right' in the United States, which has exported its 'culture wars' to Africa.

The chapter begins with an overview of the current state of the HIV/AIDS epidemic in Africa, and situates AIDS in Kinshasa in relation to Structural Adjustment and economic crisis. An ethnographic vignette illustrates now-common themes that emerged from the outset of the epidemic. It also suggests the politics of international foot-dragging and misdirection which have left the bodies of women and youth as sites of struggle. I go on to cast a backward glance at lingering historical discourses on the sexuality of Africans that re-emerged in response to AIDS. Then I examine strong cross-cutting currents of HIV/AIDS politics and religious practices that flow between leaders in the US and sub-Saharan Africa, particularly in respect of gender and sexuality. These are related to discourses of 'tradition', the struggle to eliminate AIDS, and to gain and consolidate human rights in Africa and the US.

Recent discourse and practices of many African evangelical Christian leaders in Kinshasa and elsewhere perpetuate stigma and blame; and spread witchcraft accusations, especially against children, increasing misery. As in the US, religious fervour in Africa appears to distract many people from analysing the causes of their poverty and oppression. In closing, I return to consider policy and activism, stressing the need for international support for expanded antiretroviral (ARV) drug treatment, for strong public health systems and protection for human rights. This contribution encourages researchers to ask where the religious leaders and congregations they study stand in respect of human rights and the politics and process of societal transformation now widely recognised as necessary to end the AIDS pandemic.

AIDS: the disease

The drums of affliction continue to resound across Africa. To the bitter suffering of poverty and hunger, AIDS deaths and attendant social dislocation add a fog of fear, mistrust, and superstition, exacerbated by lack of confidence in biomedicine. Over the years, medical science has achieved the means to prevent much of this infection, suffering and death. Gains made in treatment prolong lives but there is still no cure, and treatment must continue lifelong. Despite success in expanding treatment and reducing incidence rates, in 2011, 23 million Africans lived with HIV, more than 1.2 million people died from AIDS and related causes, and 1.5 million became infected with HIV (UNAIDS 2012: 36–7). The earlier that infection is detected and treatment with antiretroviral drugs (ARVs) begun, the more likely that treatment will allow infected people to live healthily for many years without hospitalisation, and render them 96 per cent less likely to transmit the virus to others (Cohen *et al.* 2011). Early treatment of HIV-positive pregnant women before delivery virtually eliminates transmission of the virus to their infants and increases the chances of giving birth to a full-term, normal birth-weight baby.

ARV treatment accounts for as much as half the decline in new infections. UNAIDS and WHO now recommend that treatment commence as soon as HIV is detected and, urgently, *before* the level of CD4 T (immune) cells declines below 350 copies per cubic millilitre. While lifelong therapy remains expensive, drug costs had dropped to as little as $100 per person in 2011 for some WHO-approved regimens. 'Treat-to-prevent' is a cost-beneficial strategy. It not only eliminates much pain and suffering; mathematical modelling shows that the expenditures are recouped by costs avoided by societies and families later on. Yet due to a dearth of resources, few African countries are able to commence treatment at this level. Many people still do not know that they are infected, while more than half of Africans, especially people living in urban peripheries and in rural areas, lack access to ARVs. Some come too late to be saved.

Given the limited reach of biomedical health services in most of Africa and the fact that people are most apt to transmit HIV when their 'viral load' is high during acute primary infection, that is, in the early months before HIV is detectable by commonly used tests, other preventive measures are needed. Circumcision offers men about 60 per cent protection from infection, but they still need to use condoms to protect both themselves and partners. Condoms, regularly used, and changes in sexual behaviour that reduce risk remain the most effective non-medical ways to prevent infection.

None of this is easy. People who have engaged in risky behaviour and do not know their HIV-status must reflect upon their risks, use condoms, then get tested for HIV and, if found positive, obtain ARV treatment. Some risky sex is linked to livelihood strategies, particularly sex work, migrant labour, and long-distance trade. Too few condoms are available. Their use, especially among couples who are emotionally involved, requires overcoming many constraints; few women can refuse unprotected sex to a steady partner. Gender inequality continues to undermine the coverage and uptake of services. Recent public health advice links HIV prevention and AIDS care to reproductive health care for women; failure to take seriously the structural, ideological and interpersonal violence that causes both men and women to engage in sex with more than one partner contributes to the continuing incidence of new infections. Thus, without societal transformation, '[t]he full potential of the recent breakthroughs in HIV prevention and treatment will not be realized' (UNAIDS 2012: 58).

Structural adjustment and AIDS

In the 1980s, as HIV spread with gathering momentum, Structural Adjustment Programmes (SAPs), a concerted move to 'roll back the state', reduced millions of Africans to dire poverty. Most African governments succumbed to pressure from the conservative 'Washington Consensus' of the Reagan and Thatcher governments along with the institutions of international finance, to carry out SAP-mandated budget cuts and institute user fees for services. With many health workers and teachers made redundant, already deficient levels of public biomedical health care, education and social services diminished (Schoepf *et al.* 2000). Underpaid public-sector health workers who remained struggled to make a living; some charged fees for themselves. Only government and business elites and their relatives could access adequate care. International assistance went primarily to non-governmental organisations (NGOs), including churches and other faith-based organisations (FBOs). In 2007 WHO estimated that FBOs operated from 30 to 70 per cent of health services in Africa, resulting in narrowed access not only to curative, but also to preventive services, including family planning and reproductive health. Staffing shortages limit the capacity to deliver health services, partly due to the ongoing brain drain of trained medical personnel, which AIDS and the professional brain drain have made worse (Mills *et al.* 2011). At present, many HIV programmes are unable to ensure consistent, uninterrupted treatment of patients already enrolled, let alone reach all the new people in need. International assistance to low- and middle-income countries has fallen in recent years, and while these countries have increased their domestic outlays, the global AIDS budget is inadequate (UNAIDS 2012).

Restricted access to quality affordable public biomedical health care and education creates barriers to understanding biomedical concepts of AIDS' causes and prevention. Fund-starved public education fails to impart crucial concepts of scientific reasoning and evidence-based understanding. Few young people can obtain secular secondary education where biology, including sex and reproduction, is competently taught. Such credibility as biomedicine enjoyed by dint of its cures was undermined by AIDS, feared as a death sentence. Rumours and persistent cosmological beliefs related to constructions of sexuality, reproduction, health and gender, along with pluralistic health-seeking practices, make biomedicine just one among several sources of authority. All these conditions contribute to the spread of HIV.

AIDS in Kinshasa

Zaire's (now Democratic Republic of Congo or DRC) economy, in crisis from the mid-1970s, collapsed in the 1980s and has yet to recover. An estimated 40 to 60 per cent of urban men, and even more women, were without waged employment. The majority resorted to the informal sector, but macro-level crisis rendered the already crowded informal sector increasingly more precarious for many small operators. Trade over long distances within Zaire and across its borders fostered multiple-partner sexual relationships. Women who formerly relied upon steady contributions from male partners, or from their extended families, reported these resources dwindling. By the late 1980s, many poor children ate just one day out of two at home, and were sent out to forage in the streets; adolescent girls were sent to peddle sex. Powerless to control their reproductive bodies, girls and women were vulnerable to HIV infection. Along with HIV and AIDS, these social forces created stressors that gave rise to fear and anxiety, reduced women's social supports and undermined their sense of self-worth.

Early in our research, women told us that gender inequality, poverty and powerlessness placed women at risk for AIDS. A population-based epidemiological survey found that young women between the ages of 15 and 19 were 2.0 times, and those aged 20 to 24, 2.5 times more HIV-infected than young men of the same age. As elsewhere, poor women engaged in sex work were the most vulnerable, with 27 per cent of a cohort working in Matonge, Kinshasa's central entertainment district, infected in 1985 and 35 per cent in 1988. This compared with 13.9 per cent of young women employed at the city hospital and 6 per cent of women giving birth there. Both the hospital and the household survey found that 39 per cent of women with HIV or AIDS were married, as were 61 per cent of the female partners of male AIDS patients.

In the time of AIDS, conditions beyond the control of many women deprive them of agency. They have enlarged their caring roles, perforce. The severe diarrhoea and the mental illnesses of AIDS sufferers are particularly onerous, as most women care for sick husbands, children and other relatives in homes without running water, indoor toilets or soap. One Kinshasa study found that 71 out of 80 poor HIV-positive women assisted by a local NGO reported that caring for sick spouses with insufficient food and medicines left them exhausted, isolated, and extremely stressed, with little energy to care for children, while stigma left them socially isolated. Only one-quarter reported help from family or others; most were refused (Kipp *et al.* 2006). AIDS support groups provide some overburdened women with a venue to share their troubles and obtain emotional solace. The material resources of small support groups are often overwhelmed by growing need, however, as Catholic women in Kinshasa told Lourdes Cottingham in 1994 (letters in files of the author). Competition over meagre resources may lead to conflict (Rukarangira wa Nkera 2002). Such groups do not result in women's 'empowerment', since their endeavours fail to alter the distribution of material resources or to engage members in critical analysis of the sources of their oppression. AIDS has punched holes in the informal social safety nets on which poor people rely and churches have not stepped in sufficiently to fill the need.

Most of the more than one million people of DRC living with HIV/AIDS are in dire straits. Churches own half of all hospitals, where they provide fee-for-service care unavailable in the public health system. Quality varies markedly, some good, some very poor. Some offer compassionate support and care for AIDS sufferers, but few offer ARV treatment. Even supposedly free care requires fees for tests, syringes and, often, inducements to health workers, as well as costs for transportation and for food needed to render drugs effective. Only 30 per cent of *Kinois* in need were receiving ARV treatment in 2012; nationwide, the figure was only 12 per cent (IRIN 2012a).

Christian leaders in Kinshasa have been active from the outset in interpreting the causes of the HIV/AIDS epidemic. Some responded to suffering with unflagging compassion, offering succour to the sick, orphaned and bereaved. A small survey of HIV-positive pregnant women showed that some churches (denominations not specified) assisted them in disclosing their infection to others (generally *not* to spouses for fear of rejection). Belief that although God sent HIV infection, he had the power to cure their infection comforted some women, most of whom were not receiving ARV treatment (Maman *et al.* 2009).

Some churches sought to provide preventive education. For example, in 1987, the Catholic Diocese of Kinshasa issued a series of pamphlets drafted by Dr Rukarangira, Co-Director of CONNAISSIDA, to guide weekly meetings of its 2,000 base communities. The fourth week included information about condoms and advised that, 'Although the Church advises faithfulness, if you can't be faithful, don't also risk your life; use a condom.' Soon afterwards, however, the Pope visited Africa and forbade condom use. Other churches' ideology and activities are also less than constructive. Many pastors and lay Catholic men claim that AIDS is sent by God (or the devil) to punish 'sinners' who contravene their moral codes, and mark sufferers as stigmatised 'Others'. Conservative African priests and pastors assured married women that fidelity would protect them from AIDS, and some proposed to exorcise the 'satan-inspired sins' of sexual transgressors (Schoepf 1993). 'Traditional healers' claimed that since biomedicine could not cure AIDS, it must be an old African disease rooted in 'witchcraft' or 'sexual pollution', afflictions which they claimed they could cure. These claims were not accepted without question, however. Many early sufferers were members of the university-educated elite, for whom biomedical explanations were uppermost.

Religion, gender and HIV risk

The CONNAISSIDA Project experimented with community-based critical consciousness-raising methods for HIV/AIDS prevention from 1987 (Schoepf 1993). One experience demonstrated the constraints of religion and the limits of women's pragmatic agency, about which many middle-class professional women also spoke (Schoepf 1988).

When male deacons of the Baptist Church in a mixed-income neighbourhood near the university refused to allow us to hold workshops at the church for sex workers living nearby, we met in the walled garden of a colleague. Before the second session, a delegation of three rotund matrons awaited us on his veranda. 'We are Deaconesses and we want you to hold workshops for the Mothers' Club at the church.' Eighty women took part in weekly sessions for six weeks. One asked, 'Is AIDS sent by God?' I answered with a question, 'Would a God who sent His only Son to earth to forgive us our transgressions act in vengeance?' The women decided that to the contrary, rather than attributing blame, God would act with compassion and succour the afflicted. Towards the end of the workshop, the deaconesses said, 'Teach us to do what you do so we can work in our community.'

The following week, at a festive meal to thank us for the workshops, the pastor's benediction echoed a recent radio broadcast by Kinshasa's Protestant bishop who assured women that faithfulness to their husbands would protect them from AIDS. Too polite to contradict authority, the women understood his error. Many husbands who traded between Kinshasa and Bandundu had wives and lovers in several places. They and other Kinshasa wives were fearful of AIDS, but although some could negotiate condom protection, most could not. One who tried had been threatened with an end to financial support for their household; another husband threatened his wife with expulsion from the family home. Some women found ways to address the condom issue indirectly, for example, slipping condoms in the valise they packed for a husband's journey or persuading husbands to use condoms for family planning. One-third of husbands swore that they had no outside partners, and wives believed them.

Armed with information gleaned from interaction with professionals, these women's pragmatic knowledge withstood the church leaders' moralist discourse. They and the women with whom they shared their new knowledge fastened onto their role as mothers to protect their children from HIV/AIDS. While Christian prohibitions inhibited them from speaking directly to their children about sex, parents found other ways to warn them, including urging them to listen to a popular singer's cassette of explicit advice then playing across Kinshasa. Numerous parents in our elite networks invited CONNAISSIDA researchers to provide sex education to the young people living in their homes.

Many people gave up hope in the 1980s, as erosion of the state, with economic crisis and structural violence, gave rise to social and domestic anomie. Religious effervescence burgeoned as some sought salvation and solace in prayer groups and sects. Social support, especially among women, helped them to cope with suffering, deprivation, and grief. Some women in Kinshasa induced husbands to take part in prayer groups, hoping that 'born-again' men might resist the temptations of drink and extra-marital sex. They prayed that their daughters would abstain from sex until they could find faithful spouses among the congregants. Many young men were unemployed and too poor to support families; when accidents happened, even among 'born-agains', few accepted responsibility for girlfriends' pregnancies (Schoepf 1993; Ngondo 2001).

In the 1990s, widespread destitution and frustration with the Mobutu regime led to city-wide looting and violence in Kinshasa and other cities by the military, youth gangs, the unemployed and destitute, which inflicted more damage on the economy (Jewsiewicki 1992; Devisch 1995). Charismatic Catholics took centre stage with a discourse of fellowship (Ngirabakunzi, pers. comm. 2004). Evangelical religious leaders, followers of the American preachers of the 'prosperity gospel', promised a new community whose faithful could enter the kingdom of heaven without worrying about the poor (Jewsiewicki 1992: 67). Membership in Pentecostal and independent charismatic 'healing' churches in Kinshasa increased from 3 per cent of inhabitants sampled in 1968 to 16.3 per cent in 1996 (de St. Moulin 1996: 205); in poor zones it had risen to more than 18 per cent by 1998, and it continues to grow. Women, hoping to experience emotional release and to rekindle social solidarity, as well as to keep husbands faithful, formed the majority of adherents. Some pastors were leaders of the Mobutu regime; they and many others made small fortunes from contributions of the credible. Biaya noted that while enthusiastic worship can be a positive experience, too often it is embedded in political messages that are anti-woman, anti-science, anti-social justice, bellicose, chauvinistic and anti-democratic. In this case, joyful experience becomes grounds for political manipulation, as 'the Pentecostal movement in Kinshasa reinterpreted structural violence so as *to obscure class interests, especially the interests of ruling class members turned pastors*' (Biaya 1997: 366, italics added).

What scholars earlier signalled as the twilight of the Mobutu regime was a prelude to its overturn in 1997 by rebels from the east and to continuing violence in 'Africa's First World War'. Regime change failed to bring economic redress or an end to corruption, as new leaders continued to 'eat' foreign aid, including donations for AIDS treatment, and to skim lucrative contracts for mineral extraction by transnational firms. Armed violence continues in the east, and with it rape, used as a weapon of war.

Sex and colonial Christian imaginaries

The view of 'dangerous women' has roots in conservative Christian moralism introduced with colonial rule. It intertwines with neo-traditional gender relations to add theological support for elder male dominance in family, property, and society. Indeed, Christian churches' support for what Terence Ranger (Hobsbawm and Ranger 1983) terms 'invented tradition' has a venerable history in Belgium's colony of the Congo and in the Mobutist regime, especially in respect of gender subordination and sexual morality, as Obbo (Chapter 2 in this volume) relates for Uganda.

Whence the stigma? Stereotypes underlying the racism that pervaded much early writing on AIDS in Africa have a long history in Western thought. Sexualisation of a despised and scapegoated 'other' in Catholic Europe by church and secular officials blamed the Jews for the bubonic plague epidemics that raged from the fourteenth century. Sartre (1946) linked stereotypes of Jewish 'hyper-sexuality' in Europe to periodic brutal pogroms and the ease with which the Nazis were able to carry out genocide. European interest in the sex life of Africans can be traced in the written record at least as far back as the Elizabethan period, as in Shakespeare's *Othello*. Europeans viewed African women and men through lenses distorted by phantasmagorical racist stereotypes that linked sexuality to colour, class and 'primitivity', the antithesis of 'civilised' whites. 'Wild eroticism', first constructed as a positive but patronising trope of the 'noble savage', subsequently turned negative as Christian puritanism took hold. The sexuality of black Africans, on the continent and in the American diaspora – and to a lesser extent of all peoples of colour – was constructed as 'natural' and 'excessive', rather than socially regulated.

During the European scramble for Africa, the colonial imagination stigmatised African women, with Congo as the realm of '"the loosest and corruptest women in the world"' (Monti 1988: 72), uncontrollable by the colonial 'civilising mission', and 'fulfilling secret wishes' (Corbey 1988: 86). Considerable fantasising was involved, but also the power of command, as women, children and 'savages' were linked ontologically, 'primitives' contrasted with 'civilised' European men. Portrayals of Africans as lazy, diseased and degenerate served to justify enslavement, forced labour, land expropriation and harsh plantation systems in Africa and in the New World, beginning with the slave trade and colonial conquest. In the territories of King Leopold's brutal 'Red Rubber' system of wild rubber collection, soldiers of the Crown and transnational concession companies raped and murdered with impunity. Racism permeated the colonial medical enterprise, with syphilis constructed as an 'African disease' rooted in 'hyper-sexuality'. In the 1880s, African women in Kinshasa were blamed for its spread and threatened with execution.

Especially in respect of gender relations, some 'customs' were invented out of whole cloth as the colonial state and Catholic Church extended their rule. While white men employed *ménagères* to satisfy their sexual urges, women's sexuality was stigmatised. When European women came, black men were feared as potential rapists. Girls were taken to mission farm-schools, put to work growing food for the missions, taught domesticity and advised that Christian women owed obedience in the church and to their husbands. Tracts reprinted in the 1970s drew upon St Paul's letter to the Ephesians (3:22) admonishing women to submit to their husbands, for just as Christ is head of the Church, so the man is the head of the family and must be obeyed. In daily life in Kinshasa in the twenty-first century, moralising discourses of femininity continue to denigrate unmarried women and proclaim marriage as the sole respectable status, with St Paul's letter brandished to support women's obedience. Few male social scientists contest these views (Mianda 1995; Ngondo 2001).

Discourse on AIDS in Africa

Although discourses of racism changed form across the decades, the enduring colonial tropes of 'super-potent' black men and 'lascivious women' remain so much a part of Euro-American culture that many are unaware of their effects. Early portrayals of AIDS in the West as a 'disease of homosexuals' led to confusion in Africa, where overt homosexuality was a rarity. Since little risk came from that quarter, most leaders and publics were unconcerned. The first Africans to be diagnosed with HIV were wealthy heterosexual men seeking treatment in Europe. International biomedical and popular journalistic accounts re-created colonial 'ethno-pornography'. Some mistakenly constructed 'heterosexual AIDS' as a uniquely African epidemic and characterised the sexuality of Africans as 'promiscuous' and different from that of peoples elsewhere. With prostitutes designated as 'a reservoir of infection', some claimed that no line could be drawn between prostitutes and other women. Sex in Africa was treated as an instrumental relationship, a mechanical act devoid of sentiment, unrelated to love and intimacy, to procreation as a social and psychological process surrounded by values and cosmology, but also related to power and mastery, submission and fear.

Western mass media seized upon the theme of 'disordered' sexuality and dubbed Kinshasa 'the AIDS capital of the world'. *Kinois* were particularly offended by the exotic 'customs' invented to explain the spread of the virus from monkeys to humans. These imaginaries contributed powerfully to shaping African responses. In defence of African personhood and culture, students designated AIDS (SIDA) as a '*Syndrome Imaginaire pour Décourager les Amoreux*' (an imaginary syndrome to discourage lovers). Encapsulating popular resistance, the phrase continues to resound across Africa as 'an American invention', along with conspiracy theories of many kinds that contribute to denial of risk.

Targeting prostitutes as a 'risk group' fuelled African men's constructions of AIDS as a disease of 'dangerous women' from whom men required protection. Many blamed women for spreading HIV while denying their own role. The racism and moralising texts were 'words that kill', as resistance to stigma by both leaders and publics fostered denial, delayed understanding of the danger to individuals and families, and hampered prevention, worsening the spread of infection. Interviews made clear that moralist control of sexuality for HIV prevention was by adult men, acting to strengthen their control over women and youth. As products of colonial religious education, many male leaders of government and the universities shared stigmatising views of female sexuality. Wealthy, high-status men promoted abstinence for youth (that is, for young men; not for the adolescent women whom they sought as partners), and fidelity for married women, while their own entitlement to multiple partners as a prerogative of wealth and power continued undiminished (Biaya 1997; Schoepf 1988, 2002), vouchsafing their 'pride in possessing an active penis and sexual rights over subordinates' (Mbembe 1992: 9).

From the US to Africa

Conservative US leaders have helped to shape discourses and practices among Africa's evangelical churches around morality, sexuality and gender. In 1983, at the outset of the epidemic, the Reagan administration, heavily influenced by the 'Christian Right' with its strong condemnation of homosexuality, turned its back on the burgeoning epidemic. It refused to regulate the US blood bank industry and stinted on federal funds for biomedical research, treatment and prevention. It also avoided the growing AIDS epidemic in Africa. American evangelical pastors claimed that God was using AIDS to punish sinners. In 1986, the US Surgeon General broke his five-year silence with a report that called for comprehensive sex education and condom use as protection against HIV. Conservatives condemned the report and vilified its author as 'pandering to the immoral'. Similar ideology continued in the teachings of US evangelical leaders whose influence in Africa grew markedly with poverty in the 1980s.

A significant reversal came during the presidency of George W. Bush (2001–8), when neo-conservative security advisers convinced him that AIDS could result in political destabilisation and a terrorist threat in failed African states. News stories of AIDS in Africa, especially of 'innocent' women and children, focused the attention of the American public and garnered bipartisan sympathy for sufferers and orphaned survivors. Bush, an evangelical Christian, made it a priority to reshape the relationship of religion to politics, providing faith-based organisations at home and abroad with government money. His evangelical Christian political base found support for AIDS programmes in Africa an opportunity to advance their social agenda and to roll back international advances that favoured women's health and reproductive rights, including condom promotion and family planning.

At the United Nations Special Session on Children in May 2002, the US joined with Libya, Indonesia, Iran, Iraq, Sudan, Syria and the Vatican in attempts to block a consensus on sex education for youth (two-thirds of whom are sexually active before the age of 18) and on the health benefits of contraception. The US repudiated commitments to international health and poverty reduction made at the 1984 Cairo Conference on Population and Development and the 1995 Beijing Platform for Action on Women's Rights. At a thirty-nation ministerial meeting of the Fifth Asian and Pacific Population Conference in Bangkok in December 2002, US officials demanded deletion of a reference to 'consistent condom use' to fight HIV/AIDS and other STDs, and issued an official statement that 'condoms are simply not 100% effective'. The Bush administration mounted a worldwide campaign to enlist other governments in restricting information about sexuality and condoms for HIV prevention.

In 2003, the US Congress appropriated $15 billion for five years for the President's Emergency Fund for AIDS Relief (PEPFAR) for treatment and prevention in fourteen countries of Africa and Haiti. Ten billion dollars of the amount was new money, while $5 billion came from established health programmes, principally from family planning. PEPFAR came with strings attached, as Americans of the Christian Right set out for Africa to proselytise their version of morality, using Uganda as a beachhead. After heated debate on prevention policy, during which Uganda's First Lady, Janet Museveni, a born-again Christian, testified to the US Congress in support of a restrictive abstinence-only policy, conservative Christian legislators ear-marked one-third of the $1 billion prevention allocation for programmes to promote abstinence-only for youth and faithfulness in marriage ('A and B'). PEPFAR funds could not be used to promote condoms to youth in schools, or for social marketing campaigns that target youth and encourage condom use.

In his plenary address to the International AIDS Conference in 2004, Ugandan President Museveni urged countries to employ abstinence-only education and exhortations to monogamy, pledging to institute this as Uganda's mass HIV prevention strategy (Schoepf 2004). Uganda received PEPFAR grants of $90.8

million in 2004, $148.4 million in 2005 and $169.9 million in 2006, including $15 million that year to an interfaith coalition for abstinence promotion and care. Evangelical Christian NGOs in Uganda that had ignored AIDS for more than a decade began to carry out abstinence-only programmes for youth with US funds, to promote misinformation, and stigmatise people with HIV. Awards to FBOs totalled $552 million in 2006 and $586 million in 2007 (IRIN 2012a). US missionary medical networks active in Africa, such as the Christian Medical and Dental Association (CMDA), also opposed both condom education and outreach that empowers sex workers to protect themselves. Some groups require Bible-reading in their sex education classes. The US Constitution's ban against the establishment of religion prohibits federal assistance to organisations that engage in 'inherently religious activities'. Nevertheless, USAID declared that the ban did not apply to foreign aid. Meanwhile, many African NGOs that actually provided services to vulnerable people were starved for funds.

Churches' influence in moulding behaviour varies. Some researchers who establish relations of confidence with Pentecostal informants find that not all are able to conform to the churches' strict moral code. Common lapses in abstinence and fidelity are not likely to include condom protection (Gusman 2009). Similarly, emphasis on fidelity leaves uninfected partners in 'stable couples' without protection and helps to explain the epidemiological shift now registered in such countries as Uganda, Zambia and Zimbabwe, where 'discordant couples' account for between 30 and 65 per cent of new infections. It also leaves vulnerable many women who struggle to survive without the support of a steady partner.

In 2005, in the wake of criticism by human rights groups, President Museveni addressed Catholic bishops from ten sub-Saharan countries in pragmatic terms, calling upon them to drop opposition to the use of condoms in order to save lives. Still, damage was done to Uganda's nascent 'condom culture' developing among youth and others with multiple partners. It inhibited the dialogue that couples need to engage in when only one is infected. New infections rose, especially among discordant couples. Two studies found that 43 per cent of married HIV-positive people had uninfected spouses, but few used condoms.

Despite its shortcomings in respect of prevention interventions, by 2008, PEPFAR provided ARV therapy to two million Africans, about the same number as the Global Fund to which the US was the largest contributor. Congress re-authorised the programme for another five years, with $48 billion to 2013. By the end of President Bush's time in office in January 2009, he could claim PEPFAR as a major foreign policy success, in contrast to the two disastrous wars he began. AIDS policy is not a stand-alone issue, for it is bound up both ideologically and practically with reproductive health policy. President Bush also reinstated a 'gag rule', initiated by Reagan, later rescinded by Clinton (and rescinded again by Obama), that eliminated PEPFAR funding for reproductive health providers who offer abortion information using *other, non-US government*, funds. This ensures that poor women will be even less likely than before to obtain HIV prevention advice, as well as contraceptive services that can save their lives. As predicted, in 2004 the policy forced closings of scarce reproductive health services, especially in rural areas where they are often the only clinics available and maternal mortality rates are high. Issues related to protection from HIV infection are also those of sexual and reproductive health: the right to knowledge, the power to use it, and access to effective technologies. Abstinence-only sex education, combined with lack of access to contraception, leaves people vulnerable to HIV infection, STDs, and unplanned and unwanted pregnancies.

As noted above, under Bush, PEPFAR funds could not be used for contraception or abortion, or even to support other activities in clinics that provided abortion advice. Providers who refused to sign a pledge restricting prevention assistance to sex workers were forced to close for lack of funds. The $48 billion PEPFAR re-authorisation of 2008 continued these policies of its predecessor. It eliminated the one-third 'A&B' rule, but required administrators to report to Congress when funding for restrictive programmes fell below 50 per cent, effectively *increasing* such funding, for administrators were likely to follow the restriction in order to fly below the radar of conservative legislators. In sum, the Bush policy shifted funds from and restricted family planning and other reproductive health services, added to women's burden of preventable suffering and death, and violated women's most basic human rights.

Policy reversal followed the election of President Barack Obama in 2008: Congress re-authorised PEPFAR, and the US continues as the largest contributor to AIDS treatment and prevention in Africa. In May 2009, President Obama launched a six-year, $63 billion, Global Health Initiative (GHI) that incorporates AIDS treatment and prevention into a broader health agenda, with health systems' strengthening at its core. The GHI stresses comprehensive prevention education and integration of HIV and reproductive health services, including increased access to family planning and measures to address women's inequality at national and local levels. Reversing anti-woman health policies is a major achievement of the Obama presidency, guided by health rights and social justice advocates.

In 2010 the Obama administration's struggle to implement science-based policies encountered entrenched opposition from the Christian Right. Bankrolled by multi-billionaires, and supported by Rupert Murdoch's Fox News media, the mainly white Tea Party wing of the Republican Party captured the political initiative. Claiming America as 'a Christian country', the Tea Party counts as supporters not only many evangelicals such as Baptists and Pentecostals, but also many Catholics and some members of mainstream Protestant churches. Its candidates swept Congress and state governments, making it impossible to enact Democrats' policies in support of reproductive freedom, gender equality and sexual health in the US and abroad. Congress decreased funding for PEPFAR and the

Global Fund annually from 2010. It also eliminated international family planning assistance from the 2012 budget.

The US electoral campaign of 2012 witnessed a vigorous assault by Republicans of the Christian Right on American women's reproductive rights in national and state governments. More than half of all states restrict access to abortion, insurance coverage for contraceptives, and other reproductive health care. The Republican Party seeks a constitutional ban on abortion and many male lawmakers oppose birth control. This concerted 'war on women' is the context in which to view the Obama administration's AIDS policies in Africa, for while the President won re-election, the Democrats do not hold legislative power, including the power of the purse. In the face of the economic recession, President Obama's 2013 budget request to Congress proposed a $563 million reduction in overall funds for PEPFAR (3 per cent of the $6.4 billion total), counting on 'greater efficiencies' to treat more than 4 million people in fifty-eight countries and to prevent 12 million new infections. It included a somewhat larger contribution to the Global Fund ($1.65 billion), however, an amount that would complete Obama's pledge of $4 billion from 2011 to 2013. Both PEPFAR and the Global Fund have made great strides and both need to do more to combat HIV/AIDS. The US provided 54.2 per cent of total AIDS funds. While some African governments have stepped up their expenditures, most lag behind on their 2001 Abuja Declaration commitment to spend at least 15 per cent of their national budgets on health. Funds, trained personnel and community involvement are essential to controlling the epidemic. AIDS treatment is complex and requires resources and logistics beyond the health centre level. UNAIDS calculates that universal access to AIDS treatment, prevention, care and support will require $22 to $24 billion by 2015.

Drug prices are an area in which to make cost savings. Prices have declined in recent years, with most of the first-line ARVs consumed in Africa coming from manufacturers of off-licence generics. According to UNAIDS, they are still too high to be sustainable. Pricing by multinationals under World Trade Organization rules enforced by the US keeps many second-line medications out of reach and will lead to treatment interruptions. These prices are not within the control of African or other governments of poor and middle-income countries; they require concertation on trade policy by the G20 nations, especially the United States, where lobbyists for the pharmaceutical industry control so many legislators that President Obama was unable to bargain down domestic drug prices in the context of health care reform, let alone institute a single-payer health insurance system.

Putting AIDS in perspective, current US military expenditures amount to $1.9 billion *each day*. Billions more that could fund health care are lost to Africa by the illicit transfer of funds by national elites and multinational corporations who drain resources from Africa as in centuries past.

Sexual politics and the Christian Right

In Africa, new organisations of the Christian Right, funded from the US and Europe, expanded their operations, with broadcasting networks that take the sexual politics of America's culture wars to the continent. Tele-evangelists and media commentators, including pastors Pat Robertson and Rick Warren, spread aggressive homophobia, and attack women's health and reproductive rights (Kaoma 2012). Evangelical preachers use interactive media to produce and reproduce discourses of male dominance and gender inequality and to break down the separation of church and state. African counterparts include numerous political leaders who call upon both 'traditional' and Christian patriarchal ideology in support of male domination, enforced heterosexuality and against reproductive rights, including both contraception and abortion. Although politicians frame their crusade as a return to 'authentic African values', anthropologists know these claims to be untrue, with examples of male–male sexual and domestic relations such as 'mine marriages' between men and youth, and socially accepted 'woman-woman marriage' documented in many countries. While colonial laws forbade the practices, many Africans (and sometimes even students and religious within Christian institutions) ignored these strictures that arrived with the Bible.

Several networks of US neo-Pentecostals, such as the 'Dominionists' and the 'Transformation Network', support African churches to reinforce their theocratic politics. They assert that men are created to rule over women, promote miraculous healing and blame poverty on 'demons' and 'evil powers', particularly lesbian, gay, bisexual and transgender people and abortion (Kaoma 2012: 3). Dr Kaoma, an Anglican priest from Zambia who led research on religion and sexual politics in seven countries, believes that Africa is a pawn in the battle the US Christian Right are fighting at home. Welcomed by some prominent African political and religious leaders, they advocate for constitutional changes to outlaw homosexuality, same-sex marriage and abortion, proclaiming these to be 'un-African'. Family Watch International claims that the United Nations has been taken over by homosexuals and terms family planning 'an assault on natural African family values' (Sharlet 2008). In a region with the world's highest maternal mortality, attacks on family planning are deadly.

Across the continent, neither government nor churches – mainstream or evangelical – have made sexual abuse of women and girls an active concern. They have ignored the role of violence – rape and coercion – especially unwanted sexual relations in marriage, in exposing women to HIV infection. Few men are prepared to institute policy measures to respond to the risk to girls and women coerced or enticed into sex. Only where stranger rape is rampant, as in the civil war in eastern Kivu, is there an outcry. Yet sexual coercion and violence within marriage appear to cause more HIV infections than stranger rape. Many men argue that couple relations are private matters, and some women support them. But as women farmers in Zimbabwe reminded social workers in 1983, this is *not* a traditional pattern; formerly families and communities protected women from abuse (fieldnotes, Harare, July 1983). Today, violence is not only a concern for families, however: under international law, states are responsible for the protection of women's bodily integrity.

Once they agree to abandon the notion that wife-beating is a time-honoured tradition, churches can help to create norms of protection; Gusman (2009) writes of youth in Uganda, 'the Joseph Generation' who rebel against the hypocrisy of their elders and use their born-again faith to help them live differently. Younger evangelical leaders and congregants are debating issues around AIDS and social justice that may result in less prescriptive rhetoric (Robbins 2004; Czeglédy 2008). Yet, as a whole, their teachings and practices join those of a global 'war on women' whose heartland is the US.

In central Mozambique's rural born-again churches, patriarchal Paulist doctrine merges with local gender practices. Married women are taught by women elders to submit to husbands' decisions, to care for them without complaint, and to maintain silence in cases of spousal violence. Churches also incorporate local gerontocratic control of young women's bodies and sexuality (Igreja and Dias Lambranca 2009).

Similarly, Pentecostals in Harare deny women control over their bodies in the same terms as Prairie Muffin.com, an American website that prescribes attitudes and conduct for 'born-again' women. With contraception considered the 'devil's work' that 'breaks the altar of motherhood' (Mate 2002: 560), protection from HIV in marriage is impossible. Women are told not to be too demanding sexually, lest they sap a husband's masculine vitality. If her husband does not satisfy her, a wife should not resort to masturbation or sex toys, as these are a sign of possession by Satan, as is 'chronic sexual insatiateness'. Gender equality should apply in the workplace, but not at home, where women should be submissive to husbands, the undisputed heads of the household, who should make all financial decisions. The fatigue of the 'double day' and of frequent pregnancies is not to be mitigated by calling on husbands for assistance. 'Submission in obedience to God's Law' should enable a virtuous wife to accept her lot with good grace, and overcome marital problems. Avoiding confrontation, she must 'hope God will moderate their conjugal relations and remove the threat of brute force' (Mate 2002: 566). Like Biaya, Mate points to a political consequence of Pentecostals' ideology: 'equating poverty with the work of the devil makes it impossible for people to critique poverty as a social, political and economic process connected with structural relations and an ideological basis' (Mate 2002: 552).

Christian moral panics

Africa has no monopoly on claims of mystical or 'supernatural' influence in human affairs. The huge success of Hollywood cinematographic portrayals of witches, demons, vampires, ghosts and 'supernatural' beings of many kinds shows the broad interest of the American public in such fantasies. Across sub-Saharan Africa, many continue to believe in 'sent sickness' and witchcraft, especially in the case of afflictions not cured by biomedical intervention.

During the past twenty-five years, as deepening mass poverty, civil wars and the deadly ravages of AIDS have eroded the solidarity of extended families, Christian effervescence, especially the expansion of conservative evangelical and fundamentalist churches, has provided many poor, frightened and suffering people with hope of salvation and a better life (Corten and Mary 2000; Devisch 1995). Miraculous healing through the 'laying on of hands' is a central tenet of the revivalist 'healing churches', a sign of their pastors' power and grace, their ability to ensure deliverance from evil and suffering (Aguilar Molino 2005; Fancello 2008). How many people have been prevented by religious leaders and traditional healers from seeking HIV testing to learn their status, and from accessing antiretroviral treatment to prolong their lives, is not known. Promises of miraculous 'cures' have attracted thousands.

Some pastors have tried to prevent access to antiretroviral drugs, urging sick people to rely on confession, exorcism and prayer. Belief in divine healing can act as a barrier to ARV adherence (Wanyama *et al.* 2007). One recent example is the rush to obtain a herbal concoction devised by a retired evangelical Lutheran pastor near Arusha who demanded that his patients discard their antiretroviral medications (Lyimo 2011). While AIDS activists warned people not to do so, it was not until July 2012 that the Tanzanian government announced that the herbs had no curative properties. Advocates believe that many have died, while others have become poor or heavily indebted as a result of their quest for a cure (IRIN 2012b).

Sufferers and their families may seek to avoid the shame and stigma of sexual transgression by claiming bewitchment (Rodlach 2006). Accusations sometimes result in ostracism or killing of the accused. Witch-hunting resonates with older beliefs, but it is by no means reserved to 'traditional healers', nor should it be labelled 'indigenous'. Some evangelical and 'revivalist' churches whose pastor-prophets claim revelation from the Holy Spirit have added fuel to the fire. Despite their rejection of the 'evil spirits' of traditional religion, these pastors have re-created demons, witches and others believed to exercise 'satanic powers' and to lead people astray.

In the past, African healers identified malfeasance, but did not actually name witches. It was illegal to do so in the Belgian Congo and violators might be prosecuted. The statute remains but is not enforced by the courts. Impoverished and demoralised by decades of privation and violence, many families cannot feed their own children or those entrusted to them. Some 30,000 Kinshasa children were estimated to be homeless, both subjected to and committing acts of violence, many in the search for food. Biaya (1997) links the plight of these children to the destitution that followed on Structural Adjustment measures and political conflict that made Kinshasa a site of evangelist fervour from the 1980s. Children and youth are accused of 'occult practices' and 'mystical harms' (Yengo 2008). Whether the parents (or often, foster parents) are destitute or slightly better off but insecure, witchcraft accusations allow them to slough off unruly, deformed or otherwise 'abnormal' children, and orphans whom extended families do not wish to support (Schoepf 2002; Aguilar Molina 2005).

Instead of offering protection, some Pentecostal pastors in Kinshasa have added to the violence against children and youth rejected by their families. While individual priests and pastors of other churches have sheltered abused children endangered by accusations of witchcraft, Kinshasa and other African cities have witnessed an epidemic of accusations against children that have led to harsh mistreatment, torture and even murders of those accused, without drawing judicial response (Biaya 1997; Tonda 2000). Pentecostal pastors' exorcism of these supposed 'evil-doers', to whose families they promise 'deliverance' for those who confess and accuse others, includes food deprivation, social isolation and torture (Biaya 1997; Cimpric 2010). While some 'delivered' children are re-integrated into families, most live on the streets in precarious conditions, subjected to violence from older children, adults and police (Aguilar Molina 2005; Cimpric 2010).

In addition to the researchers cited, several international NGOs, such as Human Rights Watch (2006), Save the Children, and UNICEF, advocate for the accused children and point to the violation of international human rights law to which governments are pledged to respond. One anthropologist, however, claims that since these children are seen by families and neighbours as perpetrators, rather than victims, the NGOs are guilty of ethnocentrism, for they do not understand 'African culture' (De Boeck 2000). He proposes that the exorcising pastors actually save the children from violence. This claim seems myopic, since in Kinshasa, Pentecostal and other revivalist pastors control nearly half the forty independent television channels and hundreds of radio stations that broadcast their anti-sorcery crusades. Their media also air soap operas and comic strips produced in Nigeria and Ghana that reproduce, legitimate and amplify the designation of scapegoats supposedly responsible for ever-present misfortunes.

The Catholic Church is not immune to 'witch-finding'. In terms reminiscent of the 1980s witch-hunting by priests among the Lele of Kasai (Douglas 1997), Behrend describes a movement of charismatic Catholics in western Uganda's Tooro District, the Uganda Martyrs' Guild (UGM), which grew from thirty members in 1982 to 10,000 in 2002. Founders of the movement were two American religious; from about 1995 the UGM began to fight 'evil' in the public arena, ridding the villages of supposed witches, vampires and cannibals (Behrend 2007: 49–50). Using these campaigns, the Catholics sought to regain adherents lost to the evangelicals and born-agains. As in the seventeenth-century witch craze in Salem, Massachusetts, and in Bandundu in Congo in the early twentieth century, Behrend shows that Ugandan Christians' fight against 'the occult' reproduced the very evil it purported to vanquish, in effect 'reinstating the occult powers they fight against'. Similarly, two years of interviews in Kinshasa by Aguilar Molina (2005) and a long-term study in rural Mozambique by Igreja and Dias Lambranca (2009) find that born-again pastors *reinstate* the 'satanic practices' of traditional healers who invoke magic and sorcery.

Discourses of culture and entitlement

Each of the organisations and ideologies examined above is guilty of human rights violations for attempting to limit the freedoms, scope of action, and access to resources, even to life, of variously, women, children and sexual minorities. Protection from diseases like HIV/AIDS and protection of sexual and reproductive health are human rights enshrined in international covenants and treaties that have the status of law. Public health experts now agree that structural transformation is critical to ending the AIDS pandemic. 'The full potential of the recent breakthroughs in HIV prevention and treatment will not be realized if social, legal, gender and economic inequalities continue to undermine the coverage and uptake of HIV services' (UNAIDS 2012: 58).

Many American and African leaders who support ultra-conservative policy agendas fail to recognise these rights, however, and enact laws to restrict them. Whether local religious and civil leaders draw upon 'traditional', Christian or 'modern' authority, they act in opposition to the numerous pan-African and UN charters supporting women's rights as human rights. An international coalition of women's organisations decries 'the safeguarding of "traditional values" at the expense of women' and seeks to hold the United Nations Commission on the Status of Women to its responsibility for implementing the consensus agreements (ISIS International 2012).

Some anthropologists view promotion of human rights as an ethnocentric, un-African stance. However, many Africans are engaged in advocacy for these rights. For many, constructions of rights are broader than those envisioned in the West, where political and civil rights predominate. Sudanese scholars An-Na'im and Deng (1990) and their collaborators examine human rights from a cross-cultural perspective. They are especially sharp in their criticism of anthropologists who take an extreme relativist position, which they see as redolent of colonial notions of 'primitivity'. Cultures change and new normative consensus can arise out of struggles engaged in by groups seeking to overturn the hegemonic power of wealthy interests in favour of greater equality and rights. The question is who has the right to change culture.

Conclusion

Both women and men with HIV/AIDS experience fear of sickness, pain, death, and grief, but biology and socially constructed gender roles and relations result in somewhat different experiences. The gender-specific stresses of HIV/AIDS fall most heavily upon poor women and their children. The macro-level forces of Structural Adjustment, with privatisation and cost–recovery in health and education that restrict access to services for the poor, have made survival more difficult and stressful, especially for poor women and girls, and even more so for women with AIDS. Analysis of AIDS in Africa underscores how male control of sexuality renders girls and women vulnerable to HIV. With notable exceptions, however, the discourses of most African leaders at national and local levels with respect to gender and power relations have changed very little in response to HIV/AIDS. They draw support from the influence of evangelical leaders from the United States whose presence in Africa grew markedly with poverty in the 1980s and with US government-funded AIDS prevention in the years of the Bush administration's PEPFAR programme. President Obama's government has made important modifications to PEPFAR, and the US continues as the largest contributor to AIDS treatment and prevention in Africa. Yet US government policies continue to be held hostage to the conservative 'Christian Right', with its attacks on reproductive freedom and sexual health in the US and in Africa.

Instead of contributing to the social transformation needed to end the HIV/AIDS epidemic, conservative colonial Christian patriarchy, resurgent in 'born-again' practices, recreates and reinforces 'neo-traditional' gender relations. Although Pentecostal churches claim to break with tradition, their discourses confer theological legitimacy on earlier patriarchal claims.

Religious leaders who deploy witchcraft accusations and moralist discourses of stigma, restrict knowledge and substitute biblical injunctions for science, add to the burden of preventable suffering from HIV/AIDS. The consequences for human rights must be weighed in the balance when the effects of religious institutions are evaluated. Churches that equate poverty with 'the work of the devil' and preach belief in supernatural or 'occult' causes of misfortune create an ideological smokescreen that makes it impossible for people to understand how poverty, inequality and structural violence result from socio-political and economic processes. Those who preach the 'prosperity gospel' absolve the successful of concern for the poor. As in the US, so in Africa, religious conservatives' focus on 'social issues' – chiefly, promotion of hetero-normativity, male dominance and control of women's sexuality – allows the true causes of misfortune to escape popular critique and collective action. Other churches provide the solidarity needed to encourage HIV testing and support for people living with AIDS. Hopefully, more will do so in the future, as treatment restores people to health and fewer families claim their illness is due to bewitchment (Pfeiffer 2011).

I do not claim that the conservative US Christian Right has *caused* many of Africa's churches to wield moralist discourses of stigma, much less invented domestic violence or patriarchy. Rather, I hope to have traced some of the ways in which US evangelicals, US-inspired SAPs, and early PEPFAR funds and personnel helped to strengthen, sometimes even to launch, counter-productive responses to AIDS in Africa and the US that impede HIV prevention and deprive girls, women and homosexuals of their human rights.

Understanding how persistence and change in ideologies and structural relations reproduce and create different vulnerabilities to HIV, it is unwise to advance the interests of the powerful – be they religious, or 'traditional' authorities or 'healers' – in allocation of the resources that accompany HIV prevention. Without returning to the colonial denigration of African religions or assertions of 'primitivity', the issue of how these contemporary beliefs and their attendant harms in Africa and the US are changing, and might be helped to change further, is a worthwhile subject for investigation.

The international community, led by the US as the world's wealthiest nation, must increase contributions for AIDS prevention and treatment without moralist restrictions. In the US, as in Africa, this depends upon political forces in which conservative Christian churches play a critical role. Given the many linkages between ideology and material circumstances, crucial to hope in the future, anthropologists can become advocates not only for generous AIDS funding, but for expansion of science-based education, for female equality and for an end to the massive drain of resources from Africa.

References

Aguilar Molina, Javier. 2005. *The Invention of Child Witches in the Democratic Republic of Congo, 2003–2005*. Kinshasa: Save the Children.

An-Na'im, Abdullahi Ahmed and Francis M. Deng (eds). 1990. *Human Rights in Africa: Cross Cultural Perspectives*. Washington, DC: The Brookings Institution.

Asamoah-Oyadu, J. and J. Kwabena. 2007. 'Broken calabashes and covenants of fruitfulness: cursing barrenness in contemporary Africa', *Journal of Religion in Africa* 37: 437–60.

Behrend, Heike. 2007. 'The rise of occult powers, AIDS and the Roman Catholic Church in Western Uganda', *Journal of Religion in Africa* 37: 41–58.

Biaya, Tshikala K. 1997. 'Kinshasa: anomie, "ambiance" et violence', in George Herault and Pius Adesanmi (eds), *Jeunes, Cultures de la Rue et Violences Urbaines en Afrique*. Abidjan: Institut Français de Recherche en Afrique (IFAN), 329–82.

Cimpric, Aleksandra. 2010. *Children Accused of Witchcraft in West Africa: An Anthropological Study of Contemporary Practices*. Dakar: UNICEF; WARO.

Cohen, Myron S., Ying Q. Chen, Marybeth McCauley *et al.* 2011. 'Prevention of HIV-1 infection with early antiretroviral therapy', *New England Journal of Medicine* 365(6): 493–506.

Corbey, R. 1988. 'Alterity: the colonial nude', *Critique of Anthropology* 8(3): 75–92.

Corten, André and André Mary (eds). 2000. *Imaginaires Politiques et Pentecôtisme: Afrique/Amérique*. Paris: Harmattan.

Czeglédy, André P. 2008. 'A new Christianity for a new South Africa: charismatic Christians and the post-apartheid order', *Journal of Religion in Africa* 38: 284–311.

De Boeck, Filip. 2000. 'Le deuxième monde et les enfants sorciers en République Démocratic du Congo', *Politique Africaine* 80: 32–57.

de St. Moulin, Léon. 1996. 'Kinshasa, trente ans après: une enquête sur la perception sociale de la justice', *Zaire-Afrique* 36(305): 197–220.

Devisch, René. 1995. 'Frenzy, violence and ethical renewal in Kinshasa', *Public Culture* 7: 593–629.

Douglas, Mary. 1997 'Sorcery accusations unleashed: the Lele, revisited, 1987', *Africa* 69: 177–93.

Fancello, Sandra. 2008. 'Sorcellerie et délivrance dans les Pentecôtismes Africains', *Cahiers d'Etudes Africaines* XLVIII(1–2), 189–90; 11–34.

Gusman, Alessandro. 2009. 'HIV/AIDS, Pentecostal churches and the 'Joseph Generation' in Uganda', *Africa Today* 56(1): 67–86.

Hobsbawm, Eric and Terence Ranger (eds) 1983. *The Invention of Tradition*. Cambridge: Cambridge University Press.

Human Rights Watch (HRW). 2006. *What Future? Street Children in Democratic Republic of Congo*. New York: HRW.

Igreja, Victor and Béatrice Dias Lambranca. 2009. 'The Thursdays as they live: Christian religious transformation and gender relations in postwar Gorongosa, Central Mozambique', *Journal of Religion in Africa* 39: 262–94.

IRIN. 2012a. 'HIV effort needs government and donor commitment to succeed', *PlusNews*, Kinshasa, 4 May.

IRIN. 2012b. 'Tanzania: popular herb cure-all "ineffective"', *PlusNews*, Dar-es-Salaam, 2 August.

ISIS International. 2012. 'Feminist and women's organisations say NO to safeguarding "traditional values" at the expense of the human rights of women!' 27 March. www.isiswomen.org.

Jewsiewicki, Bogumil. 1992. 'Jeux d'argent et de pouvoir au Zaire: la "bindomanie" et le crépuscule de la Deuxième République', *Politique Africaine* 46: 55–70.

Kaoma, Kapya John. 2012. *Colonizing African Values: How the U.S. Christian Right Is Transforming Sexual Politics in Africa*. Boston: Political Research Associates. www.publiceye.org.

Kipp, Walter, Thomas Matukula Nkosi, Lori Laing *et al.* 2006. 'Care burden and self-reported health status of informal women caregivers of HIV/AIDS patients in Kinshasa, DRC', *AIDS Care* 18(7): 694–7.

Lyimo, Joseph. 2011. 'Do not drop ARVs, official advises', allafrica.com/stories/201103140857.html (accessed 14 March 2011).

Maman, Suzanne, Rebecca Cathcart, Gillian Burkhardt *et al.* 2009. 'The role of religion in HIV-positive women's disclosure experiences and coping strategies in Kinshasa, DRC', *Social Science and Medicine* 68: 965–70.

Mate, Rekopantswe. 2002. 'Wombs as God's laboratories: Pentecostal discourses on femininity in Zimbabwe', *Africa* 72(4): 549–68.

Mbembe, Achille. 1992. 'Provisional notes on the post-colony', *Africa* 62: 3–37.

Mianda, Gertrude D.M. 1995. 'Dans l'ombre de la "démocratie" au Zaire: la remise en question de émancipation Mobutiste de la femme', *Canadian Journal of African Studies* 29(1): 51–78.

Mills, Edward J., Steve Kanters, Amy Hagopian *et al.* 2011. 'The financial cost of doctors emigrating from sub-Saharan Africa: human capital analysis', *British Medical Journal* 343.

Monti, Nicholas. 1988. *Africa Then: Photographs 1840–1918.* New York: Alfred A. Knopf (Borzoi).

Ngondo a Pitshandenge, Séraphin. 2001. 'De la nécessité d'un plaidoyer en faveur de la femme congolaise', *Congo-Afrique* 354: 197–222.

Pfeiffer, James. 2011. 'Pentecostalism and AIDS treatment in Mozambique: creating new approaches to HIV prevention through antiretroviral therapy', *Global Public Health* 6(S2): S163–73.

Robbins, Joel. 2004. 'The globalization of Pentecostal and Charismatic Christianity', *Annual Review of Anthropology* 33: 117–43.

Rodlach, Alexander. 2006. *Witches, Westerners and HIV/Aids: Cultures of Blame in Africa.* Walnut Creek, CA: Left Coast Press.

Rukarangira wa Nkera, Alphonse. 2002. 'Les groupes de soutien des personnes vivant avec le VIH et le sida à Kinshasa'. Rapport au Département de la Santé Publique, République Démocratique du Congo.

Sartre, Jean-Paul. 1946. *Relexions sur la question juive.* Paris: Morihien.

Schoepf, Brooke G. 1988. 'Women, AIDS and economic crisis in Central Africa', *Canadian Journal of African Studies* 22(3): 625–44.

Schoepf, Brooke G. 1991. 'Political economy, sex and cultural logics: a view from Zaire', *African Urban Quarterly* 6(1–2): 94–107.

Schoepf, Brooke G. 1992. 'Women at risk: case studies from Zaire', in G. Herdt and S. Lindenbaum (eds), *The Time of AIDS: Social Analysis, Theory and Method.* London: Sage, 259–86.

Schoepf, Brooke G. 1993. 'Action-research on AIDS with women in Kinshasa', *Social Science and Medicine* 37(11): 1401–13.

Schoepf, Brooke G. 2002. 'Mobutu's disease: a social history of AIDS in Kinshasa', *Review of African Political Economy* 93/94: 561–73.

Schoepf, Brooke G. 2004. 'Museveni's other war: condoms in Uganda', *Review of African Political Economy* 100: 372–6.

Schoepf, Brooke G., Alphonse Rukarangira wa Nkera, Claude Schoepf, *et al.* 1988. 'AIDS and society in Central Africa: a view from Zaire', in Norman Miller and Richard Rockwell (eds), *AIDS in Africa: Social and Policy Impact.* Lewiston, NY: Mellen Press, 211–35.

Schoepf, Brooke G., Claude Schoepf and Joyce V. Millen. 2000. 'Theoretical therapies, remote remedies: SAPS and the political ecology of health in Africa', in Jim Y. Kim,

Joyce V. Millen, Alec Irwin and John Gershman (eds), *Dying for Growth: Structural Adjustment and the Health of the Poor*. Monroe, ME: Common Courage Press, 91–125; 377–96.

Sharlet, Jeff. 2008. *The Family: The Secret Fundamentalism at the Heart of American Power*. New York: HarperCollins.

Tonda, Joseph. 2000. 'La violence de l'imaginaire des enfants-sorciers', *Politique Africaine* 75: 48–65.

UNAIDS. 2012. *Together We Will End AIDS*. Geneva: UNAIDS. July, 36–7.

USAID. 2012. *Better Health for Development: USAID's Global Health Strategic Framework*. Washington, DC: United States Agency for International Development.

Wanyama, J., B. Castelnovo, B. Wandera *et al.* 2007. 'Belief in divine healing can be a barrier to antiretroviral therapy adherence in Uganda', *AIDS* 21(11): 1486–7.

Yengo, Patrice. 2008. 'Le monde à l'envers: enfance et kindoki ou les ruses de la raison sorcière dans le bassin du Congo', *Cahiers d'Etudes Africaines* XLVIII(1–2) 189–90; 297–323.

4

From an Activist's Point of View: Experiencing Transnational Dynamics among African Migrant Communities in the UK

IJEOMA AJIBADE

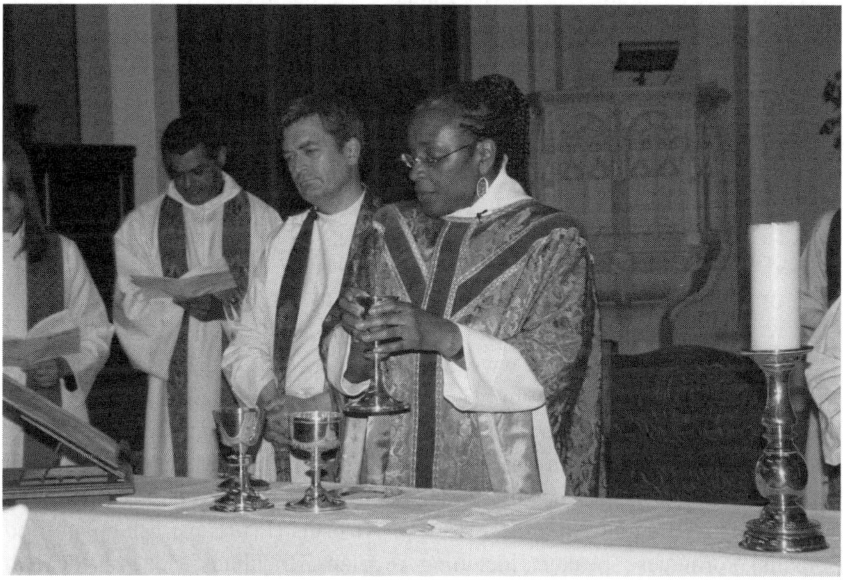

Remembering that there is unity in all our diversity (Holy Communion at St Philip's Church, Earls Court, London)

Proceedings of the British Academy **194**, *69–78*. © The British Academy 2014.

Introduction

My aim for this essay is not to provide a detailed academic narrative about the subject of transnational dynamics, but to explore my personal experience of where such dynamics are taking place within the UK African diaspora and to illustrate the connections to Africa that emerge from this. My aim in doing this is to explore what I have seen in practice and in this way contribute to this book by providing a perspective that is rooted in practical experience. I would describe myself as an activist. I am a self-supporting priest at a church in the diocese of London and a chaplain at Southwark Cathedral in the diocese of Southwark. My service in both of these churches is voluntary and therefore provides me with great freedom to both shape my ministry within the church and work with a range of other religious and secular organisations. This freedom to respond and work with others is vital for me as an activist. The organisations that I work with are focused on a range of different fields including HIV services and prevention, international development, and lesbian and gay human rights. Although these are all separate specialisms, there are ways in which they overlap and connect, especially when considering the delivery of services at community levels here in the UK and in Africa. My activism takes place through these organisations at both community and regional and international levels.

Experiencing transnational dynamics on HIV and human sexuality at community and national levels: the Naz Project London (NPL)

The Naz Project London (NPL; www.naz.org.uk) is a charity that seeks to improve the sexual health of people from black and minority ethnic (BME) communities in the UK. I have worked with the organisation for some years as a board trustee. NPL provides sexual health and HIV prevention and support services to South Asians (including Bangladeshis, Indians and Pakistanis), Muslims (including Middle Easterners and Africans), Horn of Africans (Eritreans, Ethiopians and Somalis), Portuguese speakers (including Angolans, Brazilians, Mozambicans and Portuguese), and Spanish speakers (mainly Latin American).

HIV, sexual health and the community at Naz

Through its work the organisation challenges the myths and prejudices that exist about sexual health and HIV within BME communities and works to ensure that these communities have access to care, support, and culturally and linguistically appropriate information. At the Naz Project we aim to educate and empower our communities to face up to the challenges of sexual health and the AIDS pandemic, and to mobilise support for people living with HIV. In that sense part of what we do is to nurture community leadership, so that the communities themselves take the responsibility for providing information and support, and educating people about sexual health.

The Monya project is an example of the work that NPL does. Monya is a Swahili word for 'strength'. In 2007, there was a call for a specific HIV prevention programme for migrant African men who have sex with men (MSM) in the London Borough of Newham. The project became a meeting point for migrant African men to access sexual health services that are sensitive to their needs. At the end of the third year of the project we had a total of fifty men accessing services. This is an example of one of our many projects and a setting in which transnational dynamics take place through learning and sharing together.

Within NPL the diverse communities work together to provide needed services and in doing so they are able to improve not just the sexual health of their own specific ethnic community, but also at a cross-cultural level they improve the sexual health of people beyond their ethnic and cultural grouping. Transnational dynamics lie at the heart of this process and through research and dialogue move beyond the BME community to influence wider UK sexual health policy through the relationships that NPL has with the UK government, the UK Department of Health and the National Health Service.

HIV, sexual health and the individual at Naz

It is also clear to me that NPL is a place where cultural and religious conflict around sexuality is articulated and experienced, but done so in such a way that an individual is empowered to find a way to reconcile their cultural and religious needs with their sexuality and sexual health needs. Some of these experiences are reflected in our impact assessment reports (NPL 2010: 9).

> Hearing South Asian parents talking about their experience of 'coming out' as a parent of a gay or bisexual son made me realise that 'coming out' isn't just our journey as young gay men. Our parents have also got to make a journey which they may find more difficult than ours. Coming to NPL opened my eyes to 'coming out' and talking about it in an appropriate and accessible manner with my parents.
>
> (Juned, 25, Bengali; NPL 2010: 10)

> I gave an interview for the Tonight Programme on BBC Radio 4. I talked about reconciling my faith with my sexuality and gave a lot of personal information about how difficult and isolating I found it. Without the support of NPL, I don't think I would have ever considered giving a personal interview that would be listened to by millions.
>
> (Amit, 24, Indian; NPL 2011: 7t)

Across the different cultures and groups the Naz Project is able to develop a strong sense of acceptance and community cohesion amongst its service users, staff and volunteers. For some people this culturally appropriate support actually leads to a sense of empowerment and in some cases may lead to community activism and leadership outside the Naz Project, such as participating in Pride, in fundraising activities or other forms of community outreach.

It is clear that the organisation provides the space in which transnational dynamics take place. Not only is this evidenced in the services provided to specific cultural groups, but it can be evidenced through the work that takes place across and within the different ethnic groups. Through this process individuals are able to negotiate both their sexuality and HIV in a way that takes account of their conservative cultures. This process of learning and change is not limited to the specific communities involved, but has an impact on the host country through the UK public policy process.

The African Health Policy Network (AHPN)

This national organisation has a different focus, but once again transnational dynamics can be experienced in a number of ways. The AHPN (www.ahpn.org) seeks to formulate and promote policy around sexual health, HIV and other health issues for the African diaspora in the UK. As the organisation seeks to develop policy responses on HIV, the importance of faith within this is a key factor. The organisation often finds that it has to negotiate different positions on morality and sexuality because of the pandemic and confront African religious groups with issues that are often considered taboo and are not discussed in places of worship. This interaction is focused on both African Muslim and African Christian communities. Migrant faith communities then find that they need to respond. Even where they are of a conservative background they are challenged to both understand and respond to the issue of HIV and human sexuality, not only because of the needs of the African community in the UK, but also because of wider debates that take place within the UK such as on equality and more recently on gay marriage.

Faith plays a key role in everyday life for Africans. It is for them a form of identity, and for new African migrants, participation within their faith community is one of the key ways of integrating into life in the UK. For many people, participation in the life of a faith community is vital for their well-being and it is the basis from which relationships are formed. It is recognised that if faith communities can address the stigma and discrimination surrounding HIV and recognise that HIV exists in their respective communities, not only will this develop support for people living with HIV but it could also assist with the implementation of prevention strategies at local levels and help raise awareness about HIV. Particular emphasis is placed on the role that religious leaders could have in achieving this. In 2011 the House of Lords Select Committee on HIV and Aids stated that 'faith and religion play a strong role in the lives of many people. It is essential that faith leaders engage with HIV as an issue and provide effective and truthful support and communication around the subject' (2011: 32–3).

Before Africans living with HIV can receive appropriate support within their faith communities there is a need for faith leaders to understand HIV. It is recognised by policy makers in the UK that African religious leaders are in a key position to:

- assist in HIV primary prevention by addressing some of the myths that surround HIV
- ensure that places of worship are places of welcome and acceptance for people living with or affected by HIV
- respond to the spiritual needs of people living with HIV
- contribute to decision-making on HIV at local levels
- create safe space in which the challenges of living with HIV can be discussed (African HIV Policy Network 2009).

The AHPN recognises that it is therefore crucial to engage faith leaders in the HIV response because of the authority they hold within their communities and their regular involvement and relationships with people, especially at key life stages.

I have worked to support the AHPN as they seek to engage and educate a range of African religious leaders and church-going Africans across a number of different denominations. We have developed toolkits on HIV for both Christian and Muslim faith communities, as well as providing a range of campaign materials and workshops.

In 2009 I worked with the AHPN to develop a course on HIV for Anglican clergy. This course considers the issue of HIV from a theological and ethical perspective in order to enable clergy to develop a greater awareness about HIV and how it affects people, but also for clergy to consider how they might wish to engage with the issue of HIV at both a local and a global level. In 2011 we organised a similar session, this time with a particular focus on the role of the church in responding to the HIV pandemic and to show religious leaders how the church is involved in the global HIV response. My work is not limited to religious leaders and their congregations. I also speak to clinicians and health-care workers about religious belief, especially on the issue of treatment adherence, HIV and the question of miracles. This follows on from the reports at the end of 2012 about some churches that were alleged to have been encouraging people to stop taking their HIV treatment. Thus, in a range of ways, African religious organisations in the UK are challenged to address their positions on morality and sexuality by engaging with organisations such as the AHPN, because of the need to respond to the pastoral concerns of the people they serve.

As an activist I feel that the process of transnational dynamics is very much part of this work and it often takes place without me or other activists being aware of what is happening. So, for example, within the HIV course for clergy we acknowledge that people have a wide range of views about sex and sexuality, and different theological understandings, but as part of the course, we emphasise the complexity of HIV and the fact that it affects people from all walks of life. We emphasise that HIV is global and is no respecter of religion, politics or ideology. As we do this, the clergy and religious leaders from the different theological traditions can see that HIV and AIDS is more than just a health issue, that it is deeply complex and that there are no easy responses to the HIV pandemic. It is then the responsibility of the individual clergy to think about what they believe about sexuality and their theology and how they might then respond from their theological position.

In training clergy and developing policy we have extensive local and global networks. Transnational dynamics also take place through these partnerships and networks. I find that I am often liaising with people from a range of global networks and organisations both in the global South and in the global North. This engagement leads to exchanges of ideas, awareness of different practices, access to research and access to dialogue that may be taking place within the global South or North. This for me is a lived example of how I experience transnational dynamics. The discourse takes place at community level here in the UK within the African community, but it is also influenced by discourse happening in Africa and at the international level.

Experiencing transnational dynamics on HIV and human sexuality at international levels

At the global level I encounter transnational dynamics in two key areas, one being HIV and the other being the movement for lesbian, gay, bisexual, transgender and intersex (LGBTI) human rights. These two movements have some overlap because the struggle for access to HIV treatment and prevention for men who have sex with men is also a justice issue. The World Bank (2001) reports that the effectiveness of HIV prevention is undermined by the criminalisation of homosexuality and by the lack of adequate HIV prevention for men who have sex with men. At the heart of the debates about the response to HIV, and questions about sexuality and human rights, are for me also questions of politics, power and theological conflict.

HIV

In April 2011 I was privileged to attend the UN Civil Society Hearing on HIV and AIDS. It took place in New York and for me was an occasion to see transnational dynamics at work in a very obvious way. The aim of this meeting was for civil society organisations from around the world to have an opportunity to deliver strategic messages which would then be used to influence the development of a new UN declaration on HIV and AIDS, and to feed into the policy development process. It was also envisaged that in this way civil society organisations from across the world would have an opportunity to build stronger partnerships with their own country governments, as well as with each other, through the sharing of civil society perspectives and positions on both the local and global HIV response.

Prior to the hearing day, a series of pre-meetings were held and these meetings provided an opportunity for exchange of ideas, for learning, and also a place for developing global civil society priorities. It was interesting to see this movement and process at work. The way in which the dialogue aimed to be as balanced as possible, with both southern and northern voices being listened to and valued, was deeply fascinating and a key example of the way in which transnational dynamics take place. It also provided a very good opportunity to hear about work that is being undertaken within the respective countries and regions, and it provided an opportunity to discuss the complexities involved in responding to the pandemic on the ground. Despite the diversity of the geographical regions which delegates had come from there was a strong consensus in the room about the main priorities. In the midst of this global meeting the transnational dynamics led to a strong consensus about action and priorities.

As a faith leader, I recognise that key populations – men who have sex with men, sex workers, and intravenous drug users – are particularly affected by HIV. HIV is not a moral issue and therefore I believe that working with and supporting these groups is critical in the HIV response. The Civil Society Hearing showed that the marginalised of this world are strong. They organise, they advocate and they challenge governments and the powers that be. There is a passage in the Bible that describes them. They are people 'of whom the world is not worthy' (Hebrews 11:38). Transnational dynamics are seen in minority groups that organise themselves and support each other, as in the Naz Project London. There is a level of solidarity that empowers individuals and enables them to lead their lives and manage their health and well-being. They organise themselves – often transcending national boundaries – and as faith leaders and people within academic institutions who have our own power and responsibilities we must show solidarity and support them.

Human sexuality

When it comes to dialogue about sexuality, in my experience the dialogue and the dynamics are far more polarised and difficult. The situation in Uganda which led to the death of David Kato shows transnational dynamics of a different kind, with the struggle for gay equality in the US finding a new arena in Uganda. These struggles are also taking place in other societal institutions such as churches, often with churches from the global South taking a more conservative approach to sexuality than churches in the global North.

The situation in Uganda has shown how polarised the debate about human sexuality has become. There are claims from African political and religious leaders that homosexuality is un-African and is imported to Africa from the global North. Accusations are made by activists from the global South against conservative churches from the global North stating that some of these church leaders have actively supported and inflamed anti-homosexual persecution in Uganda. An example of this is the current case brought by Sexual Minorities Uganda and the US Centre for Constitutional Rights against the US church leader Scott Lively.

Despite accusations from religious leaders within the global South that homosexuality is a Western influence and un-African, it isn't. There are a range of lesbian and gay voices showing strong locally led activism on this issue from a variety of civil society organisations based in the global South. There is also a history of LGBTI activists from the global South lobbying the Commonwealth to encourage decriminalisation of homosexuality. There is a vibrant LGBTI movement of activism in the global South even though religious and other societal institutions are in conflict and are divided over the issues. The key question in the midst of these dynamics is 'how will it be resolved?' I think that these dynamics can be harnessed to enable us to find resolution at both community and national levels.

For me as an observer of all these different kinds of dynamics, one of the key issues is finding resolution at community level, because this is where the impact of homophobia and violence against LGBTI people is experienced. It is felt by the LGBTI individual as they seek to go about their daily life and find that they are discriminated against, harassed or persecuted. As a priest and an activist in understanding the gospel the key issue for me is one of life, of human flourishing and recognising the Imago Dei (the image of God) in my fellow human being. I think that the recognition of the humanity of others and the need for compassion is actually lost within the North and South dynamic when it comes to homosexuality. In some way it needs to be regained, but new organisations are emerging which may make it possible to draw on the global dynamics to find a way forward at community level.

The Kaleidoscope Trust

An organisation set up with this compassion at its heart is the Kaleidoscope Trust (www.kaleidoscopetrust.com). This charity has been set up in the UK to work globally to promote diversity and respect for all regardless of sexual orientation. The aim of the organisation is to deploy resources and expertise to support people at community level who are working for LGBTI human rights within their own countries. The Kaleidoscope Trust hopes to encourage dialogue and cooperation between countries and will include capacity building at community level in countries where hostility towards gay men and lesbian women is particularly severe.

As an organisation, through the process of transnational dynamics the Kaleidoscope Trust aims to facilitate network development between countries that share historic, cultural or other affinities. Through opinion forming and dialogue Kaleidoscope hopes to change negative attitudes towards sexual diversity by facilitating debate at all levels including the media, political arenas and in public life. Kaleidoscope hopes to use transnational processes to improve life and indeed protect the life of many people who are currently threatened. This will not be an agenda led by the global North but a process of dialogue and campaign led by activists in the global South. The role of the Kaleidoscope Trust will be to lend capacity and show solidarity with LGBTI activists outside the UK in the global South and to build capacity so that people can struggle for human rights in their own countries with the support and resources of Kaleidoscope.

Within this global movement for change the issue of faith has deep significance. My role within this organisation is to develop faith-based responses to religious-inspired homophobia. This work is at a very early stage and will involve transnational dynamics through discussion with religious leaders in the global South but also with a range of NGOs such as faith-based development agencies. The aim will be to facilitate dialogue and some form of reconciliation and to demonstrate some of the wider implications of the criminalisation of homosexuality, showing that such moves can undermine health and development in the global South. It is hoped that our work in this area will also show how criminalisation contradicts the Christian ethos of love and justice.

Conclusion

My practical experience as an activist working across a range of religious and secular organisations illustrates that within the issue of responding to HIV and debates about human sexuality, there is much social change that is brought about by transnational dynamics. People may not always voice their opinions about these issues but will act on them within their personal lives and within their local communities. In a sense the different organisations that I work alongside subvert conservative agendas in a way that might not be readily apparent. They do this by empowering individuals to reflect on their personal experiences and their needs and to then reconcile all of this with their religious and cultural beliefs. Together with others in the community and as part of movements for social change individuals are able to negotiate their conservative cultures or religions and find new ways of living within them.

References

African HIV Policy Network. 2009. *HIV and Faith: Discussion Paper, Engaging Muslim and Christian Leaders on the Issue of HIV*. http://idoitright.co.uk/wp-content/uploads/2011/09/HIV-and-FAITH-discussion-paper.pdf (accessed 8 June 2012).

House of Lords Select Committee on HIV and Aids in the United Kingdom. 2011. *No Vaccine No Cure: HIV and AIDS in the United Kingdom*. House of Lords, 1 September.

Naz Project London. 2010. 'Annual impact statement'.

Naz Project London, 2011, 'Annual impact report'.

World Bank. 2001. *Global HIV Epidemics among Men Who Have Sex with Men (MSM): Epidemiology, Prevention, Access to Care and Human Rights*. June. http://siteresources.worldbank.org/INTHIVAIDS/Resources/375798-1103037153392/MSMReport.pdf (accessed 10 September 2011).

5

Global Moralities, Local Responses

Interpreting Sexual Morality and Social Belonging in Uganda

JOANNA SADGROVE

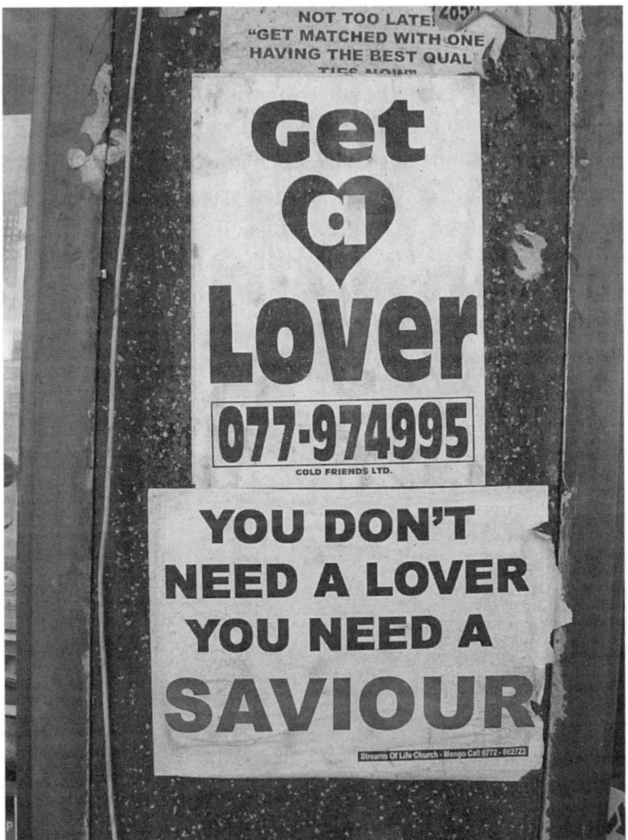

Dissonance of the morality discourses circulating in Kampala

Proceedings of the British Academy **194**, *79–103*.

Introduction and methodology

HIV PREVENTION IN UGANDA and across Africa has created a complex discursive environment in which competing recommendations and codes for the sexual behaviour and morality of young people exist side by side, influenced by a range of transnational processes, influences and actors. This chapter draws on a study which analyses the behaviour and understandings of a Pentecostal born-again peer group within the broader context of social debates about sexual morality, HIV prevention and concerns about public respectability and morality in Uganda. The study explores how elite young Ugandans, experiencing the comparative freedom and independence of university life, learn to navigate dissonant transnational moral discourses in a national climate of HIV prevention. The experiences of this group of students at Makerere University offer some illumination as to how this transition is negotiated. In order to present themselves as being accountable to a particular discourse, young people frequently employ secrecy and discretion about sexual behaviour in order to preserve public perceptions of oneself as a respectable, 'good person'.

The study is very much about the behaviour of (peer) groups and the importance of social reference groups with regard to the identity, self-esteem and self-fashioning of individual students at Makerere University. Peer group inclusion (a 'place to belong') and social networks prove critical incentives for born-again church membership and heavily influence decisions to become born-again amongst students. Peer groups also set the moral standards around which members configure understandings of 'good' and 'bad' behaviour. Yet whilst different groups posit different standards, frequently these standards are subsumed under wider social discourses within Uganda concerning publicly 'respectable' behaviour and what it means to be a 'good person'. This is particularly true for sexual behaviour; discretion and concealment of sexual activity are necessitated by wider discourses about respectability and morality – to be a 'good person' is to be discreet in matters of sex. Further, concealment functions as a means of maintaining the image of one who conforms to expected standards of any given public discourse around sexuality (such as the abstinence required of a born-again Christian) when private activity may counter what is visible in public – to be a 'good person' means not getting caught doing anything that might suggest otherwise. The focus on respectability and moral character and the recourse to secrecy and discretion to preserve public image can be usefully analysed by reflecting on histories of honour in Uganda and elsewhere.

The ethnographic data on which this chapter is based were collected over a twelve-month period in 2005–6. During this period I lived in one of the most exclusive student hostels just outside the Makerere University campus. The hostel housed over 300 students in *en suite* rooms, each of which accommodated one or two people. Room rates were comparatively high, attracting students from economically privileged and primarily urban backgrounds. I knew around 100 of these students by name. During a year at the hostel I socialised with its members daily, in a number of different social contexts, and was accorded an excellent opportunity to experience and observe the concerns, routines and social behaviour of young people at Makerere University. Many of the students who lived in the hostel were members of one of Kampala's biggest Pentecostal churches – Watoto Church Central – and it is on their experiences that this chapter is predominantly based.

I became acquainted with church members by attending weekly cell groups which met around the hostel. Attending cell group meetings formed a major part of my research, enabling me to get to know born-again students and form relationships with them outside of the formality of church environments. Cell groups hosted discussions about the tenets of salvation and the experiences of being born-again and living on campus. These group discussions revealed common concerns about university life, family life, possibilities and options beyond university, and Uganda's political situation. Cell group data were supplemented by both daily informal discussions around the hostel, church and university campus and a series of twenty-five repeat, in-depth, semi-structured interviews with born-again respondents. These interviews took place once I had spent time getting to know members through the cell groups and around the hostel, so engendering trust. The interviews took place over a number of sessions, during which I would repeat certain questions, which would sometimes evoke conflicting responses on different occasions. In addition to the data gathering, a follow-up visit in 2009 allowed me to discuss and interrogate the findings of the study with some of the participants involved, to deepen understanding.

The transnational aspect

In one sense, this chapter deals with 'soft' transnationalism. It understands the heterogeneity of Uganda's sexual moral codes (and subsequent struggles on the part of state and church leadership to bring them back under control) to have arisen in no small part out of the chaos of a relatively unstructured response to HIV, in which numerous actors from different parts of the country, continent and world came to Uganda – both in body and ideology – to assist in the fight against AIDS. It is out of this mêlée that we first witnessed the catalysation of a more deliberately transnational conservative Christian ideological influence within Uganda through the funding of PEPFAR programmes (Epstein 2005; Sadgrove 2007; Gusman 2009; Schoepf, Chapter 3, and Müller, Chapter 14, this volume). This ideological voice found a sympathetic welcome from certain religious leaders whose own attitudes towards 'family values' found financial clout and the power, authority and confidence that comes from being recognised, resourced and backed by a transnational network. This focus on family values constituted a nationalising response on the part of an alliance of church and state leaders in Uganda, seeking to reclaim control over sexual subjectivities and sexual citizenship. Yet responses 'from below' – as young Ugandans in particular responded to the growing power of this ideological voice – drew on different registers, particularly the importance of discretion about sexual behaviour to notions of respectability and social acceptability.

The ethnographic data on which this chapter is based speak to a number of debates explored within this volume. Specifically, they illuminate some of the limitations of the type of 'conservative' moral discourses that have emerged in the coalitions between transnational actors (particularly the US religious Right) and African religious and state leaders, on the actual behaviour of consumers of these discourses. Ethnographic approaches which seek to look beyond discourse reveal the ways in which alternative authoritative registers and behavioural codes are drawn on to navigate prescribed behaviour in and beyond the environments in which such prescriptions are authoritative. This creative utilisation of often diverse cosmological, cultural and historical influences speaks to simplified understandings (often fuelling the rationales of human rights interventionists) of the 'African context' as at the mercy of heteronormative, heterosexist transnational and local actors at the expense of a much more diverse moral landscape. The implications for the behaviour of young people as they seek to navigate the 'triangle' of transnationalism, conservativism and contestation (Beckmann *et al.*, Chapter 1, this volume, p. 4) with regard to sexuality in Africa are laid bare. Therefore, I argue against the analytical dangers of conflating discourse about behaviour with actual behaviour, particularly amongst those groups who have most to gain by appearing as the discourse dictates – Pentecostal born-again Christians. Analysing the behaviour of Pentecostal Christians illuminates something of the nature of this contestation in two ways – first in the ethnographer's contextual obligation to examine the various value systems with which that of conservative Christianity is competing in Kampala's moral market-place and locate points of overlap and disjuncture. Secondly, it enables analysis beyond the discourses and theologies that are articulated in Kampala's Pentecostal churches and groups to explore the gaps between 'top down' instructions and proscriptions for sexual behaviour and practices and understandings about the value of such proscriptions on the ground.

Rethinking honour

I have found the concepts of honour and shame useful lenses for understanding the ways in which the contested sexual moral landscape within which Ugandans find themselves is navigated – both by religious and state leaders and by the student body at Makerere University. As Iliffe's history of honour attests, honour is a critical if dynamic aspect of the moral and social context into which transnational discourses are received (Iliffe 2005). The heterogeneity of transnational influences, generated by the demands of response to an HIV/AIDS pandemic and a rise in mobile technologies facilitating new kinds of transnational networking within Kampala, have challenged and reshaped notions of honour in multiple ways. This is particularly true of the ways in which notions of honour and shame underpin, construct and seek to control masculinities, femininities and sexualities (Lindisfarne 1994).

Perhaps nowhere are new articulations around honour and shame more apparent than in certain born-again churches, including the church under study (not least because this church is itself 'transnational' as a Pentecostal Assemblies of God church with historical roots in the US Pentecostal tradition, run by a charismatic and influential Canadian pastor). Notions of what Iliffe (drawing on Stewart) considers 'domesticated' forms of honour in the twentieth century shift from hegemonic forms concerned with prestige and prowess (*ekitiibwa* in Luganda) to those which have at their core concern for moral character and respectability, strongly evident in talk about 'good' men and women (Iliffe 2005: 4–6). The concern with 'moral character' and the prevalence of assertions about character, discipline and conduct (*mpiisa* and *muntu mulamu*) in everyday (Luganda) discourse in Kampala are striking, particularly within the Pentecostal churches. This discursive emphasis on moral character alone makes the concept of honour critical to an analysis of the ways in which transnational moral discourses are received by Ugandans. With specific reference to Pentecostal churches, it is clear that such churches offer alternative masculinities and femininities by challenging what Lindisfarne describes as 'hegemonic masculinities' (based on competition over resources, particularly women), intimately tied to patriarchal honour codes. Instead, more nuanced alternatives construct the honour of men, as well as women, around 'moral strength of character' rather than the need to compete over and control the behaviour of women (Lindisfarne 1994: 85). Lindisfarne's comments about the limited capacity of many men to embody hegemonic ideals of masculinity lend a useful framework for analysing the constructions of male and female sexuality within born-again discourse. This may explain the popularity of such models to those men who may have reduced ability to embody or perform more 'hegemonic' forms of masculinity – those who have proved less successful in controlling women's sexuality. For women new discursive tools provided by the Pentecostal church enable a more pro-active preservation of their own honour, itself constructed around the primacy of being a 'good' (*muntu mulamu*), respectable woman which continues to entail pre-marital chastity and marital fidelity. Drawing on the reification of women as chaste, the discourse of the church offers a platform from which born-again women can confidently reject the sexual and predatory advances of men. However, this reification of the chaste woman also poses a profound challenge in contexts where there is genuine affection, attraction and desire for a sexual expression of that attraction, as we shall see.

Beyond the power of church discourses, it is evident that alternative, local (as opposed to transnational) codes for shaping behaviour as honourable or shameful hold enduring power in framing behavioural decisions. Such codes exalt concealment and discretion and are drawn on in cases where the boundaries around varying codes for honourable (sexual) behaviour in particular social settings are transgressed. Secrecy and discretion are considered, outside of the born-again discourse, as highly moral ways of avoiding the risk of publicly offending others and shaming oneself (see also Haram 2005). The public delivery of uncomfortable truths (such as admissions of adultery, an HIV diagnosis, even financial poverty) and loss of face are intimately intertwined with individual and collective shame in ways which still have social power. An understanding of historical notions of honour and the ways in which honour and morality are linked helps to explain the persistence of the tacit moral acceptability of secrecy and concealment by many Ugandans.

Histories of honour

Many of the aspects of social life in Uganda resonate with Iliffe's characterisations of 'honour cultures', where honour is understood at its simplest as 'a right to respect'. Iliffe argues that prior to the advent of world religions, honour represented 'the chief ideological motivation of African behaviour'. Therefore, 'understanding African behaviour, in the past and the present, must take account of changing notions of honour' (Iliffe 2005: 1). In accounting for the changes wrought by the advent of the historical transnational moments of colonialism and world religions, Iliffe refers to the hypocrisy in areas of life where notions of honour conflicted with the moral teachings of world religions and the demands of an institutionalised state. In the case of corruption, he draws attention to the need for ministers to 'observe, at least outwardly, an alien code of official behaviour', drawing attention to the disjuncture between what is displayed outwardly and what is done in private (2005: 342). Certainly there is considerable evidence of this acute disjuncture between public and private in the negotiations of many Ugandans as they inhabit and move across different social contexts in contemporary Kampala.

Iliffe's attention to the ways in which European colonialism domesticated African notions of honour through the development of 'respectability', shifting emphasis from 'rank and prowess' to 'virtue and duty' or 'moral character', lends a useful framework for understanding the pervasive concern with respectability as it is re-emphasised and re-articulated in discourses about sexual morality in the context of HIV prevention (2005: 5). It is also highly useful to an understanding of the concerns of young Ugandans and how they approach intersections between discourses about sexual morality.

A further way in which the notion of 'honour cultures' acts as a useful context in which to analyse and understand present-day religious and social identities within Uganda, is in the demonstration of the necessarily social aspect of the notion of respectability. Throughout Iliffe's study, and with reference to a diverse set of groups from all over sub-Saharan Africa, each with their distinct criteria for honour, recurrent characteristics include the fact that respectability 'demanded peer recognition in a public sphere of associations' (Iliffe 2005: 254). This study clearly demonstrates the continuing importance of peer recognition within the public sphere for university students within Uganda. Most or all people believe that they have a right to respect as individuals, but they can enjoy and confer it only as members of groups. The groups determine the criteria of honour, but any society is likely to contain several such groups with different criteria, so that honour is a contested category (Iliffe 2005: 4).

The broader study from which this chapter draws explores the social nature of honour by examining two distinct and divergent peer groups at Makerere University to compare sexual attitudes and behaviour among members. Each group has different criteria for peer inclusion and social status (honour). The first group, which places significant emphasis on material accumulation, encourages women to extract resources from men by promising but withholding sexual contact until a projected date in the future. These women are known as 'de-toothers' and they seek to manipulate hegemonic notions of masculinity that encourage competition between men for women, based around male financial prowess and gift giving (see Sadgrove 2007; Mills and Ssewakiriyanga 2005). The second group comprises 'born-again' members of a big Pentecostal church in Kampala with alternative codes for masculinity and femininity, as outlined above. Yet despite the very divergent criteria for honour and group inclusion, discretion and secrecy are carefully employed by individuals of both groups to ensure their continued acceptability within their particular group and their conformity with overarching 'Ugandan' criteria for respectability.

Discursive economies: talking about sex in Uganda

Because of the diversity of the national and international response to HIV in Uganda, prevention interventions have evoked a complex and heterogeneous discursive economy for talking about sexual behaviour. It is possible to identify elements of four distinct discourses within which sexual behaviour and the value of different types of behaviour are interpreted by young people in Uganda. Two of these discourses are heavily influenced by Western approaches to and understandings about sex, and both are criticised by religious and some state leaders in Uganda for appearing to separate questions about sexual behaviour from concerns about 'morality'. Each discourse configures the relationship between sexual behaviour and morality in different ways and with varying degrees of urgency. The other two discourses, informed by 'traditional' and conservative Christian values respectively, are explicitly moralising, ascribing values of 'good' and 'bad' to certain expressions of and contexts for sexual behaviour. These discourses can be explicit in blaming, shaming and stigmatising those who appear to have behaved in ways which are constructed as 'bad'. All of these discourses overlap and diverge at different points and young people must mediate between their often conflicting expectations. Frequently, this mediation entails that young people switch accountability from one discourse to another in response to different audiences with different expectations: peers, parents, church authority figures, HIV prevention workers.

The following section sketches out the shapes of these discourses. In doing so, particular attention is paid to the traditional-moral and the Christian-moral because they frequently overlap with and enforce the behavioural proscriptions of the born-again Christian students considered within this study. Further, these discourses have particular authority in constituting the notion of the 'good', 'moral' person, itself crucial to the self-fashioning exercises of young Ugandans. The traditional-moral and Christian-moral discourses heavily inform popular Ugandan conceptions about what constitutes 'good', moral conduct with which people wish to be identified and around which public respectability is commonly configured.

(Western) public health campaigns

As the introduction to this volume argues, sex and sexuality have, in the era of AIDS, become 'scripted through the imperative of disease intervention' (Beckmann *et al.*, Chapter 1, this volume, p. 18). This has resulted in the exportation of a heavily biologised model for the interpretation of sex and sexuality by Western actors. This model therefore carries specific understandings about disease aetiology to contexts which often have different ways of framing the causal relationships between the body and mind and the body and the community. Such biomedical discourses, whilst jarring with certain local understandings about sex and sexuality, underpin the (Western) public health campaigns to encourage sexual behaviour change publicly propagated by the major hospitals, clinics and many medical professionals within Kampala. This discourse aims to 'get the nation talking about sex'. It considers sex in terms of risk, health and disease, and focuses on making sexual behaviour safe, often through the use of condoms. Whilst considering sex in terms of risk and safety, this discourse does not proscribe sex itself. Implicitly individualist, again belying its Western roots, this approach relies on the 'production of a modern subject; knowledgeable, rational, responsible and in control' (Jassey and Nyanzi 2007: 11). Within this discourse:

> Individuals are treated as if they are independent of the socio-economic contexts in which they live and regarded as rational actors in the transmission cycle of the disease.

> Disease control efforts therefore are heavily focussed on educating the actors about the disease and their responsibility to prevent transmission. The assumption is that informed individuals make rational choices that will protect themselves and others.
> (Chan and Reidpath 2003: 40)

Whilst not explicitly communicating through the language of 'morality' or the production of the 'moral person', this discourse does have a directive and places preference on sexual behaviour which is sanitised and accordingly 'low risk'.

Knowledge of the means by which HIV is transmitted is extremely high in Kampala, particularly amongst the university student community. Yet, despite fluency and basic understanding of the biomedical model for thinking about sex and disease, it is clear that there are limitations as to its perceived explanatory utility, as well as considerable gaps between articulations of the discourse and behavioural responses to it. In an informal conversation about HIV/AIDS and its means of transmission, a 21-year-old male student recited the received biomedical wisdom: 'HIV is the virus that causes AIDS; it is transmitted through the exchange of certain bodily fluids, particularly semen and blood but also vaginal fluids and breast milk; it can be protected against by the use of condoms.' However, at the end of his recitation, he suggested that whilst all this might be true, it cannot explain why one person may become infected whilst another might not. Implicitly he is referring to the complex nature of risk and chance on which the biological model rests, based on a myriad of invisible and often incalculable factors. These include viral load at the time of intercourse, immune response and the general health of the individual who is exposed including the presence or absence of immuno-compromising factors. Biomedicine cannot personalise infection, as other frameworks (including witchcraft) can. 'If you or I get HIV, ourselves,' he concluded, 'well, that's just a curse or something.' Such accounts, which are by no means uncommon, suggest not only the limitations of biomedicine but the cosmological richness and breadth of interpretative frameworks for thinking through sex, AIDS and morality, and a certain pragmatism based on utility, which drives a syncretic picking and choosing across seemingly antagonistic frameworks (see also Iliffe 2006).

'Modern' romantic love (and sexual liberalism)

A second discourse which influences young people in Uganda is that of 'modern' romantic love, promoted most evidently by various forms of popular Western media – novels, magazines, films, television series, and popular music. This Western notion of romantic love is commonly understood by students at Makerere University as 'real love'; a type of love that is deemed difficult to find in the Ugandan setting with its accordant socio-economic dynamics which frequently condition the nature of sexual relationships amongst students. Whilst tending to be implicitly hetero-normative, this discourse does not explicitly place value on certain expressions of (heterosexual) sexual behaviour over others, and generally does not consider questions about risk or disease. Decisions about and expressions of sexuality are the individualised concern of two consenting adults acting behind closed doors.

Within Uganda, this discursive framing of sexuality is frequently branded as 'permissive' by religious and other leaders. Tensions regularly arise between Western-media-promoted 'permissive' sexual relationships in which sex is the concern of two consenting adults, and enduring social criteria for (particularly female) respectability and honour in Uganda, premised on sexual restraint and abstinence outside marriage.

The individualised nature of this discourse often conflicts with the desires of parents and kinship groups who consider sexual relationships between young people as a community concern. The difficulties that young people face in navigating between social expectations of peer and family groupings and the impact of media-based concepts of 'modern', 'romantic love' are recognised in literature on HIV prevention across Africa. As Smith suggests in his study of young Igbo relationships:

> The whole concept of romantic love is tied up with a growing emphasis on individuality, as male-female relationships are more likely to be seen as private and personal rather than subject to collective surveillance and regulation. However, these changes are occurring with considerable tension, as collective family and community interests in reproductive relationships influence the way in which young Igbos behave in pre-marital relationships.
>
> (2000: 100)

Whilst young people in Uganda are keen to take advantage of differing concepts of relationships and romantic love, they also still feel strongly bound by social and parental expectations. Frequently these social and parental expectations are represented in and correlate with the overarching criteria for respectability which emerge from a synthesis of 'traditional' and Christian moralities. In the case of young born-again Christians, questions about intimate relationships are often further complicated by the fact that people must mediate between the conflicting desires of parents and born-again peer group members. Tensions between the 'private and personal' nature of male-female relationships and the pressures posed by 'collective family and community interests' were repeatedly reflected by born-again women in their consideration of the 'right' marriage partner. The born-again Christian peer group expects born-again Christians to have relationships with and marry other born-again Christians. Parents were often reported as rejecting the born-again movement and its members outright. In a discussion about 'why born-agains keep quiet in the face of evil', four born-again women suggested that although they wanted to marry born-again men, they had to be discreet about these relationships in front of their parents:

> I fear rejection. If I wanted to get married I know that in church I shouldn't court a non-believer. I want to get married to a believer but I can't take this boy to my dad as he's a born-again and my dad's an Anglican. What if I argue with my dad and

> then the next day the born-again guy chucks me? I can't argue with my dad and he refuses born-agains.
>
> (Female, 23, 3rd year management student, 15.06.05)

Accordingly, relationships that run counter to the expectations of family and peer group members are frequently hidden from those who might disapprove. This implies that whilst young people are keen to take advantage of individualised concepts of romantic love, public approval remains extremely important when it comes to relationships between young men and women. It is therefore better to hide those relationships that will not satisfy concerned social others than deal with the consequences of disappointment and shame. The individualised ideals of modern, romantic love are frequently untenable for young people in Uganda, who will tend to bow to the expectations of peers and parents and wider social ideas about 'good' partners.

In reflecting on the feasibility of 'romantic' love, one male student suggested that concerns about 'class' will prove more important than 'love' within relationships between female students and potential life partners. In a statement that relates to the role of money in romantic relationships, the impact of being born-again on such dynamics and the link between money and perceptions about social hierarchy, he suggested:

> No woman on campus would go out with an uneducated man, even if they're in love. It's cause of money. It's not explicit, but it's still very much a factor for girls; they're still part of that culture and it's very strong. Money is a key player, even in salvation. Salvation won't challenge that any time soon. It's very deeply rooted. You see your parents not associating with certain people. We imagine ourselves as better or worse than them. How culture views who we end up with has to be dealt with in choosing a partner. Class is defined by money.
>
> (Male, 21, 2nd year statistics and psychology student, 19.01.06)

Prevailing understandings about money and class, informing notions of what makes a 'good' life partner, are inherited from the attitudes of parents. These understandings can also be read as having their roots in understandings of honour, particularly those notions which are constructed around material display. Such concerns about family honour and approval will frequently trump 'romantic love' as a motivation for a long-term relationship. In the short term, the considerable tensions between the expectations of 'romantic love' and those of parents or peers entail the concealment of relationships which would be frowned upon by social arbiters.

'Traditional' sexual mores

The third discourse evident in Uganda's public sphere and impacting upon the interpretations and meanings assigned to sexual behaviour amongst young people has been claimed by its advocates as 'traditional' sexual mores. 'Traditional' sexual mores are invoked to support and bolster HIV prevention campaign messages which promote pre-marital chastity and abstinence – as well as those which reject the viability of same-sex identities. They also act as a means of critiquing and commenting on the processes of social change that have taken place across Africa over the last 100 years. As the lively debates in the literature suggest, an examination of sources which describe 'traditional' or historical sexual mores in the face of considerable social change will always entail a certain idealisation of a lost past. Constructing ideals in this way plays a role in explaining, critiquing and evaluating social change. Such ideals have also been manipulated by church and state leaders to fuel the nationalising project based around the rejection of what are deemed 'Western' understandings about sexuality and sexual morality.

There are limited anthropological sources which consider pre-marital sexual morality and behaviour in Africa and many of the sources which are commonly cited are dated (Ahlberg 1994; Setel 1999).[1] Given the rapid change over the past century, the existing sources should be recognised as representing fragments within a dynamic synthesis of values and influences. This synthesis informs the ways in which historical and traditional understandings are to be (re)constructed and used in the pragmatic process of value construction in contemporary Uganda, making it difficult to evaluate the veracity of ethnographic sources as records of coherent (historical) codes for sexual behaviour. However, amongst the ethnographic body of literature which exists, it is possible to draw attention to the function and importance of sex in some of the societies in Uganda, as sources suggest and allow, to enable a better understanding of some of the material contained within this chapter.

Historically, moralising over sexual behaviour was primarily the responsibility of parents and kin members and was often linked to material prestations in the form of bride wealth. Parents were invested in controlling the sexual behaviour of their daughters because bride wealth commonly relied on virginity and chastity. Frequently, taboos existed concerning communication between parents and their children with regard to sex, and where this was the case other systems were in place to ensure that virginity was maintained and that adolescent socialisation was controlled through the 'close monitoring and regulation of female sexuality' (Parikh 2005: 131–2). Amongst the Basoga and the Baganda, such controls included the 'Sôngá'/'Ssenga', a paternal aunt who held particular responsibilities regarding

[1] Aside from the ongoing problem that sexual behaviour is of a nature that eludes scholarly methods of study, Ahlberg accounts for the absence of early anthropological literature on sexual behaviour in Africa as rooted in Victorian sexual double standards, which demanded chastity amongst 'virtuous', biologically asexual women, whilst sanctioning unchastity amongst men, socially licensed to use lower-class prostitutes to satiate their biological and 'natural' sexual desires. The result of this double standard was a silence surrounding sex and sexuality. It was within and out of this context in which sex was a taboo subject that anthropology was developing and emerging as a scholarly discipline.

the nurture and socialisation of young women during adolescence. These responsibilities included attempting to ensure virginity at marriage and instructing women about matters pertaining to marriage and running a household (Standing and Kisekka 1976; Kinsman *et al.* 2000; Davis 2001; Parikh 2005). Amongst other groups in Uganda and East Africa, ethnographic research, whilst reflecting the heterogeneity of sexual norms, frequently suggests 'prestige and value attached to the virgin bride. Extra bridewealth was paid, cattle were slaughtered in her honour, and there was corresponding shame where this was not the case' (Heald 1995: 496). Aside from the ideals of pre-marital virginity and avoidance of pre-marital pregnancy, other values include modesty about nudity and discretion regarding the discussion of sex, including often strict taboos around inter-generational communication about sexual matters. As expressions of a societal morality, information about the value of sex must be understood as embedded within the prevailing values of community life and at the heart of the social rules of 'respect'.

> Many – if not most – East African societies can be dubbed 'respect cultures', and the respect draws its power from that accorded to sexuality. There is a preoccupation with the control of sexuality, so that the controls surrounding sex, and the self-control that one must exercise with regard to it, epitomise social and moral behaviour.
> (Heald cited in Haram 2005: 58)[2]

As part of the discussion on 'traditional' morality, it is therefore important to recognise that sexual behaviour reflects a specific category around which morality – and correspondingly honour – is constructed for young people. 'Sex' is a category of experience and behaviour which stands in a class apart from other behaviour which may also be subject to social proscriptions. Because of the links between 'respect' and moral sexual behaviour, traditional codes for sexual morality, historically informed by and fused with Christian sexual mores, intimately inform enduring criteria for being 'good', 'respectable' people in Uganda. Within Ugandan society, presenting as a 'respectable', 'good' person carries with it long-term implications with socio-economic weight.

It is around the discussion of what makes a 'good' person that we witness a particular merging of religious, political and 'cultural' understandings of the HIV pandemic and approaches to its prevention. Appeals to 'time-tested culture', and reflections on the 'culture of free sex' (generally understood as being Western in origin) as a causal factor in the HIV pandemic in Uganda are commonly heard, natural explanatory categories for understanding HIV. Significantly, the *New Vision* newspaper, commonly recognised as the Ugandan 'government's mouthpiece', is a key carrier of these nationalising messages, which seek to reclaim the national

[2] Haram suggests that one's sexual conduct in particular is strongly linked to daily interpretations of 'respect', 'discipline' and 'shame', suggesting that sexual behaviour is a central reference for the construction of one's social identity as 'respectable'.

honour of Uganda by locating the source of the 'moral decay' so commonly associated with HIV/AIDS outside of Uganda itself, as the following citations attest. As the 'culture of free sex' is targeted as the cause of the spread of HIV, 'tradition' and 'culture' (located within Uganda) are suggested as idealised models for sexual behaviour which could end the HIV pandemic. This 'culture of free sex' emerges from contact with the West. The West itself is imagined as:

> A place where permissiveness in moral matters holds sway. This is an area in the world where people have cast off their moral moorings, where situational ethics is the way [. . .] In such a situation, anything goes. That is why one reads of so much sexual perversion in the West: people having sex with animals and corpses; of bishops molesting minors; of men wedding men and women wedding women under the stupefied gaze of so-called men of God.
>
> (*New Vision*, 16.07.02)

It is interesting to note that the terminology and metaphor of 'moral decay' and 'the battle for the soul of Uganda' which we see in relation to this contest over national selfhood is almost verbatim what we see discussed in relation to homosexuality later in the decade (Sadgrove *et al.* 2012; see also Müller, Chapter 14, and Ehrisman, Chapter 13, this volume).

In the majority of these cases there is an implicit if not explicit belief that things have broken down, 'decayed' from an idealised and constructed past:

> The cure to the root causes of all African problems is therefore to go back to the beginning and trace how our forefathers did it. The majority were morally upright! [. . .] In old Africa, pregnancy outside wedlock was an abomination, thieves were hanged and bringing up children was a collective responsibility of the entire community. Today all that is given lip-service. These values were lost during colonisation and are almost extinct with the advent of neo-colonialism and globalisation.
>
> (*New Vision*, 12.07.05)

With specific reference to HIV and sexual behaviour in Uganda, condoms are associated with immorality and, as a result of both religious organisations' and government campaigns, abstinence and marital fidelity are seen as the upright solutions to the problem, grounded as they are in 'African family values' and 'old Africa'. Aside from the influence of 'the West', the 'curbing' of sex outside of marriage as the model scenario with which to stop the spread of HIV is also commonly countered against the triumph of instinct over reason; the 'animal' nature of unbridled sexuality, symptomatic of moral degeneration and associated with HIV prevalence in Uganda. In press accounts concerning sexual activity, particularly those which take a pro-abstinence line, moral degeneration and the subsequent permissive sexuality (sanctioned if not fuelled by the availability of condoms) has been accused of driving young people 'into acting like a beast' (*New Vision*, 21.11.02), stooping 'to the level of goats' (*New Vision*, 23.01.07), being led 'by instinct and not by reason' (*New Vision*, 03.07.03). Moral sexual behaviour within this traditionalist discourse is therefore associated with restraint and control, and seen as something which separates human beings from animals, representing 'reasonable' over instinctive behaviour. Such negative judgements over extra-marital sex represent the most conservative end of the HIV prevention spectrum. Yet these associations have implications for the openness of discussions about and reports of sexual behaviour in a climate in which one's moral self-fashioning, entailing at its core sexual restraint, has implications for social status, as this chapter argues.

In seeking to explain the high prevalence of HIV/AIDS in Uganda and the 'moral decay' which is often implicitly associated with it, a common target is the influence of Western values and lifestyles coupled with 'a breakdown in cultural norms' (*New Vision*, 02.10.02, 30.03.04). The remedy to this situation is commonly deemed to be the revival of African cultural values and practices which, historically, controlled and restrained the sexual activity of people both prior to and outside of marriage: 'parents should groom their children into our African norms and culture that curb sex outside marriage' (*New Vision*, 10.02.03, 02.12.03).[3]

This nationalising discourse around 'traditional' sexual moral codes, in part a response to the perceived imposition of 'Western' morality, posits a moral Ugandan self against a Western, morally degenerate other, further exacerbating the concern with presenting as 'respectable' people for many young Ugandans. In turn, this increases the need to conceal socially unrespectable behaviour.

Conservative Christian morality

The final discourse which heavily dominates the public space in which messages about sexual behaviour circulate is that of conservative Christian sexual morality. This discourse echoes that of the 'traditional' by emphasising pre-marital abstinence and monogamy within marriage, and conflicts with the Western discourses in rejecting condoms outright. The traditional-moral and conservative Christian-moral discourses are, at many points, presented as mutually reinforcing. The *New Vision* newspaper and many leaders in Uganda (religious and political) use these points of reinforcement to strengthen their messages, as the evidence attests. This is not a contradiction but evidence of the convenient elision between traditional and conservative Christian discourses in a pragmatic alliance. The overlap falls in the emphasis on sexual restraint, pressure for pre-marital virginity and call for fidelity within marriage. This elision is used by conservative leaders despite the fact that the roots of the traditional-moral discourse and the conservative Christian

[3] The revitalisation of 'traditional codes of morality' has been part of Museveni's approach to HIV/AIDS in Uganda since 1988 when, in his address on World AIDS Day, he suggested the revival of 'traditional codes of morality', promoting 'old corporal punishments' as an effective way to deter prostitution and adultery: 'we should emulate the social behaviour of our ancestors which forbade immorality and irresponsible communal sexual lifestyles' (cited in Putzel 2004: 25).

discourse are distinct. Arguably, the conservative Christian discourse is ultimately premised on the notion of the fall and a concept of a society which has fallen out of relationship with God and must continually strive to make amends. The (reclaimed) traditional moral discourse has its roots in memories of Ugandan custom and history. Notably, the selection of traditional-moral aspects which are mobilised in the fight against AIDS are all too frequently those which do not antagonise the tenets of conservative Christianity.

Within Uganda, the conservative Christian discourse is intimately linked with and further enforced by the popularity of born-again churches and their preaching on sexual behaviour. At the international level, this discourse is supported by conservative Christians within the US administration who imbue its ideological positions with considerable political and financial backing. This backing means that the conservative Christian discourse has also become heavily entrenched in the national HIV preventative public health campaigns. The overlap between internationally backed conservative Christian discourses and national HIV prevention strategies in Uganda has increasingly drawn attention to what is perceived by many in the field of HIV prevention as the merging and confusion of morality with health safety. In recent years, it is the US government's role in HIV prevention in Uganda that has attracted a significant proportion of the media and scholarly attention dedicated to Uganda, HIV prevention and the politics of international donor funding (Epstein 2005; Susser 2009).

The impact of the born-again churches on the public debates about sexuality and HIV prevention has been aided by charismatic public figures. One of the most outspoken and well known, particularly with regard to university-level youth in Uganda, is Pastor Martin Ssempa. Ssempa is known for arguing 'that HIV decline in Uganda was due to abstinence and faithfulness arising from a remarkable commitment to Christian and moral values' (*New Vision*, 29.09.05). He has organised a number of marches and protests against condom use and in support of abstinence and was one of the co-authors of Uganda's draft AB policy. In 2002, a US-based study argued that the decline in HIV rates in Uganda was primarily linked to abstinence and fidelity behaviour, rather than condom use. It was also suggested that Ugandan demographic surveys implied that the number of unfaithful men and women had increased since 1995. Ssempa used these findings as a chance to criticise the emphasis on condoms in HIV prevention in Uganda, arguing that:

> This relaxation is because people have lost track from Museveni's original message of abstinence and faithfulness. In Kampala the original bill boards advocating for abstinence have either collapsed or rusted, and a new breed of condom promoting billboards have replaced them. The whole anti-HIV/AIDS campaign has been taken over by the commercial interest of promoting condoms.
>
> (*New Vision*, 16.12.02)

Ssempa champions the abstinence approach 'because Uganda is under attack from an agenda driven by homosexuals and western experts' (Reuters, 10.12.04) who wish to promote condoms. However, despite his hostility, he is happy to receive funds from those Western experts to allow him to continue his work and run his church and outreach organisation (Human Rights Watch 2005: 47).

The rapidly growing born-again churches and their leaders within Kampala have proved the most vocal proponents of abstinence and virginity until marriage, and their messages pre-date the apparent shift in government policy towards abstinence and fidelity over condom use. In an article in *New Vision*, a born-again member of Pastor Ssempa's outreach organisation 'Campus Alliance to Wipeout AIDS' (CAWA), which aims to change the sexual behaviour of students at university campuses in Uganda by reforming the morals of Ugandans, sums up popular associations with both condoms and the 'moral' source of the HIV pandemic:

> No one knows why the human values of honesty, respect, self-control, dignity, modesty and sexual morality have outrightly been abandoned and the human race has sunk to the status of animals that cannot control their primal urges. The condom strategy brings out an element of compromise and a weakling which may break the shield against the scourge.
>
> (23.01.07)

The associations of HIV with 'values' and 'morals' epitomise common church positions which seek to explain the prevalence of HIV in Uganda and I have heard these messages preached in a number of born-again churches around Kampala. The analogy of sexually active humans with 'animals that cannot control their primal urges' is another common position reflected in public debates about abstinence and condom use. The condom is seen to further undermine the moral fabric of Uganda by 'sanctioning' if not encouraging sex outside of marriage. These associations are reflected in Museveni's speeches on HIV/AIDS. Museveni's association of HIV with 'moral decadency' and his appeal to the churches to remedy this demonstrates the overlap between the 'religious' and 'political' spheres. In an appeal to the Roman Catholic Church to double its efforts to counter HIV/AIDS in Uganda:

> The president urged the church to use the freedom of worship to shape the morals of the people and nurture them spiritually. 'I appeal to the church to continue playing its role of shaping society, especially by protecting the people of Uganda against moral decadency' Museveni said.
>
> (*Monitor*, 27.06.05)

The influence of church positions and leaders in Uganda extends beyond the strictly religious sphere. Mrs Museveni is a high-profile born-again Christian, actively involved in HIV prevention in Uganda. The Uganda AIDS Commission's first chairman was a Church of Uganda bishop and its subsequent chair was a Roman Catholic bishop. The role of religious figures and organisations within Uganda's public debates and government institutions necessitates considerable reciprocity in and between the attitudes and policies of government in Uganda (cf. Müller, Chapter 14, this volume). In a public address to Ugandan youth, an MP suggested that 'the youth should forget about condoms and improve their morals instead':

> 'It's time for the youth of Uganda to respect their relationships and religious oaths to be free from HIV/AIDS instead of relying on condoms'. The MP alleged that condoms promote prostitution and accused organisations that give free condoms to youth of encouraging immorality.
>
> (*Monitor*, 06.01.04)

This reciprocity of values and ideological positions between religious and political leaders and the considerable public influence of religious leaders through both church congregations and their ownership of school and hospital facilities must be taken into account in an attempt to understand the significance of religious influence within Uganda's HIV prevention environment and the ongoing debate about sexual morality. The churches have institutional as well as discursive power which impacts on people's access to knowledge about HIV/AIDS in very different ways. At the time of the research, I witnessed the ways in which the distinct theologies and power structures of the Catholic and Anglican denominations impacted on their capacity to support those suffering with HIV/AIDS. Staff at a Roman Catholic hospital reported that they were unable to explicitly promote condom use to patients seeking advice about HIV, due to the Vatican position. Further, when Roman Catholic nuns and priests contracted HIV and developed AIDS, they were, said hospital staff, often hidden away from view, treated discreetly by the hospital, but frequently isolated and unable to access sufficient pastoral support. By contrast, unhampered by the centralised power structure that seeks to universalise the Catholic Church's top-down moral theology, the nearby Anglican hospital made condoms available on tables in the waiting room and its staff were able to discuss their use in HIV prevention. Further, the Anglican Church of Uganda also had influential public spokespersons who spoke about their HIV-infected status, such as Reverend Canon Gideon Byamugisha, who is now a global advocate for the cause of those suffering from HIV/AIDS and runs a vibrant ministry for those affected by HIV/AIDS in Kampala.

Aside from hospitals, the other key institutional vehicle through which the HIV/AIDS messages of religious organisations are carried is that of church-owned schools. When, in 2001, the Ugandan government launched the President's Initiative on AIDS Strategy for Communication to Youth (PIASCY), an HIV/AIDS curriculum to be implemented in all primary schools, the religious stakeholders present rejected certain aspects of the material that spoke in biomedical terms about sex, including depictions of ejaculation, correct condom use, and changes in the body during puberty (Human Rights Watch 2005). Because the churches control a considerable proportion of the schools in Uganda, and they refused to implement the curriculum in their schools as it stood, a chapter on biological sex was taken out, and replaced by a chapter that a coalition of religious leaders wrote on morality and moral selfhood.

These examples demonstrate the ways in which, outside of the influence of PEPFAR, different denominations reflected conservativising trends within Uganda to 'pull back' from the breadth of medicalised HIV prevention messages. It was, in the early 2000s, Ugandan religious leaders who explicitly voiced these concerns.

The moral conservativism around sexuality in Uganda, which draws a considerable amount of international attention, particularly in light of more recent tensions around homosexuality, is heavily informed by a complex mixing and merging of religious and traditional values with regard to perceptions of the 'morality' or otherwise of sexual activity. The Christian moralising approach to HIV prevention and sexual behaviour engages not only the Christian community within Uganda, including the rapidly growing born-again churches, but also the considerable funds of the US administration and those 'traditionalists' wishing to promote abstinence and avoid talking explicitly about sexual behaviour. This politically powerful coalition of actors ensures that messages about sex framed in terms of 'morality' and moral personhood dominate the discursive environment for talking about sex in Uganda in the wake of HIV.

Negotiating the gaps – the born-again members of Watoto Church

The public discourses in Uganda which propagate societal breakdown or decay from an idealised past (be it 'traditional' or Christian in origin) resonate in interesting and powerful ways with the theology of Watoto Church. Watoto's theology is implicitly premised on the notion of the fall of humanity from God, as described in Genesis, and promotes the propagation of a new (and compensatory) 'biblical worldview' through which the relationship between humanity and God is rebuilt. This biblical worldview is to be promoted by all born-again Christians and communicated through their public behaviour, as all are mandated to constantly reflect the characteristics of the biblical worldview in society and public life. This is communicated by constant reiteration of the behavioural expectations of being born-again – not drinking, not smoking, abstaining before marriage, dressing respectably (limiting the amount of flesh displayed by women). This emphasis on public performance further resonates with wider ethnographic evidence concerning the importance of outward appearances within Kampala and certainly Buganda, if not further afield in Uganda (Sadgrove 2007). The emphasis on public appearances (and a strong implicit separation of the public from the private) reflects thinking about the impact of changing social contexts on notions of honour over the twentieth century, in particular the focus on display and public respectability.

The born-again Christian group whose understandings and experiences inform this chapter commonly understood their religious identities as being configured around rules and proscriptions, and articulated their understandings of salvation in terms of 'do's and don'ts'. Such articulations persisted alongside other commonly cited theological understandings of 'human nature' and 'the flesh'. The flesh, which is not saved and must be struggled with everyday, allows some leeway around the problem of behavioural expectation. In response to an interview question about how behaviour had changed since members had become born-again, the majority of respondents suggested that born-agains still sin, and cited theological ideas of sin and repentance as existing to counter the problem. But alongside these understandings, there was still an immediate association between becoming born-again and ceasing certain forms of behaviour: not doing the 'don'ts' and publicly rejecting the other influential discourses of 'the world'. This reflects the strength of the morally proscriptive ideological discourse of Watoto Church in people's discussions of their behaviour and the behaviour change implications implicit in becoming born-again. It also reflects the expectations of wider Ugandan society, both born-again and non-born-again, with regard to what a born-again should be and how born-agains can be recognised by their 'good', respectable (and therefore honourable) behaviour.

Doing the 'don'ts' – 'the world'

The emphasis on born-agains being 'different', and the importance of publicly expressing the difference entailed by being born-again, is further reinforced by another of Watoto Church's central tenets. Watoto's theology is exclusive of and intolerant towards every other worldview. The community that Watoto aims to create through its social groups is defined in contra-distinction to everything else that goes on outside of those groups (except, of course, where the tenets of other worldviews support those of the 'biblical worldview'). Everything beyond the Watoto group's boundaries is described as 'the world' and is constructed alongside Watoto's idealised 'biblical worldview', based around the preaching of pastors and understandings and interpretations of the Bible:

> We need a new worldview that leads to life and God's pleasure. So there's a constant tension for a Christian; first to act the way of the word and second to act as a Christian in the world. We need to guard against spiritual schizophrenia. We have dual personalities. We live in two worlds. We have compartmentalised our lives. We are Christians at church but different in the world. We allow prevailing cultures to dominate the way we live, rather than our Christian worldview. The Christian worldview is the only one to provide the solution to our fractured world.
>
> (Pastor Gary Skinner, 13.03.05)

The tensions of the 'two worlds', and having to mediate between them, link clearly to some of Iliffe's reflections on the challenges that arise when notions of honour and those of world religions come into conflict. Iliffe draws attention to the importance of outwardly observing one code for behaviour whilst privately drawing from another frame of reference (2005: 342). There was certainly evidence of such pragmatism from many of the born-again students I lived with, and it is clear from broader ethnographic evidence that this employment of discretion is itself constructed as an honourable way of handling discursive tension, as it prioritises preserving social relationships above causing upset and possible offence and recognises that 'to shame another is to shame oneself' (Iliffe 2005: 50).

In reality, of course, born-again Christians are dealing with more than two worlds. They are having to negotiate multiple discourses about sexuality, as we have seen, and the often conflicting expectations of family and peer groups – born-again and non-born-again. The overlaps between the Christian-moral and the traditional-moral discourses with Watoto's theology, based around abstinence and fidelity, have been considered, and find sufficient overlap and complementarity, despite having different roots, to be articulated and utilised by Watoto Church members where useful. However, if we explore the impact of the biomedical discourses around HIV/AIDS on church members, it is clear that Watoto's emphasis on abstinence, and on behaving as a born-again at all times, makes it very difficult for church members to speak openly about their sexual behaviour and any struggles they may be having (for more details see Sadgrove 2007). The discourse of 'modern' romantic love finds mixed traction with the born-again Christian group. Many of its vehicles – TV shows, pop music – are, within Watoto's discourse, unavailable to church members as instead they are directed towards Christian TV shows, music and movies, so that their minds are not contaminated by 'the world'. Yet, romantic notions of love and attraction are clearly a struggle for some church members who rationalise their sexual relationships through a mixture of a romantic notion of love fused with a Christian rationale, as this female born-again respondent suggests of her relationship with her non-born-again boyfriend:

> My boyfriend's not born-again. He's a Christian but needs to be born-again so he can understand me more fully. It's a problem. He pressures me for intimacy, I refuse, I give in and then think 'What have I done?' I've stopped feeling guilty. You try hard, but then you have to keep the relationship and he's a human being and I also feel stupid. That's one thing I've been compromising with God. But it's not by mistake I have him. God sent him, but it's confusing. I just pray all this leads to a long-term relationship.
>
> (Female, 21, 1st year urban planning student, 15.07.05)

Born-again Christians find their own syntheses between their born-again identities and what those identities entail in terms of public behaviour, conditioned by the fact that they live, engage, interact with and are equally influenced by 'the world' and the social landscapes of campus. Frequently, as group members switch accountability between competing social dialects and discourses around campus, these syntheses involve discretion and secrecy about behaviour which would be negatively judged by the audience with whom the group member is engaging. Methodologically, it was my task to get beneath the very dense performative discourse of the born-again students to reveal the inconsistencies in behavioural reports which emerge in response to the expectations of different interlocutors. I did this by ensuring that respondents were witnessed in as many different social contexts as possible. Doing so made it possible to chart the ways in which narratives often altered as social expectations and audiences shifted. Born-again Christian members find their own ways of managing Watoto's constructed boundaries between multiple social realities with their distinct values, behavioural norms and respective peer group pressures, just as those historically handling the tensions between older systems of honour and the demands of an institutionalised state did. Frequently their strategies are based around ensuring that proscribed behaviour is concealed from social others. But this is a struggle for many and creates a difficult tension for the born-again Christian who has to continually demonstrate at the level of public behaviour that they are 'in the world but not of the world'. As two student members of Watoto Church suggested:

> Once society knows you're born-again, there's a high expectation of your life and what you do. People fear to be branded a hypocrite. You fear society knowing that you're indulging. This can make your behaviour secret. If I drink I'll drink in my own room. But if you have a basically positive life, the accountability factor encourages you.
>
> (Male, 21, 3rd year civil engineering student, KPC Youth Leader, 19.07.05)

> If I live a life which isn't born-again or Christian-like, there are people who are always watching us, even in church and out. Something small can mess you up. You say you're a Christian but they find you kissing. People can't listen to you. I feel guilty when I'm wrong as a Christian and surrounded by people who aren't born-again as I'm not giving them a good example.
>
> (Female, 23, 3rd year drama student, 30.11.05)

Throughout the interviews, many respondents talked of not wanting to be seen as hypocrites. The notion of hypocrisy is closely linked to the question of social authority and status. Being born-again commands a certain amount of authority and respect within Ugandan society. Yet no one is going to accord the respect that being a born-again Christian commands within Ugandan society if that born-again is revealed as saying one thing and doing another. Neither are people going to heed the proselytising rhetoric of a known born-again 'hypocrite'. Watoto has a strong preaching on the importance of 'truth' and 'integrity' and decries the 'spiritual schizophrenia' and duplicity which often emerge when born-again Christians move from their born-again environments into 'the world'. Yet, this social authority is accorded within the framework of Ugandan social concerns with appearance and display as creating and constituting identity. The social authority of born-again Christians within Uganda rests not in an individual's 'integrity' – either living a life in line with being born-again or being honest about their shortcomings when their behaviour falls short of that lifestyle – but in the continuous public demonstration of the born-again life. Born-again authority is intimately tied to maintaining the image of being born-again, and to be branded a hypocrite is to be stigmatised.

Resonating quite clearly with wider social discourses about breakdown and decay, the theology of Watoto Church also re-affirms a concern with public appearances, already highly powerful in Kampala as a means of constituting and preserving public identity and reputation. This combination of factors militates against an open climate of discussion around sexuality, sexual and other proscribed behaviours for young members of the church, placing them unwittingly in positions of emotional and physical vulnerability. The very appeal of a church like Watoto is also what makes it dangerous.

Concluding reflections

The commonly cited 'do's and don'ts' and talk about 'good' and 'bad' people invoke and are implicated in discourses about morality and respectability, particularly with reference to sexuality and disease. Public moral credibility and a concern with public moral conduct are extremely important within Ugandan society – historically located within discourses about honour and currently exacerbated by particular state and religious leadership. Yet by examining the social values associated with the 'morality' invoked by these complex debates, we can better understand the tendencies for born-again Christians to employ discretion and secrecy about such behaviour around peer group members. Doing so positions the born-agains within wider social discourses which inform concepts of 'good' and 'bad', invoked within national HIV prevention dialogues in Uganda, and demonstrates the links between such concepts and social status. Exploring status concerns places the born-agains within networks of socio-economic activity, in which 'respectability', informed by concerns with 'moral character' and 'good' and 'bad', carries weight (Iliffe 2005: 5). This better explains the importance of discretion in what Iliffe calls a 'face to face' society within which people are watching each other and reputation can impact upon status and future opportunities in both economic and other ways.

The demands of the social discourses to which born-again Christians pay accountability are dissonant. There are points at which overarching notions of what constitutes 'respectable' behaviour conflict with aspects of Watoto's ideology; where what constitutes 'good' behaviour within Watoto's discourse contradicts that of the overarching Ugandan discourse on morality and respectability. With regard to sexual behaviour, the sanctioning of discretion as part of Kiganda moral behaviour contradicts Watoto's emphasis on being 'honest and truthful'. It was deemed by respondents more respectable not to 'call a spade a spade' or to shame social others by confronting them with information that might offend or embarrass them.

Such findings require deeper thinking about the ways in which societies produce – and transnationally export – particular kinds of ethical framework. Mbiti's distinction between static and dynamic ethics is extremely helpful in understanding the tensions between corporate and individual interests in Ugandan society, how the management of such tensions relies on and produces moral strategies of concealment, and how such moral strategies and ethical systems are antagonised by and antagonise many of the transnational morality discourses that abound within Kampala. Mbiti distinguishes between a morality of conduct and a morality of being. A morality of conduct, Mbiti argued,

> is what one might call 'dynamic ethics' rather than 'static ethics' for it defines what a person does, rather than what he is. [Therefore within such a conceptualisation], a person is what he is because of what he does rather than he does what he does because of what he is.
>
> (1969: 279)

Such understandings can be contrasted with Kantian ways of conceptualising the relationship between the individual and society, highly influential in Western ethical thinking, in which:

> Morality is conceived of as an individual, even private affair between a person and his conscience. [. . .] This has meant assuming that our ability to live moral lives is only affected by the strengths of our individual determinations and moral will, not by the organisation of social life.
>
> (Seidler 1986: 9)

It is at moments of moral collision that tensions emerge for young people in Uganda – as moral discourses premised on differing constructions of selfhood, and ethics meet. In such meetings, discretion and concealment, necessitated by social pressures to be a 'respectable', 'good' person, represent highly moral solutions to negotiating such profound disjunctures. For the researcher seeking to understand sexual and religious behaviour alike within such a context, the challenge is to start by recognising the folly of what is *said* by paying attention to the social roles that talk about behaviour plays. It is only by moving beyond moral discourses to really engage with how social contexts produce discursive performances that we can hope to reach better understanding about the impact of transnational influences on the moral landscapes and behaviours of young Ugandans.

References

Ahlberg, B.M. 1994. 'Is there a distinct African sexuality? A critical response to Caldwell *et al.*', *Africa* 64(2): 220–42.

Chan, K.Y. and D.D. Reidpath. 2003. '"Typhoid Mary" and "HIV Jane": responsibility, agency and disease prevention', *Reproductive Health Matters* 11(2): 40–50.

Davis, P.J. 2001. 'On the sexuality of "town women" in Kampala', *Africa Today* 48(3): 29–60.

Epstein, H. 2005. 'God and the fight against AIDS', *New York Review of Books* 52(7): 47–51.

Gusman, A. 2009. 'HIV/AIDS, Pentecostal churches, and the 'Joseph Generation' in Uganda', *Africa Today* 56(1): 67–86.

Haram, L. 2005. '"Eyes have no curtains": the moral economy of secrecy in managing love affairs among adolescents in northern Tanzania in the time of AIDS', *Africa Today* 51(4): 57–73.

Heald, S. 1995. 'The power of sex: reflections on the Caldwell's "African sexuality" thesis', *Africa* 65(4): 489–505.

Cohen, J. and T. Tate. 2005. 'The less they know the better: abstinence only HIV/AIDS programmes in Uganda', *Human Rights Watch*, 17(4).

Iliffe, J. 2005. *Honour in African History*, vol. 107. Cambridge: Cambridge University Press.

Iliffe, J. 2006. *The African AIDS Epidemic: A History*. Oxford: James Currey.

Jassey, K. and S. Nyanzi, 2007. 'How to be a "proper" woman in the time of AIDS', *Current Africa Issues* 34, Nordiska Afrikainstitutet, Uppsala, 11.

Kinsman, J., S. Nyanzi and R. Pool. 2000. 'Socialising influences and the value of sex: the experience of adolescent school girls in rural Masaka, Uganda', *Culture, Health and Sexuality* 2(2): 151–66.

Lindisfarne, N. 1994. 'Variant masculinities, variant virginities, rethinking honour and shame', in A. Cornwall and N. Lindisfarne (eds), *Dislocating Masculinity: Comparative Ethnographies*, London: Routledge, 82–96.

Mbiti, J. 1969. *African Religions and Philosophy*. Nairobi: East African Educational Publishers Ltd.

Mills, D. and R. Ssewakiriyanga. 2005. 'No romance without finance: commodities, masculinities and relationships amongst Kampalan students', in A. Cornwall (ed.), *Readings in Gender in Africa*. Oxford: James Currey, 90–4.

Parikh, S. 2005. 'From auntie to disco: the bifurcation of risk and pleasure in sex education in Uganda', in V. Adams and S.L. Pigg (eds), *Sex in Development: Science, Sex and Morality in Global Perspective*. London: Duke University Press, 125–58.

Putzel, J. 2004. 'The politics of action on AIDS: a case study of Uganda', *Public Administration and Development* 24(1): 19–30.

Sadgrove, J. 2007. '"Keeping up appearances": sex and religion amongst university students in Uganda', *Journal of Religion in Africa* 37(1): 116–44.

Sadgrove, J., R.M. Vanderbeck, J. Andersson, G. Valentine and K. Ward. 2012. 'Morality plays and money matters: towards a situated understanding of the politics of homosexuality in Uganda', *Journal of Modern African Studies* 50(1): 103–29.

Seidler, V. 1986. *Kant, Respect and Injustice: The Limits of Liberal Modern Theory*. London: Routledge.

Setel, P. 1999. *A Plague of Paradoxes: AIDS, Culture and Demography in Northern Tanzania*. Chicago: University of Chicago Press.

Smith, D.J. 2000. '"These girls today na war-o": premarital sexuality and modern identity in southeastern Nigeria', *Africa Today* 48(3): 99–120.

Standing, H. and M.N. Kisekka. 1976. *Sexual Behaviour in Sub-Saharan Africa: A Review and Annotated Bibliography*. London: Overseas Development Administration.

Susser, I. 2009. *AIDS, Sex, and Culture: Global Politics and Survival in Southern Africa*. Oxford: Wiley-Blackwell.

Part 2

TRANSNATIONAL POWER AND LOCAL AGENCY

6

Transnational Religious Networks Encounter Community Realities

HIV Prevention in Zambia[1]

AMY S. PATTERSON

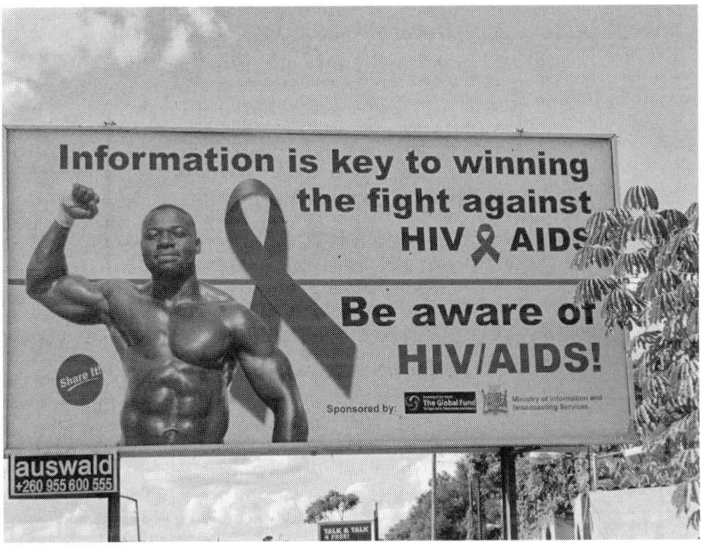

AIDS education poster along major thoroughfare in Lusaka, Zambia, 2011 (photo by author).

[1] Funding for this research was provided by the US Fulbright Africa Scholars Program, 2011. An earlier version of this chapter was presented at the conference of the Fertility and Reproduction Studies Group and the International Research Network on AIDS and Religion in Africa, Oxford, 28–30 September 2011. I am grateful for helpful comments from Ben Jones and the volume editors.

In 2003, US President George W. Bush announced the President's Emergency Plan for AIDS Relief (PEPFAR), which provided roughly $15 billion for HIV/AIDS programmes, primarily for sub-Saharan Africa. In its prevention efforts, it emphasised sexual abstinence and relationship fidelity (or 'Be Faithful') (hereafter referred to as AB). International faith-based organisations (FBOs) such as World Vision, Samaritan's Purse, Compassion International, and Catholic Relief Services that receive grants from PEPFAR have emphasised these AB messages as part of their HIV/AIDS programmes in Africa. Yet scholars know little about how these messages have been implemented in African communities. This chapter investigates that dynamic, by examining how pastors, community HIV/AIDS workers, and local populations in poor, urban communities in Zambia, a country with an HIV prevalence of roughly 14 per cent, have incorporated the AB message into their HIV/AIDS responses (Ministry of Health, National AIDS Council and UNAIDS 2011).[2] This chapter argues that there is a gap between PEPFAR's emphasis on AB prevention messages and the actual HIV prevention activities in Zambia's poorest communities. The work asserts that this 'AB disconnect' reflects the complexity of transnational governmentality and it is shaped by the extraversion strategies of African actors.

The examination of the AB disconnect in Zambia has both theoretical and policy relevance. On the theoretical side, the chapter elucidates the complicated relationship between donors and local partners. The conventional wisdom is that donors dictate policies to local partners, who implement such policies because they depend on external actors for their survival.[3] Yet, relations between external actors and local players are dynamic, and African partners are not always passive recipients. They may reinterpret externally derived policies within social contexts, emphasising new elements and downplaying others. The chapter provides a picture of the complexity and fluidity in such relations. Such a nuanced understanding also has the potential to contribute to richer, more effective policies that take into account cultural, economic and political dynamics and that acknowledge the ways that local actors utilise their dependence on external ties to gain resources and power.

The argument proceeds in the following five sections. First, I describe my methodology. Second, I highlight two theoretical concepts that inform the work: transnational governmentality (Ferguson and Gupta 2002) and extraversion (Bayart 1993, 2000). Third, I examine the role of transnational FBOs in HIV/AIDS policy making, particularly the formulation of PEPFAR's AB requirements. I argue that these requirements reflect Western ideals of individual agency and rationality as well as evangelical Christian beliefs that religious conversion can lead to moral behaviour that will alleviate social problems. I also assert that transnational

[2] To be clear, my interest in this issue does not revolve around the effectiveness of the AB strategy to limit HIV transmission or the individual-level decision to practise abstinence or fidelity.
[3] Interview, Zambian church HIV/AIDS coordinator, Lusaka, 16 August 2007.

governmentality has emerged in the HIV/AIDS field, with Western donors channelling money to local partners for policy implementation. Fourth, I examine reasons that AB messages are not fully embraced at the grassroots level in Zambia. In doing so, I demonstrate how extraversion, transnational governmentality, and Zambians' disillusionment with development explain gaps in implementation. Finally, the conclusion returns to the two theoretical concepts to raise questions for future research.

Methodology

In order to analyse the multiple layers of transnational governmentality that shape the AB disconnect, I investigate the views of transnational actors, Zambian agents who acted as intermediaries between transnational and local organisations, and grassroots organisations. For the transnational perspective, I interviewed FBO representatives and policy makers in Zambia and the United States during 2005, 2007 and 2011, and I examined documents and websites for several transnational FBOs. Interview questions sought to discern FBO participation in HIV/AIDS efforts, relations between FBOs and local partners, and support for and implementation of AB prevention messages. I also conducted roughly fifty interviews during 2007 and 2011 with such intermediary agents as Zambian pastors, HIV/AIDS educators, clinic officers, HIV/AIDS counsellors, and FBO officers. All of these individuals have some training on HIV/AIDS, and they interacted with representatives of transnational FBOs more directly than local community members did.

At the local level, I conducted focus group discussions with over fifty church-based and secular HIV/AIDS support groups in urban Zambia in 2011. Church groups were linked to mainline and Pentecostal Protestant churches, while secular groups were affiliated with the Network of Zambian People Living with HIV (NZP+). I include both church and secular groups because their community programmes are similar and because secular groups also tend to stress Christian messages (Patterson 2011b). This research concentrated on urban areas because donors in Zambia have focused their HIV/AIDS efforts in the cities, and because the urban HIV rate (20 per cent) is twice as high as the rural HIV rate (Ministry of Health, National AIDS Council and UNAIDS 2011). Many of these support groups are composed solely of people living with HIV (PLHIVs), though church-based groups often include HIV-negative members such as caregivers. Because research has demonstrated that small group discussions about HIV have more effect on behaviour change than larger media campaigns (Li *et al.* 2009), donors have increasingly turned to groups of PLHIVs to spread prevention messages through 'prevention with positives' programmes (Ministry of Health, National AIDS Council and UNAIDS 2011). Focus group discussions examined the tangible and intangible benefits of group membership, group activities, relations with donors, and group challenges. All interviewees were assured that their names would not be included in any written documents.

Transnational governmentality and opportunities for extraversion

Neoliberalism has transformed governmentality (or the multiple ways that human conduct is overseen), so that the state has ceded large areas of social policy to other actors including local organisations (such as churches and community-based organisations) and transnational actors (such as transnational FBOs) (van de Walle 2001; Ferguson and Gupta 2002). In this process, transnational actors and local organisations become partners in the development enterprise. Yet, the nature of these partnerships is complicated: on one hand, they reflect inequalities and hierarchies since the transnational organisation often has financial resources that the partner in the global South wants and/or needs. On the other hand, local organisations often have a degree of autonomy because they provide manpower, an entrée into the community, and broader legitimacy for the external partners. In so doing, they validate local participation in the broader development enterprise (Ellis 2011).

Local actors also may have autonomy in this partnership because transnational governmentality is administered through multiple levels of organisational command (Ferguson 1990). This long chain provides opportunities for players at any level to reinterpret policies and to emphasise some aspects of programmes over others. Multi-billion dollar programmes such as PEPFAR become 'large, unsupervised spaces' in which local groups can insert their own understandings of problems and solutions.[4] For example, World Vision, a Christian relief and development organisation that employs roughly 22,000 people worldwide and has an annual budget of almost $1 billion, receives multi-million dollar grants for HIV/AIDS programmes from the US government. Grants are channelled from the international headquarters in the United States to particular countries (such as Zambia), where local staff members then select Zambian FBOs with whom to work. These FBOs, in turn, often partner with churches in rural villages or urban communities (Varsalona 2008). Despite the fact that World Vision International may have specific objectives when it applies for PEPFAR funding, by the time PEPFAR money trickles down to the community level, those programme goals may change or become more nuanced.[5]

Transnational governmentality heightens the opportunity for local African partners to engage in the strategy of extraversion, or playing up the continent's

[4] I am grateful to Ben Jones for this point and for sharing this phrase.
[5] Interview, US HIV/AIDS policy maker, Washington, DC, 15 April 2005.

poverty and dependence to mobilise resources. In the case of HIV/AIDS, the external environment provides many financial opportunities since donors dispersed \$6.9 billion in HIV/AIDS money in 2011 (PBS 2011).[6] Access to these funds brings local actors opportunities for capacity building, workshop participation, income-generating projects, and sometimes, employment. As HIV/AIDS programme funding has increased, local partners have emphasised the disease at the expense of other development problems (Morfit 2011).

Three aspects of the extraversion concept are relevant in this context of high levels of funding for HIV/AIDS. First, as local actors 'skilfully exploit' their situations of dependence, they may use different types of rhetoric to appeal to Western audiences (Bayart 1993: 25–6). For example, they may emphasise the neoliberal assumption that markets will eradicate poverty and empower individuals: 'We need markets for our goods, markets with people like you.'[7] Or they may focus on religious rhetoric, including conservative views of sexuality or examples of spiritual devotion (Patterson 2011a). Such messages appeal to American evangelical churches, which have increasingly been involved in health and development issues in Africa (Hearn 2002).

Second, extraversion demonstrates the autonomy of African players in transnational governmentality. Local actors' framing of issues or their use of particular rhetoric demonstrates their conscious engagement with the external environment. African actors are not victims, despite the continent's relatively weak position in global economic and political structures. African players may even contribute to the design of institutions that advance their dependence. For example, several African experts on HIV/AIDS and African pastors gave the Bush administration input on the PEPFAR proposal, with a few African pastors, American conservatives, and some FBOs urging an emphasis on abstinence even as public health experts doubted the evidence that abstinence alone can lower HIV prevalence.[8] Many of these African participants then benefited from PEPFAR since their organisations received funding.

Third, extraversion becomes a resource some, though not all, African players can use to centralise their power and accumulate resources (Bayart 1993: 21–4). Through extraversion, relations between the West and Africa become privatised, benefiting select groups instead of the public good (Bayart 2000). Actors with access to external resources may rise in status, wealth, and political voice. Two Zambian organisations provide examples. First, the Churches Health Association of Zambia (CHAZ) had received roughly \$120 million by 2011 for its HIV-related

[6] Despite this amount, many experts on HIV/AIDS do not think global funding for the disease is adequate (UNAIDS 2011).

[7] Interview, HIV/AIDS clinic support group, Lusaka, 9 April 2011.

[8] Interview, Zambian pastor, Lusaka, 14 August 2007; interview, Zambian pastor, Lusaka, 17 February 2011.

programmes from the Global Fund to Fight AIDS, Tuberculosis and Malaria (Global Fund 2011),[9] resources that helped to increase CHAZ's voice in health policy making. Second, the Northmead Assembly of God and the Gospel Outreach Ministries (Go Centre), two Pentecostal mega-churches in Zambia, started antiretroviral treatment (ART) and HIV testing centres through PEPFAR grants. External connections with World Vision also led pastors of these two Pentecostal organisations to found the Expanded Church Response Trust, which also gained PEPFAR funding in 2008. Partly as a result of these activities, the pastor of the Northmead church was named chair of the National AIDS Council (Patterson 2011a). External connections increased opportunities for greater resources and representation, though not for all local organisations.

The local organisations examined in this chapter have little direct control over the HIV/AIDS policies or structures of donor governments or transnational FBOs. Yet because of the open spaces embedded in transnational governmentality, local players can interpret HIV prevention in ways that may differ from external partners. At times, their engagement with the larger HIV/AIDS discourse looks like weakness, while at other times, they appear to resist the narrow AB focus of PEPFAR. Yet, unlike the hidden transcripts of resistance that James Scott (1990) analyses, these actions do not appear to challenge the hegemonic structures of donor-financed HIV/AIDS programmes. Because these structures have the potential to bring power and financial resources, local actors often find ways to work within their confines.

Transnational governmentality and the AB message

PEPFAR reflects the multiple layers of transnational governmentality: it was developed by a relatively small number of actors within the White House, National Institutes of Health, the US Senate, and select evangelical Christian organisations, and its funds have been dispersed to a wide variety of US government bureaucracies, non-governmental organisations (NGOs), FBOs, and select African ministries of health. These FBOs, NGOs and US bureaucracies, in turn, channel money to local African organisations. This section analyses the official AB policy at two of these levels – the policy-making level and the highest level of implementation.

By the new millennium, evangelical Christians in the United States had become an increasingly vocal constituency on foreign policy issues such as human trafficking and debt relief, though their influence on foreign policy is often overstated (Hertzke 2004; Wuthnow 2009; see also Obbo, Chapter 2, and Schoepf, Chapter 3, this volume). FBOs such as World Vision, Catholic Relief Services and Christian

[9] CHAZ received roughly the same amount for malaria and tuberculosis programmes.

World Service, with long histories in development, lobbied for PEPFAR's passage, and they were joined by FBOs with more recent interest in development which sought greater access to government grants (den Dulk and Rozell 2011). The PEPFAR final legislation allocated 55 per cent of funds to treatment, 15 per cent to care and support of PLHIVs, 10 per cent to programmes for orphans and vulnerable children (OVCs), and 20 per cent to HIV prevention. Lobbying by FBOs and evangelical advocacy groups led to the requirement that 33 per cent of this prevention money be used for AB messages (Patterson 2006). Because mother-to-child transmission, blood safety, and safe medical use programmes are also included in prevention, programmes to stop sexual transmission of HIV received roughly 50 per cent of all prevention money. In 2005, PEPFAR recipient country teams spent 66 per cent of their sexual transmission prevention funds on AB activities, with the remaining sexual transmission funds going for HIV testing and condom distribution (Dietrich 2007). When the US Congress re-authorised PEPFAR in 2008, it changed the requirement so that 50 per cent of funding for prevention of sexual transmission of HIV must be spent on AB programmes in countries with generalised epidemics. The 2008 law continues to emphasise AB programmes, to restrict condom distribution to individuals 15 years of age and older, and to require that programmes that discuss condom use also discuss AB. In contrast, programmes that focus on A or B do not have to include discussion of condoms (Dietrich 2007; CHANGE 2011).

Three assumptions helped mobilise American evangelical Christians to support PEPFAR. First, Africans living with HIV/AIDS were often perceived to be innocent victims. This picture contrasted with the religious condemnation that PLHIVs in the United States (who were primarily gay men and intravenous drug users) experienced during the 1980s (Beckley and Koch 2002). Because most HIV infections in Africa resulted from heterosexual relations and mother-to-child transmission and because women make up the majority of HIV-positive Africans, evangelicals felt more comfortable addressing HIV/AIDS in Africa than in the United States (*Christianity Today*, 1 February 2006). As a result, FBO programmes often focused on women who were presumed to have been infected by promiscuous husbands and children who were infected *in utero*, during labour, or through breastfeeding. The 'Be Faithful' message emerged from this belief that innocent women (and their children) must be protected from philandering partners.

Second, evangelicals perceived fighting HIV/AIDS to include more than technical public health solutions such as increased HIV testing or condom distribution. Rather, they believed that the spread of the gospel should accompany technical solutions; they thought that religious adherents with sufficient faith and church support would change their sexual behaviour to limit HIV transmission. According to this view, youth should be urged to abstain from pre-marital sex, and they should receive support for such actions through church youth groups or abstinence clubs. Instead of condom distribution, HIV prevention programmes should stress the sacredness of marital fidelity and the need for holiness in sexual decisions. For conservative American evangelicals, condom use in pre-marital and extra-marital relations defeated God's plan for monogamy in marriage (Dobson 2000). Condoms were seen as a sign of spiritual defeat to worldly pressures.[10]

A video available during autumn 2011 on the website of Samaritan's Purse, a transnational FBO based in the United States, illustrates this link between spiritual salvation and HIV prevention. It begins with the statement that 40 per cent of Ugandan women are HIV-positive, with most being infected by their husbands. It then tells the story of a husband who drinks too much beer and beats his wife, but quits this behaviour when both he and his wife become 'born again' in Christ. Religious conversion gives the husband the strength to abstain from sex outside of marriage, to quit abusing his wife, and to limit his drinking (Samaritan's Purse 2008). In so doing, he does not bring HIV into the marriage.

Third, evangelicals tended to situate HIV/AIDS in the context of a highly personalised faith which revolves around the individual's relationship with Christ. Because of this focus on individualism, American evangelicals have paid limited attention to the socio-economic structures that can condition individual behaviour and limit personal autonomy (Emerson and Smith 2000; Rah 2009). One result is the belief that people can utilise information to measure the physical, emotional and spiritual ramifications of their actions. In the context of HIV/AIDS, this would mean that individuals avoid sex before marriage, sex with older partners, sex with multiple partners, and/or sex with sex workers because these actions increase the risk of HIV infection (Fenio 2009). The perspective does not emphasise the cultural or socio-economic factors that might push people to engage in such risky behaviour.

Once the AB requirement was written into PEPFAR, transnational FBOs crafted programmes to meet this policy. To be clear, not all FBOs adopted a strict AB focus. For example, the ecumenical World Council of Churches (2006) states:

> Successful HIV prevention programmes utilise all approaches known to be effective, not implementing one or a few select actions in isolation. These include promoting sexual abstinence, fidelity among married couples and the use of condoms for those who are not in a position to abstain or be faithful.

However, because PEPFAR favoured AB messages, many health and development NGOs and FBOs either had to adopt those messages or face challenges in gaining US funding. Transnational FBOs specialised in AB programmes, with 88 per cent of funding for FBOs in 2005 going specifically for AB efforts (Oomman *et al.* 2008). Four examples provide evidence of the AB focus among transnational FBOs:

- Samaritan's Purse, a relief and development organisation that started in 1970 and has been led by Billy Graham's son Frank Graham since 1978, holds

[10] Interview, transnational FBO representative, Washington, DC, 18 March 2005.

'workshop sessions based on Biblical principles with practical topics such as: HIV/AIDS basic facts, marital faithfulness, home care programmes, reducing discrimination, and overcoming the fear of testing' (Samaritan's Purse 2011).

- Serving in Mission, a century-old organisation of evangelical missionaries which works in twenty-seven African countries, trains peer educators in several African countries (including Zambia) to lead 'Life Skills' courses that emphasise abstinence in schools. The goal of these courses is for 'young people [to] hear from other young people how to live in a wise and Godly way' (Serving in Mission 2011; see also Cooper 2006).
- World Vision, which received $8.5 million for its work in Zambia between 2004 and 2008, stresses abstinence education. In 2005, World Vision Zambia trained thirty FBOs to run abstinence-only programmes, and it reached over 25,000 youth with these messages. With its 10- to 14-year-old participants, it talks about the importance of future faithfulness in marriage, while it gives general AB messages to participants in the 15- to 24-year-old group (Varsalona 2008).[11]
- The True Love Waits campaign promotes AB in conjunction with Christian conversion in several southern African countries. From 2007 to 2011, 'More than 1.6 million young people in Africa heard the True Love Waits message promoting sexual abstinence until marriage [. . .] nearly 46,000 married adults have committed to faithfulness, and more than 41,600 [individuals decided] to follow Jesus Christ' (True Love Waits International 2011).

Transnational FBOs either developed or increased their AB programming in response to PEPFAR's AB policies. But transnational governmentality provides multiple layers for policy implementation and local actors can utilise those layers as sites of extraversion. I turn now to the Zambia case to investigate this possibility.

The reality of AB messages in Zambia

Zambia provides a context with multiple opportunities for religiously based strategies of extraversion, because of its large Christian majority and its access to high levels of HIV/AIDS funding. Eighty-five per cent of Zambians are Christian (Ranger 2008), and church organisations have considerable sway in society and politics.[12] As evidence of the institutional capacity of church-based health institutions, Zambia was the first country to designate a non-state actor to be a principal recipient of Global Fund money (CHAZ was the organisation) (Patterson 2011a). Many Zambian FBOs are linked to transnational FBOs, and the country

[11] Even though World Vision stressed AB messages in Zambia, it has engaged in condom education and distribution with at-risk groups in Vietnam (Varsalona 2008).
[12] Interview, World Council of Churches official, Lusaka, 7 August 2007.

hosts a large number of transnational FBOs.[13] Finally, because of Zambia's high HIV rate, the country has received large sums of external HIV/AIDS funding. As of 2006, donors funded approximately 77 per cent of the country's HIV/AIDS response. Between 2003 and 2010, the country received thirteen HIV-related grants from the Global Fund and almost $1 billion from PEPFAR (Patterson and Stephens 2012).

HIV/AIDS programmes in Zambia are set within a context of a forty-year decline in the country's development and the stark rise in urban poverty, economic factors that push local agents to reach for external connections to survive. Upon its independence in 1964, Zambia was a highly urbanised country with modern mining towns in the Copperbelt and industrial jobs that paid good wages. State officials, external policy makers, and citizens touted what James Ferguson (1999) terms the 'myth of modernisation', or the optimistic expectation that the country would inevitably reach urban, modern life within a generation. Yet, between 1974 and 1990, the country's economy shrank 50 per cent because of declining copper prices and high external debt. Privatisation, cuts in state employment, and austerity measures exacerbated poverty, so that 64 per cent of Zambians lived in poverty by 2009 (Ferguson 1999: 10; UNDP 2011). Despite the country's economic growth in the new millennium, urban poverty remains extremely high. By 2004, 70 per cent of the Lusaka population lived in shanty compounds and 70 per cent worked in the informal sector. For urban residents, the monthly cost of food was more than double the average monthly household income (Resnick 2011).

Given the country's embeddedness in HIV/AIDS transnational governmentality and its work with a large number of American FBOs, one can certainly find evidence that AB messages are taught in Zambia. For example, the STEPS-OVC programme aims to provide HIV prevention information and behaviour change skills to 80,000 HIV-negative and HIV-positive people in Zambia.[14] One way the programme does this is by training parents and youth to discuss sex openly together and by urging churches to facilitate these discussions.[15] Yet such examples seemed unusual in community-level HIV/AIDS programmes. Below I first provide evidence from the focus groups, intermediary informants, empirical cases, and written reports for this lack of attention to AB messages. While the evidence is not comprehensive, it is from a wide variety of sources and it demonstrates a pattern. Then I analyse

[13] These organisations include International Justice Mission, Alliance for Children Everywhere, Christian Reformed World Relief Committee, Serving in Mission, Adventist Development and Relief Agency, Baptist Mission, Catholic Relief Services, and World Vision International.

[14] STEPS-OVC stands for Sustainability through Economic Strengthening, Prevention and Support for Orphans and Vulnerable Children, Youth and Other Vulnerable Populations. It is a consortium of seven NGOs, four of which are the FBOs Expanded Church Response, Salvation Army, World Vision, and Catholic Relief Services.

[15] Interview, Pentecostal church HIV/AIDS volunteer, Kitwe, 20 May 2011.

four reasons for this disconnect, situating my explanations in the context of transnational governmentality, extraversion, and Zambians' disillusionment with development.

The limited focus on AB messages at the community level

When questioned about their HIV/AIDS activities in the community, groups of PLHIVs rarely emphasised prevention of any type. Instead, members of both church-based and secular groups commented that they 'go into the community to sensitise people'.[16] Loosely defined, sensitisation included making people aware that HIV/AIDS is dangerous, discouraging community members from discriminating against PLHIVs, conducting voluntary counselling and testing (VCT), and approaching neighbours who appeared to be sick to urge them to get an HIV test.[17] In all the groups I interviewed, no one specifically mentioned AB messages as part of these community sensitisation efforts. Church-based groups were less likely to refer to any type of HIV sensitisation and more likely to emphasise home-based care programmes for PLHIVs and OVCs than secular groups were.

Many pastors, church HIV/AIDS workers, and clinic counsellors confirmed these observations. One Pentecostal pastor said that one of the biggest problems in addressing HIV/AIDS in Zambia is the silence around sex in religious communities and among highly educated individuals.[18] This silence limits discussion of AB messages. An HIV/AIDS programme director in a Pentecostal church bemoaned the fact that there is no discussion about sex in the churches or at home. As a result, youth were confused about how they should behave: 'No one wants to talk about sex with kids. It is against our cultural experiences. But we have to. It is the only way.'[19]

On the other hand, there were some pastors and officers at church-based clinics who discussed prevention of sexual transmission of HIV, though they did not always focus exclusively on AB messages. At times this led to contradictions within the same organisation. For example, one Pentecostal pastor said, 'We [the church] are about abstinence. While other places may talk about condoms, they [condoms] are not for us.'[20] Likewise, a counsellor at that same church's HIV/AIDS clinic emphasised the message of fidelity and sexual purity in a Christian devotion period with clinic clients.[21] Yet, another clinic counsellor admitted that she discusses

[16] Interview, NZP+ group, Lusaka, 22 March 2011; interview, NZP+ group, Lusaka, 23 March 2011; interview, Reformed Church group, Lusaka, 5 April 2011.
[17] Interview, NZP+ group, Lusaka, 12 April 2011.
[18] Interview, Pentecostal pastor, Ndola, 21 May 2011.
[19] Interview, Pentecostal church HIV/AIDS programme director, Kitwe, 20 May 2011.
[20] Interview, Pentecostal pastor, Lusaka, 17 August 2007.
[21] Observation by author, clinic devotions, Lusaka, 2 March 2011.

abstinence, fidelity, and condom use with clients who receive an HIV test, regardless of the outcome of the test.[22] And clinic social workers seemed pragmatic about how unequal power relations between Zambian men and women and the lack of individual agency among many poor Zambians made AB implementation difficult.[23]

Both extraversion and transnational governmentality can explain these contradictory messages. The pastor and counsellor may have emphasised AB in their interviews and public discussions because Western audiences most interested in church-based HIV/AIDS work might expect such an answer. Since this clinic receives numerous visitors from US churches, these public statements may not have been that unusual. To gain resources for their programmes, local actors may signal to their transnational partners that they share the external actor's perspective. For example, Zambian pastors often stressed that the country needed spiritual rebirth, a return to moral behaviour, and 'holiness'. HIV prevention through abstinence was just a small component of these larger messages.[24] Yet, the fact that HIV/AIDS policies are governed at multiple layers provided 'wiggle room' for local players such as the clinic staff to tailor prevention messages to their clients' situations.

Several churches that have HIV/AIDS programmes also seemed to downplay AB promotion. Many Zambian churches excelled in home-based care efforts: the Catholic diocese of Ndola alone served over 25,000 PLHIVs in 2009. But prevention messages were incorporated less frequently into many of these parish-level church HIV/AIDS programmes (Fikansa 2009). In another example, a Pentecostal church in Chingola had worked on OVC care programmes since 2002. With money from transnational FBOs, the church provided food, school fees, and mentoring help to over 400 OVCs in the area. Yet, the church had few formal programmes to discuss AB messages with these youth, as the following exchange between my informant and the pastor illustrates.

Informant: So, some of the children you have been taking care of for years are now to the point where they are interested in the opposite sex. What are you doing for them for prevention?

Pastor: We have a programme to teach them particularly about child abuse and HIV and AIDS. And their rights. Because there are some homes where you can find children being abused.[25]

[22] Interview, clinic counsellor, Lusaka, 18 March 2011.

[23] Interview, clinic social workers, Lusaka, 1 March 2011.

[24] Observations by author, Northmead Assembly of God, Lusaka, 12 June 2011, and Miracle Life Church, Lusaka, 13 March 2011. See also Ranger (2008) for more on morality themes among African evangelical churches.

[25] Observation by author, Pentecostal church meeting, Chingola, 21 May 2011.

The pastor defined HIV prevention primarily as prevention of child abuse, not as programmes that teach youth to abstain from pre-marital sex or to remain sexually faithful in their relationships. While child abuse is one means of HIV transmission (particularly between older men and adolescent girls), the pastor's answer did not acknowledge youth sexuality. The example illustrates how local actors who receive funding from transnational FBOs but who are distant from policy makers may interpret issues in ways more contextually relevant. In this case, the pastor's decision to focus on prevention of child abuse not youth sexuality may have been pragmatic and culturally situated because it did not necessitate difficult discussions about sex between youth and adults.

Public health officials, transnational FBOs, and academics working in Zambia also provide evidence that AB messages have not been fully embraced at the local level. The Ministry of Health, National AIDS Council and UNAIDS (2011: i) report that there was need in Zambia for greater attention to prevention messages, particularly those that address multiple and concurrent partners, transactional and inter-generational sex, and sex within discordant couples (these issues would partially be covered in AB messages). Along this vein, officials of transnational FBOs comment that the biggest challenge in addressing HIV/AIDS in Zambia is exposing people to prevention messages, and particularly youth to abstinence-only programmes.[26] Finally, an academic study of HIV/AIDS efforts in southern Zambia revealed that while organisations such as the Adventist Development and Relief Agency and the Catholic Church had official abstinence policies, they were not always 'successfully promoted'. And because there was a general resignation in society to the fact that men tend to have extra-marital affairs, fidelity messages gained little traction (Byron *et al.* 2006: 16).

While AB messages are apparent in the rhetoric and programmatic goals of transnational FBOs (many of whom have received large sums of PEPFAR money), there is a disconnect between these high-level objectives and community actions in urban Zambia. Often groups of HIV-positive people (who have been urged to act as HIV prevention ambassadors) do not focus on these messages, and church members are uncomfortable discussing sexuality, particularly with youth. I now turn to an analysis of why the AB messages supported by many transnational FBOs and their political advocates in Washington, DC have not been fully embraced at the local level.

[26] Interview, transnational FBO official, Lusaka, 15 August 2007; interview, expert on HIV/AIDS, Lusaka, 31 May 2011.

Analysing the low priority of AB messages at the community level

The first reason for the AB disconnect is the different definitions of prevention that transnational FBOs and local HIV/AIDS activists emphasised. Transnational FBOs (and their advocates in Washington, DC) stress prevention of sexual transmission of HIV through abstinence and fidelity. This view reflects transnational religious actors' focus on individual agency, Christian morality, and evangelism as tools to promote behaviour change.[27] In contrast, community HIV/AIDS workers in Zambia describe prevention as sharing information on the disease and encouraging HIV testing. Almost all Zambian groups stressed 'going into the community to urge HIV testing'.[28]

The country's incorporation into HIV/AIDS transnational governmentality helps explain why Zambians emphasise HIV testing in prevention. PEPFAR set specific goals for the number of individuals it aimed to put on ART medications by 2008. These goals gave donors an impetus to quickly enrol HIV-positive individuals in free ART programmes after 2004. To place people on ART, though, they needed to be tested. One community worker explained that donors used all types of incentives to urge people to get tested, to disclose their HIV status, and to join support groups (these incentives included free food supplements and income-generating projects for support groups). The process led community HIV/AIDS groups to emphasise HIV testing over other prevention messages.[29] During community meetings, HIV-positive individuals testified that ART had brought them back from the brink of death; they were now 'fit and fine looking'.[30] While inspirational, such stories drew attention away from AB strategies in HIV prevention to the promotion of HIV testing. Because the availability of ART meant that a positive HIV test was no longer a death sentence, some informants said Zambians had become complacent about HIV prevention.[31]

A perverse logic about HIV prevention emerged, illustrating how high-level policies can change grassroots dynamics and have unanticipated consequences. In terms of the AB message, because HIV testing (with a positive HIV test result) led to resources, community mobilisation has focused on prevention through testing not prevention of sexual transmission through abstinence, fidelity, or

[27] Most broadly, the term behaviour change is used to indicate any activities that prevent HIV infections. However, for religious groups involved with HIV prevention, behaviour change indicates not condom use, but abstinence and fidelity in relationships. Thus, when I refer to behaviour change in the context of these faith-based groups, I take their meaning.

[28] Interview, NZP+ group, Lusaka, 22 March 2011.

[29] Interview, NZP+ leader, Mumbwa, 15 April 2011.

[30] Interview, NZP+ group member, Kitwe, 19 May 2011.

[31] Interview, church HIV/AIDS expert, Lusaka, 31 May 2011; interview, clinic official, Lusaka, 7 June 2011.

condom use.[32] More broadly, if HIV-positive individuals can access food supplements, project monies, and free medical care, there is little incentive for poor individuals to embrace prevention messages at all. Thus, while the ART rollout had positive outcomes – by 2011, 70 per cent of HIV-positive Zambians who needed ART medications could access them and ART was readily available in urban areas – it meant the prevention discourse focused on testing not AB messages (Ministry of Health, National AIDS Council and UNAIDS 2011).[33]

Second, the AB discourse collided with the ways that Zambian PLHIVs frame their experiences with the HIV virus. Their descriptions challenged the Western public health model of public disclosure and the evangelical emphasis on spiritual rebirth and testimony. Western donors and HIV/AIDS activists have put a premium on HIV-positive individuals telling their stories, even to the point that those who publicly disclose can gain financially. These programmes emphasise disclosure of one's status and honesty about the risky sexual behaviour that led to infection (Nguyen 2010). Similarly, evangelical Christians often emphasise the role of conversion testimonies that describe how rebirth in Christ ends a life of sin (Ranger 2008). AB programmes sponsored by transnational, evangelical FBOs often include opportunities for participants to testify about how Christ's forgiveness for their past actions had given them the strength to change their sexual behaviour. Such models of public disclosure faced challenges in Zambia.

In one sense, Zambian PLHIVs were quite detailed about their lives with HIV. They described their illnesses, physical reactions to ART medications, and their experiences with stigma and discrimination.[34] But their stories of HIV infection often showed their lack of autonomy and/or downplayed personal responsibility. Some PLHIVs had no power over the actions that led to their HIV infection: they had experienced rape, spousal abuse, gender-based violence, child abuse, and unequal economic situations that made them reliant on abusive partners. These were all situations in which individuals lacked autonomy, regardless of their personal desire for sexual morality or their Christian faith (Siplon and Novotny 2007). Thus messages that emphasised choice or responsibility in sexual behaviour did not resonate with these individuals, and these PLHIVs did not emphasise such themes when they discussed HIV prevention.

Other PLHIVs with the financial resources and education to give them some autonomy did not emphasise responsibility. They did not talk about how their sexual behaviour (such as multiple partners, sex before marriage, and/or sex without a condom with a non-regular partner) may have contributed to their HIV infection.

[32] This logic in mobilisation has also led groups of HIV-negative individuals to lie about their serostatus in order to access resources. Interview, NZP+ coordinator, Ndola, 23 May 2011.

[33] Interview, transnational NGO official, Lusaka, 8 June 2011.

[34] Interview, member of NZP+ group, Lusaka, 23 March 2011; interview, member of church HIV/AIDS group, Lusaka, 11 April 2011.

For example, a spokeswoman for a church-related home-based care programme explained that she 'could have been born with it [the HIV virus]'.[35] While biologically possible, the woman's age (she was roughly 60 years old) made this seem unlikely. A pastor in a mainline church described 'turning from a past life' after his HIV test, though he was never explicit about what his past life entailed.[36]

The unwillingness to engage in public disclosure and provide testimony on one's HIV transmission is culturally situated, since Zambians sought to preserve status hierarchies and maintain community and family ties (Nguyen 2010). For example, one middle-class, educated HIV-positive woman explained that some women she knew could never disclose their sero-status publicly because poor Zambians would then look at them with disdain.[37] Silence helped to preserve their position in society. Disclosure also brought potential negative ramifications for family relations: one NZP+ activist explained that when he publicly disclosed his HIV status his family disowned him. He laughed when he explained that once he became an activist and had access to external donor resources and unique opportunities, his family welcomed him back.[38] If HIV disclosure is potentially destructive for family relationships, overt discussions of how one acquired HIV would be even more harmful (Nguyen 2010).

Because transnational governmentality provides layers for policy implementation, such culturally defined interpretations may emerge. Zambians used euphemisms to avoid direct discussions of sexual behaviour: sexual concurrency was described as 'playing' and one's 'past life' referred to past risky behaviours. While clear to Zambians, the meanings of these phrases could be obscure to Westerners.[39] Such murky terminology played a role in extraversion. It allowed local players to maintain access to external funding mechanisms while carefully framing sexual transmission of HIV in contextually relevant ways that downplayed the autonomy and personal responsibility themes embedded in AB messages. Many churches also participated in this vague discourse, mostly by limiting their discussion of sexual concurrency.[40] One highly educated HIV-positive woman said that churches 'were not doing enough' on the issue of 'playing'.[41] In doing so, these churches have ignored the fact that sexual concurrency is a major driver of Zambia's epidemic (Ministry of Health, National AIDS Council and UNAIDS 2011).

A third reason for the AB disconnect is that local players in HIV/AIDS transnational governmentality must respond to external processes in order to gain

[35] Interview, HIV-positive professional woman, Lusaka, 4 May 2011.

[36] Interview, Protestant pastor, Lusaka, 9 May 2011.

[37] Interview, HIV-positive professional woman, Lusaka, 10 May 2011.

[38] Interview, HIV/AIDS activist, Lusaka, 10 May 2011.

[39] Interview, expert on HIV/AIDS, Lusaka, 31 May 2011.

[40] Interview, Pentecostal pastor, Ndola, 21 May 2011; interview, Protestant HIV/AIDS coordinator, 10 May 2011; see also Chitando (2007).

[41] Interview, HIV-positive woman, Lusaka, 10 May 2011.

and/or maintain access to resources. Some of these processes have not focused on HIV prevention. While such responses may appear to illustrate the impotence of local players, the fact that these groups both observe external trends in development and respond to them shows a certain level of agency. Yet, these actions have consequences, as two examples illustrate. In the first, the Northmead Assembly of God in Lusaka developed HIV/AIDS programmes in the late 1990s, which included VCT, a support group for PLHIVs, a school for OVCs, and HIV/AIDS awareness programmes that emphasised abstinence. As the church gained international media attention, it was able to lobby for PEPFAR money to establish an ART clinic. By 2011, the clinic served over 2,000 clients (Northmead Assembly of God 2011). To conform to donor and state-mandated requirements, the clinic hired professional nurses, clinical officers, counsellors, data entry specialists, and a programme manager. Yet these overworked and underpaid staff members had little time for community-level mobilisation on prevention.[42] Also, the clinic-sponsored support group for PLHIVs concentrated its efforts on ART adherence messages and condom use among sero-discordant couples, not community-level AB prevention campaigns.[43] The consequence of tailoring programmes to donor funding opportunities was a decline in attention to HIV prevention and an increase in attention to treatment and adherence.

The second example shows how local organisations responded to the demand among transnational NGOs and FBOs for empowerment and sustainability in HIV/AIDS programming.[44] This trend emerged with PEPFAR's 2008 reauthorisation and the decline in global HIV/AIDS funding that was sparked by the global recession in 2008 (PBS 2011). The financial situation increased competition among local FBOs, NGOs and CBOs (community-based organisations) for global HIV/AIDS money and it necessitated that these groups distinguish themselves in order to gain the attention of transnational groups. In response, one Pentecostal church began a rotating credit society and savings association for church and community members. This effort did not specifically target PLHIVs, caregivers, or OVCs, and the church emphasised that income was important for both people with HIV and people vulnerable to HIV infection. It received financial assistance from a Zambian FBO that had received money from PEPFAR.[45] Even though it met PEPFAR's focus on sustainable programmes, the church did not concentrate on AB prevention messages.

[42] Interview, clinical officer, Lusaka, 18 May 2011.

[43] Observations by author, clinic group meetings, Lusaka, 12 March 2011, 31 March 2011 and 26 May 2011.

[44] Interview, transnational FBO official, Lusaka, 13 April 2011; interview, transnational FBO official, Lusaka, 31 March 2011.

[45] Interview, members of church HIV/AIDS group, Chingola, 20 May 2011.

Strategies of extraversion allowed these two Zambian churches to gain external resources, but these strategies may empower some local actors while disadvantaging others. In the case of the clinic, professionalisation meant that the HIV-positive church members who had initially mobilised to establish the clinic did not get jobs at the clinic. With time, a board of health and business professionals governed the clinic and represented the church's HIV/AIDS activities in the wider community. While extraversion brought resources, it empowered some Zambian professionals while it disempowered PLHIVs. Similarly, the ability of the Pentecostal church to get HIV/AIDS money for its rotating credit programme helped community members, though perhaps at the expense of using HIV/AIDS monies for people infected with or directly affected by the disease.

Finally, and perhaps most crucially, Zambians' disillusionment with development has undermined the AB message, since this prevention message has not addressed the major concerns of most HIV-positive individuals and their HIV-negative neighbours. The discourse on sexual morality, with its roots in evangelical understandings of individual behaviour, clashes with the reality of life for many Zambians. In all focus group meetings with people infected with or affected by HIV, participants mentioned a 'lack of food' as a common problem they faced (Patterson 2011b). Participants discussed how their lack of income meant they could not send their children to school or pay for housing. One man detailed how he moved from place to place after his house was destroyed in a windstorm.[46] Another father had no money to pay school fees and thus his son could not take the Grade 12 final exam for his high school diploma.[47] And I lost count of the number of people who told me both formally and informally that they had not eaten anything in the last twenty-four hours. For Zambians infected with and affected by HIV/AIDS, prevention activities of any type were often a secondary priority.

However, this priority ranking could change, if sharing HIV prevention messages meant greater opportunities for material resources. Some HIV-positive Zambians gained positions as peer educators at community clinics, where they shared their experiences with clients and community members and urged prevention (though not always through direct AB messages). In return they received small stipends from the transnational NGOs or FBOs that funded these programmes. One man described how capitalising on his HIV status brought personal empowerment:

> I started as a peer educator at a clinic, and then I was chosen to be an HIV counsellor. I was trained and did well. Then I eventually got this position as outreach coordinator for the NGO. I have a real job and am thinking of going to college now.[48]

[46] Interview, HIV-positive man, Kitwe, 19 May 2011.
[47] Interview, HIV-positive man, Lusaka, 8 March 2011.
[48] Interview, HIV/AIDS coordinator with transnational NGO, Lusaka, 8 June 2011.

Extraversion strategies are evident in the man's story: he utilised what outsiders often perceive to be a weakness (HIV positivity) as a resource to gain NGO employment. However, while it was possible for some PLHIVs to successfully use the extraversion strategy of sharing HIV prevention messages, the majority of PLHIVs (and their HIV-negative neighbours) did not consider HIV prevention efforts to be their biggest priority.

The rigid bureaucratic lines drawn in PEPFAR-funded programmes compounded this problem. For many transnational FBOs and NGOs, HIV prevention activities and economic support programmes for people infected with and affected by HIV are distinct. This delineation is evident in the separate coordinators, offices, and budget lines for each programme.[49] This outcome resulted from the political bargains needed to gain support for PEPFAR from American conservative lawmakers, who saw individual-level sexual behaviour as distinct from social structures and who were sceptical of foreign aid. PEPFAR is results-oriented, focused on short-term solutions such as distributing ART medications and exposing people to HIV prevention messages. PEPFAR officials have tended to view economic support programmes or food distribution for PLHIVs as short-term solutions, not sustainable programmes.[50] The fact that support, OVC care, prevention, and treatment all received distinct percentages of the PEPFAR budget solidified these divisions.

Yet, this policy delineation ignores how poverty can push individuals into sexual relations that make them vulnerable to HIV infection (Whiteside 2002). For example, abstinence-only education programmes for youth aged 14 to 24 may not acknowledge that many youth are already involved in sexual relationships that derive from their need to earn income. As one young HIV-positive woman argued, HIV infections are growing rapidly among youth in Zambia. This is partly because youth lack clear information about sexuality, and partly because youth seek economic opportunities, some of which may involve sexual relations with older men with income. In the informant's opinion, for AB messages to resonate among Zambian youth the messages needed to be coupled with income-generation opportunities.[51] This respondent did not distinguish between economic support and HIV prevention programmes. Because of the politically expedient programmatic divide in PEPFAR, HIV prevention efforts focused solely on sexual transmission often seemed irrelevant in poor Zambian communities.

In summary, through their different definitions of prevention, their indirect ways of discussing sexual responsibility, their response to new donor programme demands that drew attention from HIV prevention, and their emphasis on economic

[49] Interview, transnational NGO official, Lusaka, 5 May 2011; interview, Zambian FBO official, Lusaka, 31 March 2011; interview, transnational FBO official, Lusaka, 31 March 2011.
[50] Interview, transnational FBO official, Lusaka, 31 March 2011.
[51] Interview, NZP+ youth group member, Mumbwa, 15 April 2011.

support over AB messages, community HIV/AIDS groups sought to subtly shift the focus of externally designed prevention messages. In theory, local players did not disagree that sexual abstinence and marital fidelity were important prevention tools; rather, they just found these messages to be unrealistic or simplistic because they assumed socio-economic and cultural systems in which individuals have high levels of autonomy in their sexual choices. As one church HIV/AIDS worker explained: 'You just can't ask people to be perfect. They aren't saints.'[52]

Conclusion

This chapter has analysed the disjuncture between the AB prevention programmes supported by many transnational FBOs and funded by PEPFAR and the implementation of those programmes in urban Zambia. PEPFAR's requirement that a sizeable portion of money for the prevention of sexual transmission of HIV be spent on AB programmes gave transnational FBOs the opportunity to partner with local Zambian groups on AB efforts. While AB messages are conveyed in Zambia, they were noticeably absent among Zambian support groups for PLHIVs, groups that have increasingly been charged with prevention education. This AB disconnect results from different understandings of prevention, local groups' desire to develop non-prevention programmes to meet donor's demands, and the huge need for poverty reduction among many urban Zambians. AB models also faced challenges because of their assumption of personal responsibility in disclosure and autonomy in sexual choices. The multiple layers of policy implementation evident in a programme like PEPFAR created space for these nuanced interpretations.

The work raises two questions for future research. First, what are the conditions under which extraversion is most effective for gaining external financial support? Both secular and church-based support groups in Zambia stressed their poverty and dependence, and complained that they would be unable to continue their work without external funds. While most of these groups did lack capacity and resources, their emphasis on these themes highlighted their ability to play to Western assumptions, particularly the emphasis on charity-based development. Charity-based development is rooted in the idea that there is a hierarchy of deservedness, with women, children, and (often) HIV-positive people perceived to deserve more assistance than men, adults, or HIV-negative people (Siplon 2010). The expectation of Western charity was apparent when one HIV/AIDS group member said: 'If we just had a well-wisher from abroad to help us, we would be okay.'[53] How effective

[52] Interview, Protestant church HIV/AIDS worker, Lusaka, 25 February 2011.
[53] Interview, NZP+ women's group, Kitwe, 19 May 2011.

is such rhetoric for gaining external resources? This research has not investigated how Western partners perceive such extraversion strategies. Yet, if extraversion implies a relationship between the African actor and the external player, more research is needed on how outsiders perceive extraversion strategies, including the use of particular rhetoric and imagery.

Finally, what are the implications of the gap between policy requirements in development programmes such as PEPFAR and their local interpretations and implementation? From the theoretical perspective, this divide challenges the conventional wisdom that foreign aid policies are imposed on poor countries. Scholars need to better understand how transnational linkages influence not only the making of development policies, but also their interpretation and implementation. From a practical angle, does this policy gap create confusion in HIV/AIDS programming? And if so, what does that mean for local efforts to prevent HIV transmission? How might HIV prevention policies be changed so that local populations view them to be more culturally relevant or more responsive to the larger issues in their lives? This research demonstrates that HIV prevention policies that divorce poverty reduction from messages of sexual morality often do not resonate with poor urban Zambians. Because HIV prevention is essential to curb the HIV/AIDS epidemic in Africa, scholars and policy makers must pay greater attention to the disjuncture in official HIV prevention policies and their implementation on the ground.

References

Bayart, J. 1993. *The State in Africa: The Politics of the Belly*. London: Longman.

Bayart, J. 2000. 'Africa in the world: a history of extraversion', *African Affairs* 99: 217–67.

Beckley, R. and J. Koch. 2002. *The Continuing Challenge of AIDS*. Westport, CT: Auburn House.

Byron, E., S. Gillespie and P. Hamazakaza. 2006. 'Local perceptions of HIV risk and prevention in southern Zambia', Report for the International Food Policy Research Institute, Washington, DC.

CHANGE (Center for Health and Gender Equity). 2011. 'Abstinence and fidelity'. http://www.pepfarwatch.org/the_issues/abstinence_and_fidelity (accessed 22 August 2011).

Chitando, E. 2007. *Acting in Hope: African Churches and HIV/AIDS*. Geneva: World Council of Churches.

Cooper, B. 2006. *Evangelical Christians in the Muslim Sahel*. Bloomington: Indiana University Press.

den Dulk, K. and M. Rozell. 2011. 'George W. Bush, religion, and foreign policy: personal, global, and domestic contexts', *Review of Faith and International Affairs*, Winter: 71–82.

Dietrich, J. 2007. 'The politics of PEPFAR: the President's Emergency Plan for AIDS Relief', *Ethics and International Affairs* 21. http://www.carnegiecouncil.org/resources/journal/21_3/essay/001.html (accessed 24 August 2011).

Dobson, J. 2000. *The Complete Marriage and Family Home Reference Guide*. Carol Stream, IL: Tyndale House Publishers.

Ellis, S. 2011. *Season of Rains: Africa in the World*. Chicago: University of Chicago Press.

Emerson, M. and C. Smith. 2000. *Divided by Faith: Evangelical Religion and the Problem of Race in America*. New York: Oxford University Press.

Fenio, K. 2009. 'Between bedrooms and ballots: the politics of HIV's "economy of infection" in Mozambique'. Unpublished PhD thesis, University of Florida.

Ferguson, J. 1990. *The Anti-Politics Machine: 'Development', Depoliticization and Bureaucratic Power in Lesotho*. Cambridge: Cambridge University Press.

Ferguson, J. 1999. *Expectations of Modernity: Myths and Meanings of Urban Life on the Zambian Copperbelt*. Berkeley: University of California Press.

Ferguson, J. and A. Gupta. 2002. 'Spatializing states: toward an ethnography of neoliberal governmentality', *American Ethnologist* 29: 981–1002.

Fikansa, C. 2009. 'Reflections on the contradictions of ARVs from a practitioner perspective'. Paper presented at the Conference of the International Research Network on AIDS and Religion in Africa, Lusaka, Zambia, 15–17 April.

Global Fund. 2011. *Zambia: Grant Portfolio*. http://portfolio.theglobalfund.org/en/Grant/List/ZAM (accessed 17 August 2011).

Hearn, J. 2002. 'The invisible NGO: U.S. evangelical mission in Kenya', *Journal of Religion in Africa* 32: 32–60.

Hertzke, A. 2004. *Freeing God's Children: The Unlikely Alliance for Global Human Rights*. Lanham, MD: Rowman & Littlefield.

Li, L., M. Rotheram-Borus, Y. Lu, Z. Wu, C. Lin and J. Guan. 2009. 'Mass media and HIV/AIDS in China', *Journal of Health Communication* 14: 424–38.

Ministry of Health, National AIDS Council and UNAIDS. 2011. *Zambia Country Progress Report*. UNGASS 2010 Reporting. http://www.unaids.org/en/dataanalysis/monitoring countryprogress/2010progressreportssubmittedbycountries/zambia_2010_country_progress_report_en.pdf (accessed 30 May 2011).

Morfit, N.S. 2011. '"AIDS is money": how donor preferences reconfigure local realities', *World Development* 39: 64–76.

Nguyen, V.-K. 2010. *The Republic of Therapy: Triage and Sovereignty in West Africa's Time of AIDS*. Durham, NC: Duke University Press.

Northmead Assembly of God. 2011. 'Information'. http://www.northmeadassembly.org.zm (accessed 25 June 2011).

Oomman, N., M. Bernstein, S. Rosenzweig and J. Pearson. 2008. 'New PEPFAR data: the numbers behind the stories'. http://www.cgdev.org/files/15799_file_theNumbersBehind TheStories.pdf (accessed 30 May 2012).

Patterson, A. 2006. *The Politics of AIDS in Africa*. Boulder, CO: Lynne Rienner.

Patterson, A. 2011a. *The Church and AIDS in Africa: The Politics of Ambiguity*. Boulder, CO: First Forum Press.

Patterson, A. 2011b. 'Preliminary report of findings on support groups for people living with HIV and AIDS'. Report for Network of Zambian People Living with HIV/AIDS, Lusaka, Zambia.

Patterson, A. and D. Stephens. 2012. 'AIDS mobilisation in Zambia and Vietnam: explaining the differences', *Contemporary Politics* 18: 215–26.

PBS. 2011. 'Delivery of global AIDS funding drops 10 percent', *NewsHour*, 17 August. http://www.pbs.org/newshour/rundown/2011/08/delivery-of-global-aids-funding-down-10-percent.html (accessed 30 May 2012).

Rah, S.-C. 2009. *The Next Evangelicalism: Freeing the Church from Western Cultural Captivity*. Downers Grove, IL: IVP Press.

Ranger, T. (ed.) 2008. *Evangelical Christianity and Democracy in Africa*. New York: Oxford University Press.

Resnick, D. 2011. 'In the shadow of the city: Africa's urban poor in opposition strongholds', *Journal of Modern African Studies* 49: 141–66.

Samaritan's Purse. 2008. 'Beatrice's story', video clip. http://link.brightcove.com/services/player/bcpid (accessed 18 August 2011).

Samaritan's Purse. 2011. 'Samaritan's Purse HIV/AIDS education programs'. http://www.samaritanspurse.org/index.php/PFH/Our_Programs (accessed 22 August 2011).

Scott, J. 1990. *Domination and the Arts of Resistance: Hidden Transcripts*. New Haven, CT: Yale University Press.

Serving in Mission. 2011. 'Apple Project'. http://www.sim.org/index.php/project/94248 (accessed 21 August 2011).

Siplon, P. 2010. 'Can charity and rights-based movements be allies in the fight against HIV/AIDS? Bridging mobilizations in the United States and Sub-Saharan Africa'. Presentation at the Conference of the International Research Network on AIDS and Religion in Africa, Kampala, Uganda, 5–9 July.

Siplon, P. and K. Novotny. 2007. 'Overcoming the contradictions: women, autonomy and AIDS in Tanzania', in P. Harris and P. Siplon (eds), *The Global Politics of AIDS*. Boulder, CO: Lynne Rienner, 87–108.

True Love Waits International. 2011. 'True Love Waits International grows worldwide', press release, 10 February. http://www.gofbw.com/News.asp?id=12600 (accessed 24 May 2012).

UNAIDS. 2011. 'Decline in AIDS funding risks jeopardizing recent gains made by countries', press release. http://www.unaids.org/en/resources/presscentre/pressreleaseandstatementarchive/2011/november/20111127aidsfunding (accessed 4 June 2012).

UNDP. 2011. 'Zambia: country profile'. http://hdrstats.undp.org/en/countries/profiles/ZMB.html (accessed 22 August 2011).

van de Walle, N. 2001. *African Economies and the Politics of Permanent Crisis, 1979–1999*. New York: Cambridge University Press.

Varsalona, D. 2008. 'World Vision International. Report for Center for Public Integrity'. http://projects.publicintegrity.org/aids/org.aspx?id=21 (accessed 17 August 2011).

Whiteside, A. 2002. 'Poverty and HIV/AIDS in Africa', *Third World Quarterly* 23: 313–32.

World Council of Churches. 2006. 'Churches in the lead on HIV prevention reinvigoration'. http://www.oikoumene.org/fileadmin/files/wcc-main/documents/p4/contact/con-182.pdf (accessed 17 August 2011).

Wuthnow, R. 2009. *Boundless Faith: The Global Outreach of American Churches*. Los Angeles: University of California Press.

7

Condoms, Pills and Professional Identity

The Transnational ART Scale-up Project and Catholic HIV/AIDS Counsellors in Uganda

LOUISE MUBANDA RASMUSSEN

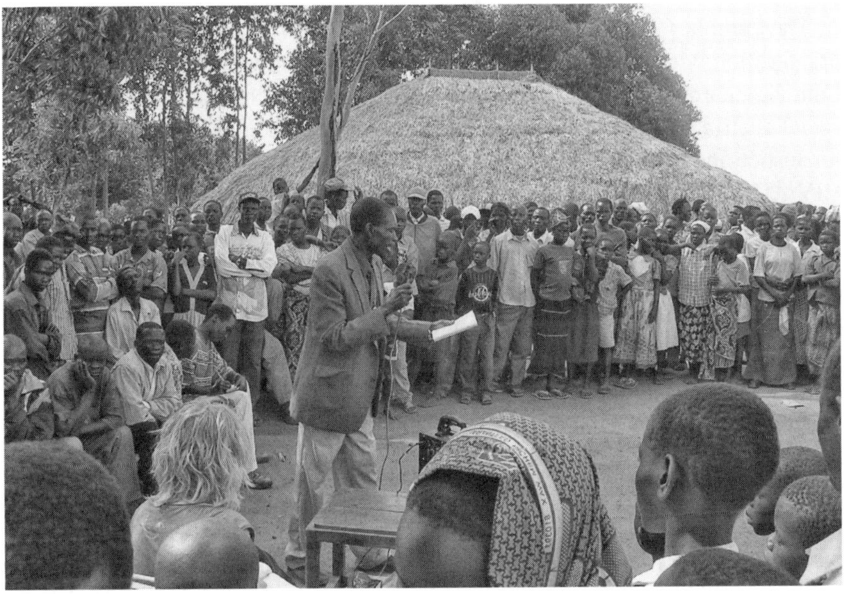

HIV prevention seminar in Arua diocese

Introduction

WITH THE INTRODUCTION OF THE (US) PRESIDENT'S EMERGENCY PLAN FOR AIDS RELIEF (PEPFAR) in 2003, the emphasis placed on abstinence and faithfulness in its funding of HIV prevention in Africa became a widely debated issue. Uganda in particular became the centre of the debate. Critics argued that PEPFAR funding conditionalities contributed to steering Ugandan HIV/AIDS policy away from the successful ABC approach towards an almost exclusive emphasis on abstinence and faithfulness (e.g. Epstein 2007; Human Rights Watch 2005). As argued in the introduction to this book, this development provides an example of how transnational connections in the realm of HIV/AIDS interventions may contribute to a conservative agenda on sexuality, and in the process empower local religious organisations that are interested in promoting sexual morality as a basis for societal transformation (see Gusman 2009).

However, what this debate tends to have obscured is that PEPFAR was an initiative meant to rapidly expand the access to antiretroviral treatment (ARV/ART), especially in African countries. From 2005 to 2008 between 70 and 79 per cent of the funds were devoted to treatment and care interventions.[1] This chapter demonstrates that in the realm of ARV treatment programmes implemented by local Catholic organisations in Uganda, the transnational dynamics at play are different and more complicated than in the case of PEPFAR's influence on HIV prevention policy.

The Catholic Church can in itself be considered the world's largest transnational organisation with its estimated more than one billion members worldwide. The Catholic Church's official prohibition of condom use, which is linked to the church's social doctrine on marriage and reproduction (see for example Pontifical Council for Justice and Peace 2004: 132–3), has also been widely debated in the context of HIV/AIDS. Many commentators assume that because of the hierarchical structure of the church, the Pope exerts an almost direct top-down influence on local Catholic organisations working with HIV/AIDS. Indeed the Catholic Church has much clearer hierarchical structures than any other world religion, with the centralised power of the Vatican, and the doctrine of Papal Infallibility constituting papal pronouncements on church doctrine as divine revelations.[2] However, ethnographic studies of local Catholic practices and identities around the world reveal a wealth of diversity (e.g. Behrend 2007; Mosse 2006; Harris 2006; Green 2003; Kassimir 1995), which serves as a warning to those who assume that the pronouncements of the Vatican can perfectly determine the experience and behaviour of Catholics (Cannell 2006: 10). Likewise my research with various Catholic HIV/AIDS initiatives in Uganda from 2006 to 2009 demonstrates diversity when it comes to the question of condom use. I experienced how there was some room for local staff to reconcile the official policy on contraceptives with local realities, as well as global demands. However, this room for manoeuvre within the transnational organisation of the Catholic Church itself took a different shape in different types of HIV/AIDS interventions.

[1] This included around 45 per cent for ARV treatment and around 30 per cent for 'care', which includes palliative care for HIV and TB patients, HIV counselling and testing and care for orphans and vulnerable children; see http://www.pepfar.gov/about/c19388.htm.

[2] See http://www.catholic.com/library/Papal_Infallibility.asp.

During HIV prevention sensitisations, local staff in Catholic HIV/AIDS projects follow the official prohibition of condom use in most cases and therefore discourage the use of condoms as a morally inferior, and sometimes also a medically inferior, method of preventing HIV infection. But, in the more private settings of counselling, and especially when counselling people who are already living with HIV/AIDS, counsellors often explicitly encourage their clients to use condoms, and in some cases other forms of contraception as well, to protect themselves and others from HIV infection/co-infection and pregnancy.

This contrast first of all directs attention to the different moral politics played out in public forums of HIV prevention versus in the more private spaces of counselling people already living with HIV/AIDS. Secondly, and of particular relevance to a discussion on transnational dynamics, the contrast draws attention to the position of HIV counsellors; the forms of expertise and professional identity that make them 'special' and the way they become part of a particular transnational bio-political project, through large-scale ARV treatment programmes. It seems that for HIV counsellors working in Catholic HIV/AIDS projects, their local professional identities and the transnational relations of the ART scale-up project structure their position on condom use much more than the official policy of the Catholic Church. To further explore this phenomenon, this chapter analyses the position and practices of HIV counsellors in Catholic HIV/AIDS projects in Uganda, focusing on the way they negotiate, take up and transform counselling techniques and notions of appropriate sexuality in the context of ARV treatment, and how these negotiations are connected to both transnational dynamics and local moral discourses.

Methodology

This chapter builds upon my master's and PhD research from 2006 to 2009 with various Catholic HIV/AIDS initiatives in Uganda. During this research I shifted between focusing on HIV prevention programmes and treatment and care programmes, which has given me insights into the similarities and differences between the two, in various types of Catholic HIV/AIDS initiatives.

In 2006, I completed an internship in the microfinance department of a Catholic AIDS-NGO in Kampala, called Reach Out Mbuya Parish HIV/AIDS Initiative. Also in 2006, for my master's thesis, I researched two HIV prevention programmes targeting men, one of which was run by Reach Out. In 2008, in the beginning of my PhD research I broadly researched the HIV/AIDS activities implemented by another Catholic NGO in Kampala, called Kamwokya Christian Caring Community (KCCC) and by the diocese of Arua in the northwestern West Nile region of Uganda. In 2009, I focused on 'treatment, care and support' for people living with HIV/AIDS, provided by KCCC and two Catholic health facilities in Arua diocese,

Maracha Hospital and Ediofe Health Centre. This focus eventually became the main focus of my PhD thesis. In this chapter, I draw on all these research projects, but in the main discussion on HIV counsellors, I primarily make use of experiences from KCCC and the AIDS clinic in Maracha Hospital.

The above-mentioned research projects have generally consisted of participant observation of everyday organisational practice, with a particular emphasis on HIV prevention seminars, counselling sessions and home visits. This was combined with semi-structured qualitative interviews with programme managers, facilitators, peer educators, counsellors, community workers and clients. All the informants mentioned in this chapter appear under pseudonyms.

Most of the organisations I have researched can be characterised as 'religious development organisations', as opposed to being church-run projects (cf. Christiansen 2010). For the NGOs and health facilities identifying as 'Catholic', there is some flexibility in what precisely makes them 'Catholic'. They operate under the authority of their respective bishops, but there are no requirements that their beneficiaries or patients are Catholic, and no absolute requirement that employees or volunteers have to be Catholic (often Catholics are preferred, but given good qualifications this preference can be overcome). The room for manoeuvre I identify in this chapter must be seen as partly connected to the larger degree of flexibility that comes with being a religious development organisation, in contrast to church-run projects.

The chapter begins with a presentation of what I have termed the transnational bio-political project of scaling-up of ART in Africa. Here I outline the Foucault-inspired theoretical perspectives I employ in analysing the ART scale-up. The following section presents the emerging ethnographic literature on HIV counsellors in Africa, which I use to complement the Foucault-inspired perspectives. Thereafter the contrast experienced between HIV prevention and HIV counselling in Catholic contexts is used as a stepping stone to pursue the main focus of the chapter: how counsellors working in Catholic HIV/AIDS projects negotiate the official policy on contraception. In the final sections of the chapter, I discuss how these negotiations are influenced by both transnational dynamics and the local professional identity of counsellors.

The transnational bio-political project of ARV treatment scale-up in Africa

The question of ARV treatment in Africa has undergone a dramatic shift in the past decade. Until the early 2000s, providing ARV treatment in Africa was considered an unfeasible, unrealistic and inappropriate solution to the AIDS crisis (see Jones 2004). However, during the late 1990s a transnational advocacy coalition lobbying for greater access to ARV treatment in developing countries began to take shape (Nguyen 2005). Eventually, the activists were successful not only in pushing for a significant reduction in the prices of first-line generic ARV medicines (Hein 2007), but importantly in framing the lack of access to ARV treatment as a humanitarian emergency (Nguyen 2009). The activists argued that access to ARV treatment constituted a right to life – a right that should not be denied to the poorest people in the world (Smith and Siplon 2006). In response to this activism, a number of large-scale funding initiatives were launched between 2002 and 2003 with the aim of achieving 'universal access' to ARV treatment. These included, among others, PEPFAR and the Global Fund to fight HIV/AIDS, Tuberculosis and Malaria.

In the context of framing access to ART as 'a right to life', major donors like PEPFAR and the Global Fund demonstrate their achievements in rolling out universal access with figures illustrating the 'number of lives saved' or 'the years of life saved' by their programme (Nguyen 2009: 209). In this way, providing ARV treatment is conceived as a way of literally 'saving lives' in Africa. Involved in this project to 'save lives' are not only such major donors, but a complex, trans-national network of non-governmental organisations, faith-based organisations, African governments, foreign donor governments, private philanthropists, Northern universities and hospitals and even the American military (Nguyen 2009: 196).

In Uganda, access to ARV treatment has significantly increased with the help of funding initiatives like PEPFAR and the Global Fund. In 2003, it was estimated that about 10,000 people were receiving ARV treatment (Meinert *et al.* 2003). By the end of 2010, 248,200 Ugandans were receiving ARV treatment, constituting 47 per cent coverage (UNAIDS 2012). Characteristic of the Ugandan ARV treatment landscape is that, unlike in for example Mozambique and Botswana, the ART scale-up has not been implemented through the national public health system, but by a wide variety of organisations and projects (Whyte *et al.* 2013). PEPFAR or the Global Fund fund most of these, but the funds are channelled through a host of different intermediary organisations to various clinics placed in government health facilities, mission health facilities and NGOs.[3] For example in the Kampala-based NGO KCCC, ARV provision was made possible in 2004 with PEPFAR funding, which was channelled through a consortium of local and international NGOs, headed by an American faith-based organisation. The AIDS clinic in Maracha Hospital was primarily funded by the Ugandan government's Global Fund-funded ART programme, which delivers ARV medicines, condoms and HIV testing kits to government health facilities, as well as some mission health facilities.

PEPFAR funding of ARV treatment programmes has to some extent been contingent upon the implementing organisations focusing on abstinence and

[3] In some clinics, the ARV medicines are even funded by different donors, leading to different types of medicines and different enrolment criteria in the same clinic (see Richey 2012).

faithfulness in their HIV prevention programmes, which has given faith-based organisations an advantage in the competition for funds. However, the transnational dynamic I wish to highlight here is how local Catholic organisations become part of a transnational bio-political project concerned with 'saving lives' with ARV treatment.

The ART scale-up in Africa vividly illustrates how life itself can become the objective of political intervention, as captured in Foucault's term *bio-politics* or *bio-power* (Foucault 1978, 2004, 2008). Bio-power is 'a power that exerts a positive influence on life, that endeavors to administer, optimize, and multiply it, subjecting it to precise control and comprehensive regulations' (Foucault 1978: 137). Foucault argued that, as opposed to disciplinary power, which has individualising effects by manipulating the individual body to render it useful and docile, bio-power has totalising effects by directing itself towards life at the mass level of the population (Foucault 2004: 246–9). With the ART scale-up, a transnational network, consisting of various actors, with no clear centralised authority, has become concerned with optimising life through the deployment of technologies that target, describe and aim to regulate specific populations (Nguyen 2009: 199).

However, it is important to keep in mind that the politicisation of certain health problems may not necessarily only reflect a bio-political ambition to optimise life at population level, but also a concern with how subjects govern themselves (Larsen 2011: 202–3).[4] Foucault coined the term *governmentality* to capture such 'contacts' between technologies of power and technologies of the self (Foucault 1988). He also used the term to describe the historical processes whereby the problematic of how to govern was increasingly rationalised (Foucault 2008: 311). With the term governmentality, this chapter traces the connections between bio-political ambitions, rationalities of government and technologies of the self as these play out in counselling practice.

To start with, it is important to notice how the bio-political project of ART scale-up in Africa is characterised by a number of specific rationalities and technologies of government, which is related to how ARV treatment works as a medical technology and to the history of having to overcome widespread scepticism about the possibilities of expanding the treatment in Africa. As a medical technology, ARV treatment is premised on following a strict treatment regimen. The treatment consists of a combination of three different antiretroviral drugs that target the replication of HIV at different stages. The purpose of this combination is to delay the emergence of drug resistance and permanently suppress the virus (Nguyen 2010: 90). However, this kind of therapy is vulnerable to interruptions, and though drug

[4] As for example the ways in which medical missionaries during colonial times viewed diseases in Africa as manifestations of larger social ills and therefore attempted to achieve not only physical transformations of the body, but also the creation of new subjectivities through evangelisation (Vaughan 1991: 73–4).

resistance is delayed, it still constitutes a risk, which entails that some patients, after some time, will have to change to another, and often more expensive, drug combination. Consequently, on the global scale there is great emphasis on taking steps to prevent the development of drug resistance, because failure to do so would eventually lead to severely reduced treatment options.

In the context of the ART scale-up in Africa, these concerns have been heightened. Among Northern donors there was initially scepticism about the viability and the risks of expanding such a complex treatment in resource-poor settings, characterised by under-funded health sectors, widespread poverty and food insecurity (Jones 2004). In particular, there were fears that expanding the treatment in Africa would lead to 'antiretroviral anarchy', thereby rapidly fuelling the production of drug resistance (Whyte *et al.* 2004: 17). Consequently, in African countries, ARV treatment has been provided in a manner where ensuring patient adherence to the treatment has been foregrounded more than any other issue (see Mattes 2011; Meinert *et al.* 2009; Nixon and Veenstra 2008; Richey 2011, 2012). This emphasis on treatment adherence, along with the transnational relations of power characterising the ART scale-up, influences the practices of and the position of counsellors in the Catholic organisations I have studied.

HIV counsellors: professionalism and local entanglements

Apart from the Foucault-inspired perspectives outlined above, the approach I take in this chapter is characterised by an ethnographic interest in how counsellors as situated actors negotiate between governmentality and varying strategies and multiple identities (Richey 2012: 828). In this respect, the chapter considers how counsellors, as 'brokers' of the ART scale-up, take up, negotiate and possibly transform techniques of HIV counselling and ARV treatment adherence (Lupton 1997: 94–5; Mosse and Lewis 2006: 5). Considering counsellors a type of 'broker' emphasises the unscripted intercultural role they perform when transforming techniques into practice and the dynamics that result from the social technology of counselling becoming part of the counsellors' own social trajectories (Mosse and Lewis 2006: 15). Furthermore, examining HIV counselling as a social technology directs attention to how the technology must be realised within social relations and highlights how the connections between governmental techniques, moral perspectives and actors are produced in practice (Jöhncke *et al.* 2004: 388).

The emerging literature on HIV counsellors in African countries suggests that counsellors, as people 'entangled' in the communities they serve, may transform and even subvert the professional and ethical principles of counselling. Especially in rural settings where counsellors are deeply embedded in dense social relations, they have to negotiate principles such as confidentiality and professional detachment with a local moral discourse, concerned with for example protecting others from HIV infection and involving the wider family in care of patients (Angotti 2010; Whyte *et al.* 2010). In this chapter my concern is not merely how such negotiations might result in counsellors subverting key principles of counselling. Rather I am interested in whether cultivating a professional identity as an HIV counsellor holds a particular potential in local moral worlds to the point where this professional authority is used to promote goals which are both relevant to the transnational ART scale-up project and to local moral discourses.

Different approaches to condom use

Before proceeding to the analysis of how HIV counsellors in Catholic HIV/AIDS projects negotiate counselling technology, and especially the official policy on contraceptives, this section outlines the contrast I experienced between HIV prevention and HIV counselling with regard to the messages on condom use.

During various forms of HIV/AIDS education and 'sensitisation' primarily aimed at preventing the spread of HIV, facilitators in the studied Catholic organisations presented condoms as a morally inferior prevention method. The message they gave was that condoms might protect you from HIV infection but not from the consequences of sinful behaviours, such as 'adultery' and 'fornication'. Instead of condom use, the facilitators promoted abstinence and faithfulness as strategies that both keep you safe from sin and from HIV infection. For example, during an HIV sensitisation in Arua diocese, a male facilitator presented methods of HIV prevention in the following way: 'Once you're married, be faithful to each other. If you're not married, abstain.' Then he said, directed to the women present: 'When your husband is not there,[5] stay very close to your church. The church also teaches that you should not commit adultery, condoms are the last resort' (Field notes, 20 May 2008). This statement reflects a rather common way that Christian moralities are combined with rationalities of health promotion in Catholic HIV prevention contexts: abstinence and faithfulness keeps you safe from HIV and it is also what the church teaches (see Rasmussen 2008).

In Kampala, I found that it was common for facilitators to discourage the use of condoms on the basis that they were both morally and medically inferior methods of HIV prevention. An example of this phenomenon comes from a Life Skills workshop in the Kampala-based NGO Kamwokya Christian Caring Community (KCCC). This was a three-day workshop for a group of young people in a poor, informal settlement in Kampala. When one of the participants asked, 'How come you don't give out condoms?', the facilitator, Bukenya, replied:

[5] In the West Nile region there is a long history of men migrating to central Uganda for work.

> The reason why we don't give out condoms and don't talk about it is not because we are against it. We are a faith-based, Christian-founded organization, if you read the bible, condoms promote promiscuity and adultery and that is against God's word . . . Plus, we didn't make them, so we don't know if they work. PSI did a study that showed that some people became pregnant and got HIV who had used a condom . . . According to my best knowledge, no one has ever used a condom completely correctly as it says on the packet.
>
> (Field notes, 18 April 2008)

Bukenya then referred to the time when the Ugandan government compounded some 30 million condoms of its own Engabu brand, because they were not 'safe'.[6] He also explained how you can 'test' the ineffectiveness of condoms by putting chilli inside. He concluded with assuring the participants that 'even on the packet it says they are not 100 per cent safe'.

The first part of Bukenya's reply was similar to the method used in the Arua example: he referred to the connection between condoms and sinful behaviour. But later he invoked the authority of medical science to indicate that, medically speaking, condoms are also an ineffective HIV prevention method. This is one of a number of examples from my research of how facilitators, in the Kampala-based NGOs, combined the authority of medical science with the moral authority of biblical teachings to craft a strong message against the use of condoms (see also Farrell 2003).

As a stark contrast to the messages on condom use provided in Catholic HIV prevention contexts, in counselling sessions in Catholic HIV/AIDS clinics, most counsellors actively encouraged their clients to use condoms and sometimes other forms of contraception as well. However, the clinics did not (officially) provide the clients with condoms or other forms of 'family planning'. There could be some differences between how explicitly condoms were encouraged depending on whether it was a pre- and post-test session or an ongoing counselling session of someone already living with HIV/AIDS. The message also depended on the client's age and marital status.

In pre- and post-test counselling sessions, especially with young unmarried clients, the message on condoms could be somewhat ambiguous. In KCCC, the Anglican counsellor, Jagwe, counselled a young girl, who was still in secondary school, before her HIV test. He asked her about what she knew about HIV/AIDS. Discussing how HIV can be prevented, the young girl said: 'you can use condoms, but it's not completely safe'. To this, Jagwe commented:

> This organization is built on a strong foundation of the Catholic Church, but as a counsellor I talk about condoms, because I know it is one of the ways you can protect yourself. But it is good that you know they are not completely safe.
>
> (Field notes, 17 December 2008)

[6] See http://www.thelancet.com/journals/laninf/article/PIIS1473-3099(05)70227-9/fulltext.

But when it came to people already living with HIV/AIDS or their partners, the advice counsellors gave was rather univocal: you should avoid unprotected sex, and therefore you should use condoms, and if you are not willing to do so or cannot persuade your partner to do so, you should abstain or at least try to reduce the frequency of sex. For example, in Maracha Hospital, in Arua diocese, the counsellor, Joyce, gave these instructions to a woman taking ARV medicine:

> Once you're taking this drug, you should not take alcohol, smoke and not play sex unnecessary, if it's with condom, it's ok. Once you have started taking this drug, you're advised to use condoms simply because if you have sex you will add viruses to yours, yet you have started taking the drugs to help you reduce the virus.
>
> (Field notes, 17 March 2009)

However, as the example with Jagwe and the young girl above also illustrates, the counsellors often had to position their recommendations of condom use against the Catholic identity of the organisation, and it was also common that the counsellors lowered their voice a bit when speaking about condoms. In Maracha Hospital, Joyce counselled an HIV-positive man, whose wife she also knew to be HIV-positive (but receiving her treatment from another clinic). Towards the end of the session, the man asked Joyce: 'Do you have condoms here?' Quietly, Joyce replied:

> Yeah, condoms are here. When condoms are brought there, they are sent to smaller health centres, because this hospital is of Catholic foundation. We normally don't give here, but for your case I can give.
>
> (Field notes, 24 April 2009)

Joyce found some Life Guard condoms in the closed closet and gave the man about ten condoms.[7]

In the Kampala-based NGO KCCC, seven of their nine counsellors were Catholic and the others were Anglican. In my interviews with them, both the Catholics and the Anglicans explained that despite KCCC being a Catholic organisation, they encouraged clients to use condoms in order to 'protect their lives'. For example, Damian, who is a Catholic, said: 'Personally, although the Catholic Church doesn't allow to use condoms, but for heaven's sake . . . for someone's life, that's why I discuss the issue of condom' (Interview, 19 January 2009). Another Catholic counsellor, Anthony, explained: 'at least we help these people who are living together to learn how to condomize, we are Catholics, but with HIV, we don't just say that you go open, when you know that you have the virus' (Interview, 2 February 2009). And the Anglican counsellor Jagwe said:

[7] As mentioned earlier, the ART programme in this clinic was primarily funded by a government programme. The locally produced Life Guard condoms were part of the ART package delivered to the clinic through the Ministry of Health.

> . . . these people are Catholic, we are Catholic-based, we don't, they don't promote like the condoms for instance, but still as we sit and discuss . . . we don't distribute, but us counsellors one on one, we tell them because we know, ehe, leave alone the religion, because Catholics don't believe in that, they have their reasons, but this is the reality.
> (Interview, 19 January 2009)

For discordant couples – when one partner is HIV-positive and the other is HIV-negative – there were many complex issues for counsellors to deal with. But committed to seeing the couples stay together, the counsellors generally encouraged them to use condoms, stressing the dangers of 'live sex'. In KCCC, they referred discordant couples to a number of partner organisations, which specialised in the matter (and who could provide them with condoms). The referral of discordant couples is a move that allows the Catholic providers to avoid getting directly involved with the tricky question of condom use, but at the same time offer potentially life-saving assistance to the couples.

The moral politics of condoms in different settings and with different audiences

The contrast between HIV prevention education and HIV counselling with regard to how condoms are dealt with first of all directs attention to the different public/private character of these interventions and to the difference between addressing the 'uninfected' and those already living with HIV/AIDS.

During the HIV sensitisation in Arua diocese mentioned above, the facilitator's comment that 'condoms are the last resort' contained enough ambiguity for the audience to question whether local Catholic Church representatives were in fact encouraging people to use condoms. The diocese's HIV/AIDS coordinator and the parish priest, who were also present during the sensitisation, had to intervene and clarify that 'as a Church we have not encouraged condoms'. This example reflects how important it is for church representatives in the public forums of HIV education carefully to manage the Catholic Church's image as a defender of moral values. This argument also has some relevance for the Kampala-based NGO KCCC. Despite the fact that Bukenya generally promoted rather fierce anti-condom messages during the Life Skills workshops, he admitted in an informal conversation with me and my assistant that he had begun to doubt if young people can really abstain, 'because I remember what it was like being young' (Field notes, 19 December 2008). In contrast to HIV prevention education, counselling takes place in a private and confidential space, where counsellors tend to display a more pragmatic attitude with regard to whether condoms might be appropriate for some people under certain circumstances. As the discussion about discordant couples above indicates, counsellors are confronted directly with the complicated realities of living with HIV/AIDS, which seems to result in them adopting a more pragmatic approach to condom use.

As such, the difference between addressing the 'uninfected' and those already living with HIV/AIDS is also important to consider. In international HIV/AIDS discourses more generally, it is possible to discern how HIV prevention is debated differently with regard to the uninfected and the infected (see Center for AIDS Prevention Studies 2005; National Prevention Information Network 2012). HIV prevention for people living with HIV/AIDS has in fact only become an international priority in recent years, under the name 'Positive Prevention' (see International HIV/AIDS Alliance 2003). International debates about Positive Prevention stress the need to balance the public health objectives of reducing HIV infections with a concern for not increasing stigma and placing blame on people living with HIV/AIDS (ibid.; Allen *et al.* 2011). In fact, some AIDS activists have argued against the idea of 'Positive Prevention' for fear that it would only further stigmatise those living with HIV/AIDS (Cairns 2008). This debate highlights how the question of HIV-positive people's sexuality is fraught with moral dilemmas.

In the local Catholic organisations, HIV prevention seminars are conceived as being directed at the 'uninfected',[8] with the objective of encouraging them to avoid HIV infection by practising an individualised form of sexual responsibility. Counselling practices for people living with HIV/AIDS, on the other hand, target their sexual responsibility from the point of view that as infected members of the community, their sexual conduct poses a direct threat to the community. Therefore, when encouraging them to protect others from HIV infection, condoms may seem a more pertinent method, despite the official policy of the Catholic Church. As a Catechist volunteering as a community counsellor in a home-based programme in Arua diocese explained: 'To those who are living positively, what I speak to them, not to have unprotected sex. I encourage them not to spread this virus. I tell them God does not like this spreading deliberately' (Interview, 30 May 2009). Likewise, counsellors and community workers in KCCC discussed how a spiritual approach of 'reconciliation' was important to help people living with HIV/AIDS overcome feelings of bitterness and resentment, which otherwise might propel them to deliberately spread the virus (Focus group discussion, 16 June 2008). Such discussions illustrate how great a threat to the community the sexual behaviour of people living with HIV/AIDS is perceived to be, and the fact that counsellors consider these potential dangers reflect their 'entanglements' in local moral worlds (cf. Whyte *et al.* 2010). In KCCC, the counsellor Rose, for example, talked about a woman she had counselled, who confessed to her that she was having an affair with a married man:

> that man has got a wife and children from another woman, and she comes 'eh counsellor, I have a boyfriend, it's a man of another woman' . . . it becomes a challenge, you can't show that you are annoyed, you just imagine what if you are the

[8] Even if there might be HIV-positive people, or some people suspecting they are positive, in the audience.

> one, it is your husband who is being taken away by such an HIV-positive woman . . . it's so challenging.
>
> (Interview, 27 January 2009)

Another important factor to consider is how the bio-political project of scaling-up ARV treatment in Uganda has engendered new difficult questions about the sexual behaviour of people living with HIV/AIDS (Allen *et al.* 2011). In the counselling of people living with HIV/AIDS, the advice counsellors give on sexual conduct is part of a larger set of 'rules' that people living with HIV/AIDS are taught to follow, particularly once they begin taking ARV treatment. These rules are common among all types of ARV providers in Uganda (see Meinert *et al.* 2009; Richey 2012). They are related to the central concern of treatment adherence and to the challenges of making the treatment effective in low-income settings. According to 'the rules', ARV patients have to take their medicine every day at the same time, come on time for clinical appointments, eat a balanced diet, avoid smoking, drinking, unprotected sex, and overworking, discuss plans to have children with their doctor and counsellor, disclose their HIV status, and maintain a positive attitude. I will discuss the rules further below, but note here that the rule that people living with HIV/AIDS should avoid unprotected sex is not only about generally protecting the HIV-negative population. As is evident in Joyce's instructions above, the rule is also connected to anxieties over ARV clients potentially infecting others with drug-resistant virus strains, and themselves becoming re-infected, which is believed to affect the effectiveness of the ARV therapy.

In this sense, I will argue that HIV prevention facilitators and HIV counsellors seem to be on a different 'mission' – that the larger goal of social transformation they identify with is rather different. If we consider the lengths that some facilitators go to to craft strong anti-condom messages, they appear to identify with a vision of transforming society along the lines of Christian values. As the coordinator of Reach Out's prevention programme clarified during a staff meeting: 'We promote values, faith, morals and young people to be focused. We are not promoting, neither fighting the use of condoms. We are working to change people's attitudes, so that they can change their behaviour' (Field notes, 17 July 2006). In contrast, counsellors seem to identify with the bio-political logic of enabling people living with HIV/AIDS to follow 'the rules' of ARV treatment as a way of both prolonging their lives and avoiding new HIV infections. It is my argument that the professional identities of counsellors and the kind of transnational linkages their work is connected to via ARV treatment programmes are an important background to this difference.[9]

[9] In most of the organisations I studied, HIV counsellors and HIV prevention facilitators were different people. But in one home-based care programme in Arua diocese, the 'community counsellors' who went on home visits also had the task of 'sensitising' their communities on HIV/AIDS. Most of these community counsellors were living with HIV. Unfortunately, I did not have the chance to participate in any of these sensitisations. But it would be quite interesting to see how they framed the issue of responsible sexuality and condom use.

The professional identity of HIV counsellors

Compared to facilitators or peer educators in HIV prevention programmes, HIV counsellors have a stronger professional identity. As counsellors they are part of a growing profession in Uganda. This is a profession which is currently trying to outline guidelines and definitions for what it means to be a counsellor (cf. Ochieng 2009). For example, during the first HIV counselling conference held in Kampala in May 2009,[10] a code of ethics for counsellors was launched. HIV counsellors receive a more standardised, and often much longer, training than facilitators or peer educators, who may not even receive any formal training before embarking on HIV prevention education.

In Uganda, training of HIV counsellors is almost exclusively in the hands of the two national-level NGOs, the well-known TASO (The AIDS Support Organization)[11] and AIDS Information Centre.[12] All the counsellors I interviewed or interacted with were trained by one of these two NGOs, in courses lasting from a couple of months to a whole year. The uniform training background manifests itself in the way that HIV counsellors across different institutions and in different parts of the country follow similar templates in their counselling sessions (for example with regard to which topics are covered in which order in a pre-test counselling session), and in the way they all, at least at the level of normative discourse, display a strong commitment to non-directive counselling methodology.

The professional identity of counsellors is enacted on a national scale through such events as the HIV counselling conference. In my experience, in organisations and clinics, counsellors also cultivate a sense of professional identity that distinguishes them from other employees and volunteers. During my PhD studies, I experienced this mostly in KCCC, which had a counselling team with nine members.[13] The counsellors for example distinguished between themselves and the lesser-educated semi-volunteer 'community health workers' who go on home visits to ARV clients. These community workers perform similar tasks to counsellors and may make use of counselling methods (some of the counsellors were in fact going to offer them a short course on counselling methods). But the counsellors

[10] The conference was funded and organised by the PEPFAR-funded SCOT project. SCOT stands for Strengthening Counsellor Training. The project primarily works on developing and harmonising curricula for HIV/AIDS counsellor training.

[11] TASO was started in 1987 and is widely recognised as the first organised group of people living with HIV/AIDS in Africa. It has since grown to become a nationwide NGO, which is internationally renowned: see http://www.tasouganda.org/.

[12] AIDS Information Centre is an NGO started in 1990. It is the largest and oldest provider of Voluntary Counselling and Testing (VCT) services in Uganda and also a major provider of VCT training in Uganda: see http://www.aicug.org.

[13] In Maracha Hospital there was only one permanently employed counsellor, and four young intern counsellors who worked on a voluntary basis.

often emphasised that they were not 'real counsellors'. Jagwe for example lamented that they did not always appropriately protect the clients' confidentiality:

> Yeah we know how to handle them so that if you, like especially community health workers, because they are not counsellors . . . you find them like, talking to those clients, like in places where . . . they wouldn't need to discuss all about that, but as counsellors, we know.
>
> (Interview, 19 January 2009)

The counsellors also distinguished between themselves and the doctors in the clinic, whose medical ethics sometimes were at odds with the ethical principles of right to self-disclosure and confidentiality they were trained to uphold. The counsellor Elisabeth narrated how a male client she had counselled for some time one day came to the clinic with his wife, to whom he had never disclosed his HIV status. She tried to get them to test together as a couple, which would entail revealing both their test results to them together. However, the man managed to dodge the counsellor's proposal and the wife was tested alone. When she was found negative, the doctor who had handled the case insisted that the counsellor should reveal the husband's positive HIV status to the woman. The counsellor refused since this would have violated her counselling ethics (Interview, 12 February 2009).

Finally, the counsellors also distinguished between themselves and the organisation's management team, who they felt often did not understand or appreciate what counselling was about, as managers expected them to produce more 'tangible' results than they believed they could deliver.

The professional identity of HIV counsellors, and the expertise that defines this profession, is central and often seems to overshadow religious ideology. For counsellors working in Catholic organisations it means that although they may identify with the church's social doctrines as Catholics, they also strongly identify with their professional tasks as counsellors. As illustrated above, their professional identity centres on ethical principles of confidentiality and self-determination and a non-directive approach to counselling. This focus may encourage counsellors to follow a more pragmatic approach towards condom use – because, as they are taught during counselling training, condom use is one method of protecting yourself and others from HIV transmission and unwanted pregnancies that counsellors should give information about, so that the client can make his or her own 'informed decision'.

The transnational linkages of the ART scale-up

As mentioned above, the counsellors in the Catholic organisations appeared to identify strongly with the transnational bio-political project of 'saving lives' with ARV treatment. I actually found it to be a central aspect of their professional identity to display a strong commitment to seeing their clients follow 'the rules' of ARV treatment, despite the potential contradiction this poses to the principles of client self-determination.

The idea of 'the rules' of ARV treatment is a way that Ugandan providers of ARV treatment have translated the demands of treatment adherence into mechanisms for governing the self-conduct of people living with HIV/AIDS (see Allen *et al.* 2011; Meinert *et al.* 2009; Richey 2012; Whyte *et al.* 2013; and Mattes 2011 on the Tanzanian context). The rules illustrate how ART providers attempt to overcome the challenges of providing the treatment in settings characterised by under-funded health sectors, widespread poverty and food insecurity, by shifting onto the individual patient a large part of the responsibility for ensuring that the treatment works as effectively as possible.

The counsellors' commitment to seeing their clients follow 'the rules' can first of all be connected to the way their own performance as counsellors was tied to how effectively they helped 'save lives' with ARVs. The statistics on 'lives saved' produced by major donors are based on cumulative statistics gathered from implementing organisations. Local implementing organisations collect data for example on adherence, enrolment and retention rates. These data are usually sent to the intermediary organisation through which they receive funds for the ART programme. In my experience, such techniques of government affect the relationship between management and counsellors in the implementing organisations. At KCCC, for example, the clinic data showed increasing mortality rates and an increasing number of clients 'lost to follow-up'. During a staff meeting, the executive director used his data to blame the counsellors and community workers for not doing their work well enough. In a context where success is measured in terms of mortality and treatment adherence rates, and where counsellors' professional status is tied to ensuring that clients do follow 'the rules' (see also Richey 2012: 838), it is not surprising that the ambition to prolong life with the help of ARVs was primarily translated into a question of enabling, teaching and even disciplining their clients to follow 'the rules' (see also Rasmussen 2011; Rasmussen and Richey 2012).

Through 'the rules' of ARV treatment, just as in HIV prevention, sexuality becomes scripted through the imperative of disease prevention (Pigg and Adams 2005: 19). The rules of sexual conduct for ARV clients revolve particularly around drug-resistance concerns. As indicated above, when counsellors encourage people living with HIV/AIDS to avoid unprotected sex, they refer to the dangers of unprotected sex for the individual client's health, as well as to the success of the global ARV treatment project, by emphasising the importance of avoiding the transmission of drug-resistant virus strains. This context provides one clue as to why many counsellors emphasise condom use against Catholic doctrine and policy. The ART scale-up project has made decisions on who sleeps with whom, when and how, and what kinds of contraceptive to use into 'a question of life and death', in ways that for counsellors in Catholic organisations even trump the social doctrine of the church (cf. Pigg 2005: 15).

In this sense, it can be argued that in the context of large-scale ARV treatment programmes, counsellors in Catholic HIV/AIDS projects identify with particular bio-political ambitions that steer them away from the social doctrines of the church. This suggests that it is the transnational relations of the ART scale-up project, in combination with the counsellors' local positions as HIV experts, that shape the counsellors' recommendations on condom use more than the pronouncements of the Pope.

Professional identities and local entanglements

I do not want to suggest that the counsellors are merely foot soldiers of a global health intervention. They themselves identify with and seem motivated by a wish to see their clients stay healthy and alive and to prevent new HIV infections. When I asked the counsellors what made them happy or satisfied as counsellors, many of them spoke of the satisfaction they felt when their clients improved and 'came back to life'. In KCCC, Anthony, for example, said:

> What makes me happy as a counsellor is to meet my clients when they are changing, you see, when I counsel someone and the next time is going down, I feel maybe my counselling did not work, but when I see these people changing and they come looking better . . . it gives me an encouragement, counselling is working in their lives, so when people change from the worst to the better, it gives me encouragement, but I don't want to hear that ah, your client died, so when I spend at least four months when I don't hear that your client died, I feel that I'm doing something.
>
> (Interview, 2 February 2009)

Some of the KCCC counsellors spoke in general terms of seeing clients improving and coming back to life, while others spoke more specifically about rising CD4 counts and the role of counsellors in making it possible for clients to realise the 'miraculous' potentials of ARV treatment. The counsellor Daniel, for example, said:

> . . . that element of accessing treatment, and this person coming forward and saying now, my health has improved, I've been able to accomplish task a and task b . . . so you feel happy actually, you feel you are contributing to someone's improvement, I think those are some of the aspects which make me feel that I'm doing some important kind of work.
>
> (Interview, 3 February 2009)

As such, we can see how the counsellors identified with the special task the transnational flows of funding, resources and ideas in ART programmes make it possible for them to take up: helping clients to 'come back to life'.

Additionally, the responsibility the counsellors felt to help clients follow 'the rules' was manifest in the contradiction they actually experienced between the non-directive principles and methods they were trained in and the reality that many clients did not reach the 'right' informed decisions. In Maracha Hospital, Joyce, who faced a significant work burden handling all the clinic's clients on her own, expressed frustration at her limited ability to get clients to follow the rules of sexual conduct. Among other things, she explained how she had counselled many female clients who claimed they were not having sex at all, only to discover later that they had become pregnant (Field notes, 5 March 2009). In KCCC, Rose explained the frustration she felt over clients who failed to make 'positive' decisions. She said: 'when I counsel someone and he does not listen, he does . . . the opposite of what we talked about, I feel discouraged'. When I asked her to clarify, she explained:

> . . . especially when they become all right, they gain the strength, when it comes to the terms of their relationships . . . especially in discordant couples. You tell them the dangers of having unprotected sex . . . the one who is negative may turn positive, and in a few months, you see the wife pregnant [laughing] then you feel discouraged . . . you talk about dangers of smoking and taking alcohol, the client will tell you, counsellor, I have left all of those, 'aha I'm going to give up smoking, I'm going to give up drinking', but when he gains strength you meet him when he is totally drunk, he's smelling of cigarettes, and you feel, you feel unhappy, I feel that he may go back to the way he was.
>
> (Interview, 27 January 2009)

The point here is thus that some aspect of their professional commitment, the commitment to non-directive counselling, was actually at odds with the responsibility they felt they had as HIV counsellors to help clients make the 'right' decisions, which could help prolong their lives, and prevent new HIV infections. I actually found that the counsellors often transformed the counselling encounter into a didactic teacher–student exercise, focusing on teaching and disciplining their clients to follow 'the rules' (see Rasmussen 2013). This reflects studies from rural Uganda and rural Malawi that found that HIV counsellors may be personally committed to the health and well-being of clients and the wider community in ways that follow local moral discourses but are at odds with key principles of counselling (Angotti 2010; Whyte *et al.* 2010). I want to suggest that it is precisely *because of* their position as counsellors in an ARV treatment programme that they feel they have this responsibility to help clients make the 'right' decisions. Being an HIV counsellor seems to grant them a particular position, characterised by both authority and compassion, which provides them with a sense of responsibility to help clients.

Consider for example the case of Rose. She is a middle-aged, Catholic woman who lives close by KCCC. With an O-level certificate and a diploma in counselling, she is among the least educated among the counsellors in KCCC (some of the others even had bachelor degrees). She began to work for KCCC in 2004, after first having left a secretarial job, which did not pay much, and then not having much luck running a small business in her neighbourhood. When I asked her what she had learnt while being a counsellor, she replied:

> I've learnt how to live in a community; I've learnt how to handle people and I have learnt more about HIV/AIDS . . . I have learnt how to socialise, and I have even gained some confidence eh? In that I can eh? That I can help someone help himself, I feel happy . . . And I have gained a lot of knowledge from KCCC. Learned different personalities and how to handle them. At least that has helped me.
>
> (Interview, 27 January 2009)

Rose's statement reflects how being a counsellor and the kind of expertise one acquires while being trained and working as an HIV counsellor can become part of the person's own agenda to gain social status and secure a more stable livelihood. More importantly, this kind of expertise seems to grant her a position as someone capable of and responsible for helping HIV-positive people 'help themselves'. In the local context, the expertise of counsellors grants them a certain position of authority and responsibility. The counsellors' authority is enacted in the didactical way HIV counsellors teach and discipline their clients to follow 'the rules' of ARV treatment, and the way clients appropriate the counsellors' advice precisely as 'rules' or 'instructions' which come with 'penalties' if they are not followed (Allen *et al.* 2011: 533).

If we see counsellors as local authorities on HIV committed to prolonging the lives of people living with HIV/AIDS and preventing new HIV infections, it is important that the local fears around the sexual conduct of people with HIV/AIDS, which I mentioned earlier, coincide with the concerns of sexual responsibility articulated by the transnationally linked ART scale-up project. In informal conversations, the counsellors expressed concern over the potential dangers of sexually irresponsible clients in the context of ART. Despite their commitment to the ART scale-up, the counsellors talked about how the scale-up had potentially contributed to an increase in HIV prevalence, because with ARV treatment people can now live for a long time without the visible signs of AIDS. The KCCC counsellor Esther claimed that in the clinic they were seeing newly tested clients who already had drug-resistant virus strains, and she reasoned it was because their partners were taking ARVs without informing them of the fact, or revealing their HIV status (Field notes, 27 January 2009).

When teaching clients that their sexual (and reproductive) behaviour is now governed by 'the rules' of ARVs, counsellors can use their authority as HIV experts and the promises of the ARV medicine to attempt to govern clients' sexuality. So why did these counsellors not instruct their clients to abstain from sex entirely? In fact, as mentioned earlier, abstinence was sometimes given as an option and so was the practice of reducing the frequency of sex (this was presented as a method to minimise the risk of re-infection), but mostly, as the interview quotes above reflect, the counsellors recommended condom use. This suggests that because of their training as HIV counsellors, and the position counsellors can acquire as enablers of the ARV treatment's life-prolonging potential, they are more committed to 'the truths' of ARV treatment and HIV prevention than to the truths of the Catholic Church.

Conclusion

Starting from the contrast experienced between HIV prevention education and HIV counselling in Catholic HIV/AIDS projects in Uganda with regard to the messages on condoms provided in these contexts, this chapter has analysed the position and practices of counsellors in Catholic HIV/AIDS projects. The chapter has considered how counsellors negotiate, take up and transform counselling techniques and notions of appropriate sexuality in the context of ARV treatment. This analysis has illustrated how despite being employed by Catholic organisations, and some of them identifying as Catholics, the local professional identity of HIV counsellors and the transnational relations of the ART scale-up project appear to structure the counsellors' approach to condom use much more than the pronouncements of the Pope and the official policy of the Catholic Church.

In a broader sense, this chapter has illustrated how the transnational flows of money, resources and ideas related to HIV/AIDS interventions may help 'create' a new category of professionals in Africa: HIV counsellors. This category, however, unfolds and takes shape in local moral worlds and in a dynamic relationship with religious discourses. Whereas transnational connections in the realm of HIV prevention are seen to strengthen a conservative agenda on sexuality, the project of 'saving lives' with ARV treatment seems rather to result in creating a subtle opposition to the Catholic Church's social doctrine.

Acknowledgements

An earlier version of this chapter was presented at the conference 'Sexuality, AIDS and Religion; Transational Dynamics in Africa', held in Oxford, 28–30 September 2011. I am grateful to the participants in this conference for the comments and suggestions they made towards the improvement of the chapter. My PhD fieldwork in Uganda was made possible with financial support from the Danish Council for Development Research, Nordic Africa Institute and University of Copenhagen's fund for Theology Students and Candidates. But most importantly, this chapter could not have been written without all the HIV facilitators, counsellors and clients in Uganda who agreed to offer their time and experiences to participate in my research. I am equally indebted to my assistants Norah Kirabo, Nelly Arikuru and Jimmy Candia for the invaluable help they provided during my PhD research.

References

Allen, C., M. Mbonye, J. Seeley, J. Birungi, B. Wolff, A. Coutinhou and S. Jaffarf. 2011. 'ABC for people with HIV: responses to sexual behaviour recommendations among people receiving antiretroviral therapy in Jinja, Uganda', *Culture, Health, Sexuality* 13(5): 529–43.

Angotti, N. 2010. 'Working outside of the box: how HIV counsellors in Sub-Saharan Africa adapt Western HIV testing norms', *Social Science and Medicine* 71(6): 986–93.

Behrend, H. 2007. 'The rise of occult power, AIDS and the Roman Catholic Church in Western Uganda', *Journal of Religion in Africa* 37(1): 41–58.

Cairns, G. 2008. 'Who defines "Positive Prevention?"' http://www.aidsmap.com/Who-defines-Positive-prevention/page/1431092/.

Cannell, F. 2006. 'Introduction: the anthropology of Christianity', in F. Cannell (ed.), *The Anthropology of Christianity*. Durham, NC: Duke University Press.

Center for AIDS Prevention Studies. 2005. 'What are HIV+ persons' HIV prevention needs?' Factsheet from Center for AIDS Prevention Studies, University of California, San Francisco. http://caps.ucsf.edu/factsheets/hiv-persons/.

Christiansen, C. 2010. 'Development by churches, development of churches – institutional trajectories in rural Uganda'. PhD thesis, University of Copenhagen, Department of Anthropology.

Epstein, H. 2007. *The Invisible Cure: Africa, the West and the Fight against AIDS.* New York: Farrar, Straus and Giroux.

Farrell, M. 2003. 'Condoms and HIV/AIDS prevention: a comparison of three faith-based organizations in Uganda', *AIDS and Anthropology Bulletin* 15(3): 6–10.

Foucault, M. 1978. *The History of Sexuality. Volume 1: An Introduction.* London: Penguin Books.

Foucault, M. 1988. 'Technologies of the self', in M.H. Luther, *Technologies of the Self – A Seminar with Michel Foucault.* Amherst: University of Massachusetts Press, 16–49.

Foucault, M. 2004. *'Society Must Be Defended': Lectures at the Collège de France 1975–76.* Ed. M. Bertani and A. Fontana, trans. D. Macey. London: Penguin Books.

Foucault, M. 2008. *The Birth of Biopolitics: Lectures at Collège de France 1978–1979.* Ed. M. Senellart, trans. G. Burchell. Basingstoke: Palgrave Macmillan.

Green, M. 2003. *Priests, Witches and Power: Popular Christianity after Mission in Southern Tanzania.* Cambridge: Cambridge University Press.

Gusman, A. 2009. 'HIV/AIDS, Pentecostal churches and the "Joseph Generation" in Uganda', *Africa Today* 56(1): 67–86.

Harris, O. 2006. 'The eternal return of conversion – Christianity as contested domain in highland Bolivia', in F. Cannell (ed.), *The Anthropology of Christianity*. Durham, NC: Duke University Press, 51–76.

Hein, W. 2007. 'Global health governance and WTO/TRIPS: conflicts between "global market-creation" and "global social rights"', in W. Hein, S. Bartsch and L. Kohlmorgen, *Global Health Governance and the Fight against HIV/AIDS.* Basingstoke: Palgrave Macmillan, 38–66.

Human Rights Watch. 2005. 'The less they know the better – abstinence-only HIV/AIDS programs in Uganda', *Human Rights Watch* 17(4).

International HIV/AIDS Alliance. 2003. 'Positive Prevention: prevention strategies for people living with HIV/AIDS'. Draft background paper. http://www.cdc.gov/hiv/topics/prev_prog/ahp/resources/other/pdf/Positive_Prevention_IHA_Marked.pdf.

Jöhncke, S., M.N. Svendsen and S.R. Whyte. 2004. 'Løsningsmodeller – social teknologier som antropologisk arbejdsfelt', in K. Hastrup (ed.), *Viden om verden*. Copenhagen: Hans Reitzels Forlag, 385–408.

Jones, P.S. 2004. 'When "development" devastates: donor discourses, access to HIV/AIDS treatment in Africa and rethinking the landscape of development', *Third World Quarterly* 25(2): 385–404.

Kassimir, R. 1995. 'Catholics and political identity in Toro', in H.B. Hansen, and M. Twaddle (eds), *Religion and Politics in East Africa: The Period since Independence*. London: James Curry, 120–40.

Larsen, L. 2011. 'The birth of lifestyle politics: the biopolitical management of lifestyle disease in the United States and Denmark', in U. Bröckling, S. Krasman and T. Lemke (eds), *Governmentailty – Current Issues and Future Challenges*. New York: Routledge, 201–24.

Lupton, D. 1997. 'Foucault and the medicalisation critique', in A. Petersen, and R. Bunton (eds), *Foucault, Health and Medicine*. London: Routledge, 94–110.

Mattes, D. 2011. '"We are just supposed to be quiet": the production of adherence to antiretroviral treatment in urban Tanzania', *Medical Anthropology* 30(2): 158–82.

Meinert, L., M. Whyte, S.R. Whyte and B. Kyaddondo. 2003. 'Faces of globalisation – AIDS and ARV medicine in Uganda', *FOLK – Journal of the Danish Ethnographic Society* 45: 105–23.

Meinert, L., H. Mogensen and J. Twebaze. 2009. 'Tests for life chances: CD4 miracles and obstacles in Uganda', *Anthropology and Medicine* 16(2): 195–209.

Mosse, D. 2006. 'Possession and confession – affliction and sacred power in colonial and contemporary Catholic South India', in F. Cannell (ed.), *The Anthropology of Christianity*. Durham, NC: Duke University Press, 99–133.

Mosse, D. and D. Lewis. 2006. 'Theoretical approaches to brokerage and translation in development', in D. Lewis and D. Mosse (eds), *Development Brokers and Translators: The Ethnography of Aid and Agencies*. Bloomfield, CT: Kumarian Press, 1–26.

National Prevention Information Network. 2012. 'HIV prevention today'. http://www.cdcnpin.org/scripts/hiv/prevent.asp.

Nguyen, V.-K. 2005. 'Antiretroviral globalism, biopolitics, and therapeutic citizenship', in O. Aihwa and S.J. Collier (eds), *Global Assemblages: Technology, Politics and Ethics as Anthropological Problems*. Malden, MA: Blackwell, 124–44.

Nguyen, V.-K. 2009. 'Government-by-exception: enrolment and experimentality in mass HIV treatment programmes in Africa', *Social Theory and Health* 7(3): 196–217.

Nguyen, V.-K. 2010. *The Republic of Therapy*. Durham, NC: Duke University Press.

Nixon, S. and N. Veenstra. 2008. 'Maintaining and developing health systems to sustain HAART', in J.M. Zuniga, A. Whiteside, A. Ghaziani and J.G. Bartlett (eds), *A Decade of HAART: The Development and Global Impact of Highly Active Antiretroviral Therapy*. Oxford: Oxford University Press, 463–75.

Ochieng, L. 2009. 'Counselling: the broader perspective'. Presentation, 6 May 2009, given at the National HIV Counselling Conference, Kampala, Uganda, 6–8 May 2009.

Pigg, S. L. 2005. 'Globalizing the facts of life', in V. Adams and S.L. Pigg (eds), *Sex in Development: Science, Sexuality and Morality in Global Perspective*. Durham, NC: Duke University Press, 39–66.

Pigg, S.L. and V. Adams. 2005. 'Introduction: the moral object of sex', in V. Adams and S.L. Pigg (eds), *Sex in Development: Science, Sexuality and Morality in Global Perspective*. Durham, NC: Duke University Press, 1–38.

Pontifical Council for Justice and Peace. 2004. *Compendium of the Social Doctrine of the Church.* Nairobi: Paulines Publications Africa.

Rasmussen, L. 2008. '"As a man this is how you should behave!" A critical look into "developing men" as a means of HIV/AIDS prevention in Sub-Saharan Africa', *Political Perspectives* 2(1).

Rasmussen, L.M. 2011. 'From dying with dignity to living with rules: AIDS treatment and "holistic care" in Catholic organisations in Uganda'. PhD thesis, University of Copenhagen, Centre of African Studies.

Rasmussen, L.M. 2013. 'Counselling clients to follow "the rules" of safe sex and ARV treatment', *Culture, Health and Sexuality* (ahead-of-print), 1–16. http://www.tandfonline.com/doi/abs/10.1080/13691058.2013.809606.

Rasmussen, L.M. and L.A. Richey. 2012. 'The Lazarus Effect of AIDS treatment: lessons learnt and lives saved', *Journal of Progressive Human Services* 23(3): 187–207.

Richey, L.A. 2011. 'Anti-viral but pro-natal? ARVs and reproductive health: the view from a South African township', in C. Browner and C. Sargent (eds), *Reproduction, Globalization and the State*. Durham, NC: Duke University Press, 68–82.

Richey, L.A. 2012. 'Counselling citizens and producing patronage: AIDS treatment in South African and Ugandan clinics', *Development and Change* 43(4): 823–45.

Smith, R.A. and P.D. Siplon. 2006. *Drugs into Bodies: Global AIDS Treatment Activism.* Westport, CT: Praeger.

UNAIDS. 2012. 'AIDS info country fact sheets – Uganda'. http://www.unaids.org/en/data analysis/tools/aidsinfo/countryfactsheets/ (accessed 29 June 2012).

Vaughan, M. 1991. *Curing Their Ills: Colonial Power and African Illness*. Palo Alto, CA: Stanford University Press.

Whyte, S., M. Whyte, L. Meinert and B. Kyaddondo. 2004. 'Treating AIDS: dilemmas of unequal access in Uganda', *Journal of Social Aspects of HIV/AIDS Research Alliance* 1(1): 14–26.

Whyte, S.R., M.A. Whyte and D. Kyaddondo. 2010. 'Health workers entangled: confidentiality and certification', in H. Dilger and U. Luig (eds), *Morality, Hope and Grief: Anthropologies of AIDS in Africa*. New York: Berghahn Books, 80–101.

Whyte, S.R., M.A. Whyte, L. Meinert and J. Twebaze. 2013. 'Therapeutic clientship: belonging in Uganda's projectified landscape of AIDS care', in J. Biehl and A. Petryna (eds), *When People Come First: Critical Studies in Global Health.* Princeton, NJ: Princeton University Press, 140–65.

8

Contested Sexualities and Shared Concerns

Power Dynamics in a Transnational Network of Faith-Based Organisations

BRENDA BARTELINK AND ERIK MEINEMA

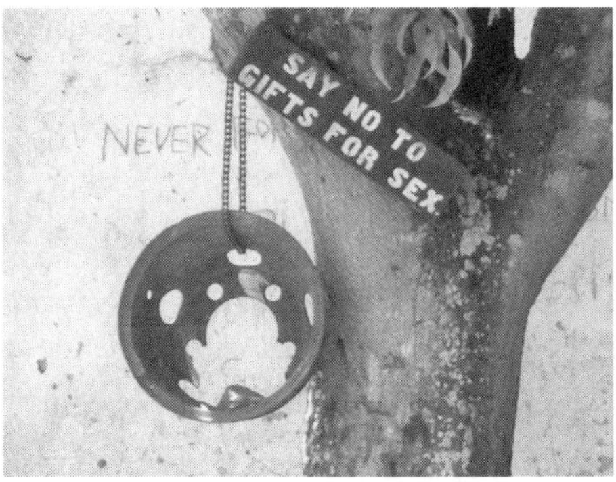

Poster just outside Kampala, Uganda, 2010 (photo by Erik Meinema)

Introduction

THIS CHAPTER FOCUSES ON HOW DIFFERENT VIEWS ON SEXUALITY are discussed, contested and negotiated in transnational networks of faith-based development organisations in East Africa and the Netherlands. HIV/AIDS has presented an opportunity for religious organisations in particular to take a more prominent role in the public sphere (see Chapter 1, this volume, p. 2). Faith-based organisations (FBOs) especially have been criticised for having a condemning attitude on sexual activity among youth. However, we argue in this chapter that the 'moralisation of AIDS and sexuality' in Africa is not only influenced by African FBOs, but also by Dutch FBOs.

In spite of their faith-based background, Dutch FBOs' understandings of sexuality and African youth are predominantly framed in a secular, liberal discourse focused on health and individual rights. Taking the Educaids network as an example, contestations over sex education seem to be demonstrating the stereotypical liberal-conservative divides that have been dominating the discourse on religion and HIV/AIDS. However, what we intend to show here is how a narrow focus on this divide among actors in the Educaids network, as well as in the wider debate, ignores the complexities of views and agendas negotiated among FBOs transnationally.

The basis of this chapter is an empirical study of the Educaids network. The Educaids network is a Christian Alliance for HIV and Education, which was initiated by Dutch development organisations to integrate prevention of HIV/AIDS in formal and informal education among partner organisations in four East African countries. Our focus is on the Shareframe project. The Shareframe project was carried out between 2008 and 2010, and comprised a series of workshops in which FBOs in Kenya and Uganda were trained in developing evidence-based sex education policies and programmes. The central questions answered in this chapter are: (1) Which understandings of sexuality are expressed by FBOs in the Educaids network? (2) How do actors in the Educaids network deal with different or colliding perspectives on sexuality and prevention of HIV/AIDS? (3) Which forums or practices prevail in the transnational network of Educaids?

Empirical data to answer these questions have been gathered in the Netherlands, Uganda and Kenya. Interviews with Dutch organisations were held in 2008 and 2009. In 2009 we stayed in Uganda for a month to do participant observation in a workshop on sexual and reproductive health and rights organised by the Educaids network (Shareframe), to visit organisations, and do interviews with the workshop participants. In 2010 the Educaids organisations in Uganda and Kenya were visited again. Over a period of four months at least two employees of each organisation were interviewed, and a total of twenty focus group discussions and additional interviews were held with young people in the target groups of every Educaids organisation. In addition Educaids texts and policy documents were analysed.

We will start this chapter with an introduction to the Educaids network, followed by an explanation of the concepts and theoretical notions we draw upon in linking the Educaids network to the wider debates on religion, sexuality and transnationalism. In the next two sections we explain the understandings of sexuality and sex education that prevail in Dutch and Ugandan/Kenyan FBOs. We then reflect on the contestations over the liberal approach to sex education introduced in the Shareframe project, and conclude with a reflection on the role of practice as a way to solve or overcome these differences within the Educaids network.

Introducing the Educaids network

The Educaids network was initiated after a conference in the Netherlands on education and HIV/AIDS in 2004. The conference was organised by three Dutch development organisations with a Protestant Christian identity: ICCO (Dutch Interchurch Organisation for Development Cooperation), Edukans (Organisation for Education and Development) and Prisma (Association for Christian Organisations in Development and Diaconate). The extent to which they identify as a Christian organisation, and how this impacts on their work, differs, ranging from liberal to orthodox Protestant. The liberal Christian perspective on development embraced by ICCO has been criticised by Prisma member organisations in the past (interview with employee of Prisma member organisation). However, recently, these Protestant Christian development organisations in the Netherlands have started cooperating and building alliances. In addition, the organisations have historically differed in their approaches to development cooperation and how they access funds.

Many of the small conservative Christian member organisations of Prisma access funds through their loyal Christian constituencies in the Netherlands. ICCO, on the other hand, was established by the mainstream Protestant churches in the Netherlands to access funding from the Dutch government in the 1960s (Bos and Prince 2000). Edukans was also founded as a result of the foreign activities of the mainstream Protestant churches. Their work is based on relations between Dutch Christian schools and Christian schools in developing countries; school actions also provide part of their funds. ICCO, Prisma and Edukans organised themselves in the ICCO alliance in 2005, together with a few smaller development organisations. In 2012 the three organisations merged their activities into the so-called 'ICCO cooperation'.

These decisions were made against the background of changes in the co-financing system of Dutch government. New requirements that have arisen in the past decade include the demand for NGOs to have support from Dutch constituencies and access to private funding in order to be eligible for government funding. The ICCO alliance was (at least partially) a strategic move to meet these new requirements. In 2004 the Educaids network was still an independent initiative; however over the years Educaids became part of the education programme of the ICCO alliance. Until early in the new millennium, ICCO, Prisma and Edukans all worked primarily through their own transnational networks of partner organisations in developing countries. The Educaids network was set up to improve the quality of HIV/AIDS education in the education programmes of partner organisations in four countries: Ethiopia, Malawi, Kenya and Uganda.

Our focus in this chapter is on the Educaids networks in Kenya and Uganda, in which predominantly ICCO and Edukans partners are involved, with only a few Prisma partner organisations being part of the network. A majority of these partner organisations are faith-based organisations, comprising non-governmental organisations with a religious identity as well as education departments of churches. At the time of our research, the Educaids networks' activities were primarily focused on training partner organisations in developing sexual and reproductive health and rights (SRHR) policies and programmes based on a public health and human rights approach. This was done through the Shareframe project that was carried out between 2008 and 2010, and is the primary focus of this chapter.

Positioning the Educaids network in the transnational social field of development

Discussions on sexuality in the Shareframe project focused on abstinence and condom use as preferred methods of prevention of HIV/AIDS. These discussions were characterised by conflicting understandings on sex education and approaches to the sexuality of youth between Ugandan/Kenyan FBOs and Dutch FBOs. However, at the same time, we have also been surprised by the creative solutions to deal with these colliding viewpoints. We aim to understand these creative solutions using theoretical notions that focus on the active role people play in making sense of and negotiating social reality.

Social life is heterogeneous and comprises a wide diversity of cultural repertoires. Different cultural repertoires are mediated, transformed and perpetuated at critical points of linkage or confrontation. These 'social interfaces', as Norman Long (2001) calls them, require some degree of common interest between the actors. However, they are also characterised by contradictory social interests and unequal power relations. Long argues that all actors should be seen as active participants who process information and strategise in their dealings with others, despite unequal power relations. Large-scale powerful social forces can only influence actors when they are transformed and mediated by these actors themselves.

At the same time, however, the critical points of linkage and confrontation are increasingly situated in a transnational context in which not all actors meet each other physically, but do exercise (discursive) influence on how views on sexuality are shaped. In the Educaids network, for example, Dutch actors have a large influence in setting the agenda for the network and determining the parameters for the sex education programmes carried out by their partners. Conceptualising development cooperation as a 'transnational social field', the Educaids network should be seen as a network in which discourses and capital are transferred and negotiated (Glick Schiller 2005). The relations between actors in this transnational social field are shaped by both conflicting and shared concerns.

The transnational social field of development has become 'one of the most pervasive, influential, and mundane areas in which sexuality is at issue' (Adams and Pigg 2005: II). Non-governmental organisations are among those actors that exercise a strong influence on how sexuality is shaped discursively. Dutch organisations in general hold a liberal view on sexuality in which free choice is emphasised. As Mepschen *et al.* (2010) have argued, this must be seen against a background in which sexual freedom has come to represent a liberated modernity against religious tradition in Dutch society itself. Notwithstanding their faith background or identity, the Dutch organisations that have established the Educaids network have mainly operated along the lines of this secular, liberal discourse on sexuality and modernity, as we will show in our analysis of the Shareframe project.

The views on sexuality held by their Ugandan and Kenyan partner organisations are shaped by their faith-based identity as Christian NGOs and education departments of churches. It is well known that many FBOs working on HIV/AIDS and sex education in Africa view sexuality within a 'conservative' moral, religious framework, resulting for example in them resisting the promotion of condom use (Chikwendu 2004; Tiendrebogo and Buyckx 2004; Parasitau 2009; Gusman 2009; Prince *et al.* 2009). The room for manoeuvre to develop more progressive policies and practices on sex education within these FBOs is influenced by internal power hierarchies, as well as by the (faith) context in which they operate.

The social interface of the Educaids network is thus characterised by conflicting conceptualisations of what sex education should be about among the Dutch and African FBOs involved. In addition, the Educaids network's transnationalism also involves different claims to power based on an unequal access to capital (Bourdieu 1986). The transfer of cultural capital (training) and economic capital (funding) from Dutch organisations to their Ugandan and Kenyan partners brings up the question of how definitions of 'good sex education' are negotiated in the context of power within the Shareframe project. However, as power is always relational, the cultural and symbolic capital that Ugandan and Kenyan FBOs exercise in the Educaids network needs to be taken into account as well.

Dutch organisations depend upon their FBO partners in Uganda and Kenya to realise their mission to improve the quality of HIV/AIDS prevention and sex education in schools. This gives Kenyan and Ugandan FBOs a power basis within the Educaids network that is closely linked to their faith-based identity. Churches and FBOs are important providers of education in both Kenya and Uganda. Moreover, Dutch organisations want to promote a more open and liberal approach to the sexuality of young people among their faith-based partners. This change can best be realised when working with precisely these FBOs who tend to promote a more conservative view on the sexuality of young people.

A third aspect of the power claims of Ugandan and Kenyan FBOs in the Educaids network is their access to the symbolic capital vested in their religious identities. Liberal Dutch FBOs (including ICCO and to some extent Edukans) have been influenced by a trend of secularisation since the 1970s. Since the late 1990s, this has influenced new religious identifications within these organisations, which got a new impetus when the competition over development funds from the Dutch government increased early in the new millennium. Dutch FBOs affirmed the importance of the role of religion for development cooperation and started to identify more strongly with their religious background by articulating partnerships with FBOs in the South (Ter Haar and Ellis 2006; Bartelink and Buitelaar 2006;

Bartelink 2009). When the Educaids network was initiated in 2005, a Knowledge Forum on Religion and Development Policy and a Knowledge Center on Religion and Development were established as well. These latter initiatives signpost an increased interest in the role of religion in development in Dutch development discourses. Like other initiatives of that kind, these have been criticised for adopting a rather narrow and instrumental focus on FBOs, as Jones and Petersen (2011) have argued.

ICCO employee Lisette van der Wel explains that Dutch FBOs tried to find an answer to the problem of staying connected to their international Christian networks (2011: 348). Van der Wel, however, points to another problem as well: Dutch FBOs also had to find ways to remain true to their Christian roots. In our view, the Educaids network responds to both problems. It connects Dutch FBOs actively to their Christian networks and offers them the possibility to affirm their religious identities through the symbolic capital of FBOs in Kenya and Uganda. In other words, the connection with a Christian network made these organisations more 'true' in their Christian identification. This provided Ugandan and Kenyan FBOs with a power basis *vis-à-vis* the Dutch FBOs in the context of the Educaids network.

Explaining Educaids' secular, liberal approach to sexuality

HIV/AIDS had become a key priority in the development policies of Dutch FBOs in the 1990s. In the new millennium these FBOs became concerned with how their faith-based partners in developing countries provided sex education (Marijnis and Ooijens 2009). While Dutch FBOs knew or expected that their partner organisations would focus primarily or exclusively on abstinence-only messages when providing sex education, they found it difficult to initiate an open discussion about sexuality with their partner FBOs:

> Let's be honest, we discovered that partners didn't work along the policies we put on paper. We are in favour of the ABC approach and what can we do if only abstinence-only messages are given [by our partners].
>
> (Interview, Educaids coordinator, May 2009)

In the ABC approach, (A)bstinence, (B)eing faithful and using (C)ondoms are presented as three equal ways to prevent SRHR problems from which youth can choose for themselves. The comprehensive sex education promoted by Dutch FBOs also includes attention to broader issues such as gender equality and respect for sexual diversity. The central emphasis on conscious and free choice, including for young people, in the ABC approach points at a specific liberal morality on sexuality that the Dutch organisations aim to introduce and promote.

In an attempt to prevent any moral disputes, Dutch FBOs in the Educaids network also referred to comprehensive sex education as a 'neutral', 'evidence-based approach'. This neutrality was highlighted by contrasting it with a 'value-based approach', which referred to sex education based on biblical values (Marijnis and Ooijens 2009). The suggestion that an evidence-based approach is more neutral than a value-based approach is problematic. Adams and Pigg (2005) argue that a scientific view on sexuality is not neutral but makes specific moral claims as well. It claims that science offers better explanations than traditional accounts of sexual health, and produces an idea of a rational individual who is responsible for his/her own sexual behaviour and therefore also for changing this behaviour when it is unhealthy (ibid.: 27).

When the terms 'comprehensive approach' and 'evidence-based approach' were used by Dutch organisations within the Educaids network, they both referred to a liberal understanding of sexuality. In this understanding of sexuality, sex education contributes to improving the knowledge and skills of individual (young) people so that they can make informed decisions in order to ensure or improve their sexual health. Thus, the emphasis on comprehensive and evidence-based approaches within the Educaids network referred to a specific morality that was introduced.

Understanding 'conservatism' among Kenyan and Ugandan FBOs

Kenyan and Ugandan Educaids partners expressed their view that abstinence is the best way for youth to protect themselves against SRHR problems. A staff worker from ZOA, the Ugandan branch of the refugee organisation that is a member of the Educaids network, explained: 'As a Christian organisation, we support Christian values. This means that we promote abstinence amongst the youth.' In their communications aimed at unmarried youth, many of the Kenyan and Ugandan partners tried to convince unmarried young people that abstinence was the best choice. Abstinence messages were often phrased in religious language. For example, during an interview, an employee of CEREDO (Catholic Education and Research Development Organization) mentioned: 'The message we give is abstinence. There is a right time for everything. First you go to school, then after university you find the woman you love [and marry her].' In using the expression 'There is a right time for everything', the interviewee is echoing the words of the Bible in Ecclesiastes (3:1–15). Thus, sexuality is connected to a specific time or phase in life, the phase of marriage. With this kind of message the staff worker tells young people that they can enjoy sex the 'right' way (only) within marriage. Similarly, an employee of an education department of the Church of Uganda (COU) in Soroti diocese explained that Bible teachings on sexuality within marriage can be compared with the 'manual of a car' which informs people how to properly operate the car in practice.

FBOs often combined religious arguments such as the ones above with health arguments when they advocated abstinence to unmarried youth. During a group discussion with a fieldworker and peer educators of the YWCA in the slums of Kampala, the fieldworker argued: 'Youth won't be able to use condoms consistently, so it's better to abstain.' Another fieldworker from the YWCA claimed that youth often forget to check the expiry date of condoms before they have sex. By arguing that using condoms in this way increases the risk of sexual health problems, abstinence is presented as a better option. A third argument we heard was the lack of availability of condoms in rural areas. Such health arguments often served the purpose of making the choice of abstinence more attractive to the youth.

Whether or not to educate on condoms is a subject of internal discussion in the FBOs that participate in the Educaids network. There are two important reasons for this. First of all, many Kenyan and Ugandan FBOs fear that by distributing information or handing out condoms they will be giving youth the opportunity to engage in sexual behaviour without consequences. Because sexual intercourse outside of marriage is seen as sinful and immoral, condom education is viewed as promoting promiscuity. While this argument is found among the FBOs in the Educaids networks, some secular organisations do follow similar lines of argumentation. This can be illustrated by the comments of a male, middle-aged fieldworker from the secular NGO Health Need Uganda (HNU): 'Culturally and traditionally we believe that [. . .] everyone is supposed to abstain or delay their time of debut of sexual intercourse. At HNU that is something that we also would want to uphold' (March 2010). Moreover, he emphasised that although HNU is a secular NGO, many of its employees are Christians. These comments clearly show that the ideal of abstinence is not limited to Christian communities and organisations, but shared by a broader public (Epstein 2005, 2007; Ibembe 2008; Kuhanen 2008). This draws into question the association between religion and conservativeness in secular, liberal discourses on sexuality.

Second, depending on where they work, organisations need to be conscious about the communities they work with. Their work is possible because of the support of churches, schools, teachers and parents. When communities oppose education about condom use, this threatens the credibility of an organisation. Because Educaids organisations need the cooperation of teachers, parents, churches and communities to execute their education programmes, the emphasis on abstinence is strategic, as well as religious. In a private meeting with the Dutch Educaids trainer that we observed, a researcher working with YWCA argued that parents do not want to recognise that their children are sexually active because 'that feels for them like they encourage their children. So that is why they look up to YWCA and expect us to use the fear-based approach.' This researcher felt that parents expected YWCA to warn youth that they can get infected with HIV/AIDS if they engage in sex, as opposed to teaching them about sexuality as positive and pleasurable (Fieldwork report, Kampala, March 2009).

Another example is related to the observation that many Kenyan and Ugandan Educaids partners execute their sex education programmes in public schools with the approval and in the presence of the teachers. Organisations are not allowed to distribute condoms in high schools, or talk about anything but abstinence in primary schools, for example (Fieldwork report, HNU, March 2009). In other words, it is not only the religious morality of FBOs that influences how sex education is given in school; it is also influenced by many other factors including governmental policies, school regulations and expectations people have of FBOs.

FBOs are often seen as a homogeneous category, in particular when presenting them as instruments in realising conservative approaches to sex education and prevention of HIV/AIDS. However, differences between FBOs do influence the available room for manoeuvre to change or stretch conservative approaches. Church-based organisations generally cannot deviate from the official positions of their church on matters related to sexuality. In a meeting between an Educaids trainer and church-based organisations, employees of CEREDO and COU quoted church policy documents on abstinence and condom use. They explained that only a pastoral letter from the bishop would allow them to take a comprehensive approach to sex education.

Ugandan FBOs with a closer link to the church or a strong faith-based identity were more often keen on working in line with the official policies of the churches. This created diversity among FBOs that were not church-based, and influenced their space for manoeuvre on controversial issues such as condom education. Secular organisations have the freedom to include condom education and administration in their sexual and reproductive health and rights policies. However, this does not mean that secular organisations in Uganda and Kenya share the liberal view on sexuality with their Dutch partners; the HNU employee who argued that his organisation wanted to uphold certain values as well is a case in point.

In this section we have argued that FBOs often combine religious and secular health arguments in their promotion of abstinence before marriage. However, conservatism is influenced by many contextual factors, too. Moreover, FBOs differ in their strategies and room for manoeuvre to stretch or change conservative approaches. The example above of a locally based secular health NGO shows that they are embedded in the same field of forces and not necessarily embracing a secular, liberal approach to sexuality.

Contestations over sex education in the Shareframe project

That liberal and conservative approaches to sex education are never static, but always open for adaptation to local circumstances, can be seen by looking at the practices of transnational cooperation in the Educaids network. A focus on the transnational transfer of views and techniques provides insights into how these views and techniques are appropriated within the local FBO context and dynamic.

The Shareframe project was a series of three workshops in which two staff members of the African organisations were trained in developing a comprehensive SRHR policy for their organisation. The workshops were organised independently in Kenya and Uganda, and each hosted by a different Educaids member in their town of residence. We observed the third workshop held in Lira, Uganda. The workshop brought together around twenty participants with two trainers from the Netherlands. The staff members of Ugandan Educaids organisations were usually lower-level, technical professionals trained as health workers or teachers. This was particularly the case for Church organisations. A representative of the management sometimes also represented the smaller and less hierarchically organised FBOs. Two of them were also ordained priests/ministers. All participants had in common that they worked on the level of implementing policies in projects, giving sex education themselves or working directly with teachers and educators in the communities.

As an example of social techniques that travel along transnational paths, the Shareframe project transferred liberal and human rights-based understandings of (young people's) sexuality through a series of techniques based on a scientific understanding of sexuality from the Netherlands to the Ugandan/Kenyan organisations in the Educaids network. Participants were literally called upon to 'break the silence' and start an open conversation about sexuality in the first workshop (Chapter 1, this volume, p. 18). The trainers asked them to name body parts associated with sex, and mention all the types of sexual acts they could think of. One of the participants later recalled that she was shocked that the trainers were so blunt in discussing these issues during this first workshop (interview participant, March 2009).

In addition to talking about sexuality, participants were also trained in reviewing scientific data about sex and HIV/AIDS. The second workshop focused on training participants in a series of research techniques that were used to talk about sexuality to young people themselves. This again involved an open conversation about sexuality, but this time with the young people in the target groups of the FBOs themselves. Participants were discouraged from introducing any of their own understandings of sexuality and supposed to listen to young people themselves. The new research skills were used to gather data about young people's views on sexuality that would be discussed in the third workshop. In this workshop the scientific evidence was used to write a sexual and reproductive health and rights policy. Initially the aim was to develop one shared SRHR policy for all Ugandan/Kenyan Educaids organisations that could be used as a basis for joint programmes and for lobbying and advocacy. In the course of the Shareframe project this aim changed into developing SRHR policies for each organisation.

The policies had to meet several requirements, among which were the following: policies were required to explain how the organisation would offer choices to young people regarding their sexual health. A reference to the ABCDEF+ approach to sex education in the policy document was required. The abbreviation refers to

Abstinence, Be faithful, Condom use, Delay of sexual debut, Equal relations between men and women, Fewer partners + an HIV test. This ABCDEF+ approach of comprehensive sex education thus also includes gender equality and the importance of HIV testing in marriage or steady relationships. In addition, the policy documents were required to explain how the organisation was dealing with sensitive issues such as pre-marital sex, contraception, masturbation, and sex between people of the same sex (PowerPoint presentation by Dutch coordinator, Shareframe workshop 3, March 2009).

These requirements for the SRHR policies show that the Shareframe project can be seen as an attempt by Dutch organisations to change the policies and approaches of Ugandan/Kenyan FBOs from a more conservative to a more liberal, evidence-based policy on SRHR. This is also confirmed by the text on the Educaids website:

> Effective education on sexuality has to be comprehensive, which means that no sensitive issues should be left out (intentionally or non-intentionally). In such Comprehensive Sexuality Education (CSE), the curriculum is based on academically developed theory and practical research evidence.
>
> (www.educaids.nl – under mission/vision, comprehensive sexuality education)

The earlier quote from the Educaids coordinator (see p. 160) illustrated that the Shareframe project was intended to introduce a more liberal alternative to conservative approaches to sexuality education that focus on abstinence education for unmarried youth. The quote shows that this alternative is comprehensive sex education based on scientific theory and research evidence. This shows that Shareframe was focused on achieving a liberal approach to sex education.

The workshops followed a specific methodology that limited the room for discussion on mutual understandings of sexuality and sex education for young people. Instead some of the discussions focused on the 'evidence-based' methodology of the Shareframe project. Initially participants were sceptical about this new approach. One of the participants who was an Anglican pastor stated that 'evidence can only be found in the Bible' (interview, Shareframe trainer, March 2009). In interviews, several participants expressed criticism of the Western liberal perspective introduced in the Shareframe project. One participant pointed at the 'disintegration of this practice [of marriage] because of Western culture' (interview informant, March 2010). A few other participants phrased this opposition against the far-reaching implications of Western liberalism in terms of a resistance against an imposed acceptance of homosexuality:

> No that cannot be, we do not go against the values we stand for. We are not going to advocate for homosexuality and masturbation, we are going to go out and condemn homosexuality and there is no question about that.
>
> (interview participant, Uganda, March 2009)

Notwithstanding the contestations, this reference to homosexuality as a symbol of the immorality of Western liberalism mainly served as a boundary marker within the Educaids network. Practices in these organisations show that Ugandan and Kenyan FBOs were willing to change their views on sex education, although within limitations.

Conservative rhetoric meets pragmatic practices

Despite the critical views on condom education expressed in the Shareframe project, in practice the FBOs in the Educaids network turned out to be more pragmatic. Even though some organisations were reluctant to give education on condom use, we have not visited one organisation that did not give any information about condoms at all. While the abstinence message is a dominant message used by the Kenyan and Ugandan FBOs in the Educaids network, this does not mean that they feel that abstinence should be the only message. Many staff members of the Educaids organisations in Uganda and Kenya we have talked to also wanted to give youth more options to protect themselves, and recognised that for some young people condoms may be the only way to prevent HIV.

This is exemplified by the comments of a male fieldworker from the secular NGO HNU on condom use. This fieldworker referred to education on condoms as teaching youth on 'disaster preparedness', implying that condom use is only allowed in case 'the disaster' of pre-marital sex is already taking place. Using a similar argument, a fieldworker from RAPADO, operating in Lira, Uganda, argued that 'it is better to have alive sinners than dead sinners', meaning that it is better to save lives by using condoms than let people die because having sex is sinful. Finally, an employee of ZOA in Pader (northern Uganda) explained that, being aware that young people are sexually active, she wanted to provide information on condom use, even though she considered herself sinful for going against Christian values.

Thus, the conservative understandings of sex education that were expressed in the Shareframe workshop turned out to be more flexible in the views and opinions of individual staff members. This flexibility and pragmatism was also demonstrated at the organisational level. While many organisations reject condom use in official policies, or focus strongly on abstinence until marriage, professionals were thus seeking ways to ensure comprehensive sex education without policy change. A good example of this can be found in Soroti, Uganda, where three Educaids organisations have a joint sex education programme. Two of them, COU (Church of Uganda) and CEREDO, are church-based, and the third one, HNU, is a secular NGO.

COU and CEREDO do not promote condom use. This is against the Christian morals of the church, and the church hierarchy in which these organisations are embedded does not allow comprehensive sex education policies. Yet, the professional staff employed within CEREDO and COU realise that it is necessary to give full information on HIV prevention to youth, and achieve this by drawing on the secular organisation HNU to deliver those parts of the programme that their own church prohibits. They rely on HNU to provide information on condom use, while they explain church ideals of abstinence before marriage. The successful cooperation between the three parties has been acknowledged, as the three organisations were selected for a follow-up training in sex education interventions after the Shareframe project ended.

While this kind of cooperation is unusual, other FBOs cooperated with third parties such as government health centres in order to ensure education about condom use for young people. These pragmatic coalitions enabled FBOs and their staff to develop their own strategies to make an open dialogue about condom use possible, without adjusting their organisational policies. As one of our Ugandan informants said: 'the church is eternal and should not give up morals to solve problems that are only temporary'. However, flexibility in practice does not necessarily jeopardise the moral power which FBOs and churches exercise in the communities, while officially embracing a comprehensive approach does.

Ugandan and Kenyan FBOs did not work exclusively according to the 'value-based' approach that was described by Marijnis (2009). However they repeatedly voiced strong reactions against (aspects of) the Dutch FBOs' liberal understanding of sexuality in the Shareframe workshops. The earlier quoted resistance against homosexuality is a case in point. In addition, we have observed many discussions on whether or not to include information on condom use in sex education, as well as on the risks of positively promoting sex to young people when talking about sexuality in an open, choice-oriented manner. Given the flexibility of individual FBO staff and the pragmatic solutions organisations had found in practice, these strong reactions may be seen as rhetorical. In our view, this rhetoric must be understood in relation to the transnational power dynamic. An experience of 'pressure' from Dutch donor organisations that wanted the Kenyan and Ugandan organisations to use the comprehensive approach invoked strong reactions. While the economic capital of Dutch organisations is needed to be able to carry out projects, Ugandan organisations tried to limit the influence of Dutch organisations by taking strong ideological positions.

Taking a conservative position served as a boundary marker within the Educaids network, limiting the power of Dutch organisations to influence the policies and practices of Ugandan and Kenyan FBOs. In addition, criticism of the liberal perspective introduced in the Shareframe workshop often underlined the importance of religious authority, highlighting the cultural and symbolic capital of FBOs in Uganda and Kenya. An analysis of the precise transnational linkages of the Educaids network shows that conservative and liberal agendas and their contestations are entangled in the transnational social field of development. Which forum prevails is to a large extent influenced by the power relations between different actors. However, as we will show in the final section, while on the policy level these conflicting agendas are affirmed, everyday practices tend to be more flexible.

The power of practice in the transnational Educaids network

The fact that all FBOs do give some information on condom use, even when they tend to emphasise abstinence, shows that practices tend to be more flexible than policy discussions suggest. These observations speak to Mosse's argument about how policy relates to practice as a model that legitimises political support and action, but does not determine practice. Instead, policies tend to be 'ignored, resisted, "consumed" or tactically used in ways that make them irrelevant in the face of more relational demands', as discussed by Mosse (2005: 16). In this section, we will show how an analysis of the practice of transnational cooperation provides us with a novel perspective on the contestations over conservative and liberal understandings of sex education.

Despite the critique of the liberal approach to sexuality in the Shareframe project, the training, in discussing sex openly with young people, also became an important new experience for the participants. In the interviews, participants from the Ugandan and Kenyan FBOs described their experiences in interviewing young people about sexuality as impressive, confrontational and 'eye opening' (interviewee, Child Restoration Outreach, Mukono, Uganda, March 2009). Conducting the research among young people created a shared concern with their sexual health among Dutch, Kenyan and Ugandan organisations in the Educaids network. Another interviewee said: 'We live in this community but we did not know that children have misconceptions on contraceptive use. We did not know until I carried out the needs assessment. To me that was enlightenment' (interviewee, ZOA, Pader, March 2009).

A concern with the influence of sexual violence, force, transactional sex and peer pressure motivated a more open attitude towards the comprehensive approach. Against the background of these examples, it was more acceptable for Ugandan participants in the Shareframe project to emphasise choice in situations of force. One of the arguments we came across in the Shareframe workshop was that:

> we should realise not everyone is Christian or lives according to Christian values. We have to decide on how we can help people. If we become very fundamentalist [silence, indicating that fundamentalism is not a preferred response] it is still important for us to take such decisions.
>
> (Shareframe workshop, March 2009)

We also mentioned earlier how condom education was acceptable as a form of disaster preparedness. This genuine concern about young people's sexual health opened up a new space for pragmatic solutions despite the moral contestations within the Educaids network. It provided these participants with examples of situations in which abstinence was not an option. In addition, it motivated professionals working in FBOs to include sensitive issues, such as giving information on condoms in one way or the other.

Dutch organisations in the Educaids network, in turn, acknowledged these strategies and the room for manoeuvre that these Ugandan and Kenyan partners had created. This also meant that they had to leave behind their initial goal, which was focused on developing human rights-based SRHR policies for each organisation. During the Shareframe project it became clear that for church-based organisations in particular, it was not feasible to hold on to this aim, because their policies were developed by religious clergy and implemented top-down. The Shareframe project, however, focused on the technical staff in the lower hierarchy of the organisations who were (usually) not able to change organisational policies. The Dutch FBOs thus suggested that organisations could write work plans to be used by the technical staff, rather than trying to get an official sex education policy accepted within their organisations. The work plans had to meet the requirements described above, but were not expected to be officially approved by higher management and policy makers in the organisation.

We have mentioned before that Dutch and African organisations need one another. This provides all actors in the Educaids network with a power basis. Ugandan and Kenyan FBOs connect Dutch donor FBOs with young people whose sexual health needs to be improved. Moreover, Dutch FBOs draw upon the symbolic capital (the religious identity and authority) of Ugandan and Kenyan FBOs. This gives them credibility in the Kenyan and Ugandan communities where projects are carried out, but it also provides them with the opportunity to strengthen their own faith-based identity in the Netherlands.

Ugandan and Kenyan FBOs, in turn, need the Dutch donor FBOs in order to access their economic and cultural capital. Their involvement in the transnational network of Educaids provides them with opportunities for funding and training. This allows Dutch FBOs to influence their policies and practices. Their power basis described above allows them to mark out the boundaries of this influence and creates room for agency and a flexible interpretation of the demands of Dutch donor FBOs.

The example of the Educaids network illustrates that transnational cooperation between FBOs on sex education cannot be explained in terms of contestations over liberal and conservative approaches to sex education only. A multi-sited fieldwork approach (Marcus 1995) is needed to understand how contestations over liberal and conservative approaches to sexuality are influenced by practice and vice versa. Our analysis illustrates that experiences of (and difficulties with) transnational cooperation are framed in terms of liberal-conservative divides, while actors at the same time exchange capital and share concerns.

A practice perspective on the Educaids network also sheds light on how development policies are produced through practical forms of transnational cooperation, rather than the other way round. In line with Mosse's argument about the relation between policy and practice, SRHR policies served as a 'metaphor' rather than as a fixed outcome of the Shareframe project (Mosse 2005). The Shareframe project created, first and foremost, a relationship of trust between Dutch organisations and their FBO partners in Kenya and Uganda. Instead of a full-fledged SRHR policy, Dutch donor FBOs accepted a work plan which explained how Ugandan and Kenyan FBOs ensured comprehensive sex education. Thus the case presented in this chapter illustrates that coherence of transnational development practice is achieved through relationships rather than through the implementation of policies (Mosse 2005).

Conclusion

In this chapter we have analysed how understandings of sexuality and sex education for young, unmarried people are contested and put into practice in the transnational social field of development. We have argued that contestations over sexuality and the strategies employed to overcome these contestations are based on conflicting power claims and shared concerns. This argument is based on a case study on the Educaids network, a transnational network of Dutch and East African faith-based organisations that aims to improve the quality of HIV/AIDS prevention education. The positioning of Dutch and African actors on sexuality is often understood in terms of a conservative/liberal and religious/secular opposition. However, the practice of transnational cooperation shows that common grounds are found as well. The pragmatic common ground that was found between Dutch and Ugandan FBOs involved a more comprehensive approach to sex education for Ugandan FBOs (including condom education and referral to a secular health organisation) and a compromise with regard to the aim of developing a comprehensive SRHR policy on the side of the Dutch FBOs. This was motivated by shared concerns with young people's sexual health problems, but must also be understood against the background of the specific power sources which Dutch and African FBOs bring to the network. The overall argument in this chapter is that a narrow focus on colliding liberal and conservative understandings of sexuality does not contribute to a better understanding of the complex nature of transnational linkages between FBOs around sexuality and HIV/AIDS. Instead, a practice perspective makes clear how contestations over conservative and liberal approaches serve the purpose of establishing and renewing relationships between Dutch FBOs and their partner FBOs in Africa.

Acknowledgements

The authors thank Anna Booij for her contribution to the data collection, Marjo Buitelaar for her inspiring and enriching reviews of this chapter at several stages of the writing process, and Pieter Nanninga for his comments on earlier versions of this chapter.

References

Adams, V. and S. Pigg. 2005. *Sex in Development: Science, Sexuality and Morality in Global Perspective*. Durham, NC: Duke University Press.

Bartelink, B.E. 2009. 'The devil's advocate. A religious studies perspective on Dutch discourses on religion and development', in C. de Pater and I. Dankelman (eds), *Proceedings of the Conference on Religious Studies and Theology Exploring Sustainable Development: Challenges for Higher Education Nijmegen*. Nijmegen Studies in Development and Cultural Change. Münster: Lit Verlag, 169–79.

Bartelink, B.E. and M.W. Buitelaar. 2006. 'The challenges of incorporating Muslim women's views into development policy: analysis of a Dutch action research project in Yemen', *Gender and Development* 14(3): 351–62.

Bos, J. and G.H.A. Prince (2000) 'Partners in development. Development work by church and other non-governmental organisations in the early days', in J.A. Nekkers and P.A.M. Malcontent (eds), *Fifty Years of Dutch Development Cooperation 1949–1999*. The Hague: Sdu Publishers.

Bourdieu, P. 1986. 'The forms of capital', in J.E. Richardson (ed.), *Handbook of Theory of Research for the Sociology of Education*. New York: Greenwood Press, 241–58.

Chikwendu, E. 2004. 'Faith based organisations in anti-HIV/AIDS work among African youth and women', *Dialectical Anthropology* 28(3/4): 307–27.

Dilger, H. 2009. 'Doing better? Religion, the virtue-ethics of development, and the fragmentation of health politics in Tanzania', *Africa Today* 56(1): 89–110.

Epstein, H. 2005. 'God and the fight against Aids', *New York Review of Books* 52(7): 47–50.

Epstein, H. 2007. *The Invisible Cure: Africa, the West and the Fight against AIDS*. New York: Farrar, Straus and Giroux.

Glick Schiller, N. 2005. 'Transnational social fields and imperialism: bringing a theory of power to Transnational Studies', *Anthropological Theory* 5: 439–61.

Gusman, A. 2009. 'HIV/AIDS, Pentecostal churches, and the "Joseph Generation" in Uganda', *Africa Today* 56(1): 67–86.

Ibembe, P. 2008. 'The evolution of the ABC strategy of HIV prevention in Uganda: state and international impact on public health', in C. Pope, R.T. White and R. Malow (eds), *HIV/AIDS: Global Frontiers in Prevention/Intervention*. New York: Routledge.

Jones, B. and M. Juul Petersen. 2011. 'Instrumental, narrow, normative? Reviewing recent work on religion and development', *Third World Quarterly* 32(7): 1291–306.

Kuhanen, J. 2008. 'The historiography of HIV and Aids in Uganda', *History in Africa* 35: 301–25.

Long, N. 2001. *Development Sociology: Actor Perspectives*. London: Routledge.

Marcus, G.E. 1995. 'Ethnography in/of the world system: the emergence of multi-sited ethnography', *Annual Review of Anthropology* 24: 95–117.

Marijnis, M. and M. Ooijens. 2009. 'The involvement of religious institutions in promoting sexual and reproductive health and rights in education', in B.E. Bartelink and U. Pape (eds), *Political, Social and Religious Dimensions in the Fight against HIV/AIDS: Negotiating Worldviews, Facing Practical Challenges*. Groningen: CDS Research Report no. 28, 167– 84.

Mepschen, P., J.W. Duyvendak and E.W. Tonkens. 2010. 'Sexual politics, orientalism and multicultural citizenship in the Netherlands', *Sociology* 44(5): 962–79.

Mosse, D. 2005. *Cultivating Development: An Ethnography of Aid Policy and Practice*. London: Pluto Press.

Parasitau, D. 2009. '"Keep holy distance and abstain till he comes": interrogating a Pentecostal church's engagements with HIV/AIDS and the youth in Kenya', *Africa Today* 56(1): 45–64.

Prince, R., P. Dennis and R. Dijk. 2009. 'Introduction to Special Issue: Engaging Christianities: negotiating HIV/AIDS, health, and social relations in East and Southern Africa', *Africa Today* 56(1): v–xviii.

Ter Haar, G. and S. Ellis. 2006. 'The role of religion in development: towards a new relationship between the European Union and Africa', *European Journal of Development Research* 18(3): 351–67.

Tiendrebogo, G. and M. Buyckx. 2004. *Bulletin 361: Faith Based Organisations and HIV/AIDS Prevention and Impact Mitigation in Africa*. Amsterdam: Koninklijk Instituut der Tropen.

Wel, L. van der. 2011. 'Integral development: religion and development cooperation in the Netherlands', in G. Ter Haar (ed.), *Religion and Development: Ways of Transforming the World*. London: C. Hurst & Co. Publishers.

9

'I Don't Want to Hear'

HIV, AIDS and the Power of Words in Bushbuckridge, South Africa[1]

ISAK NIEHAUS

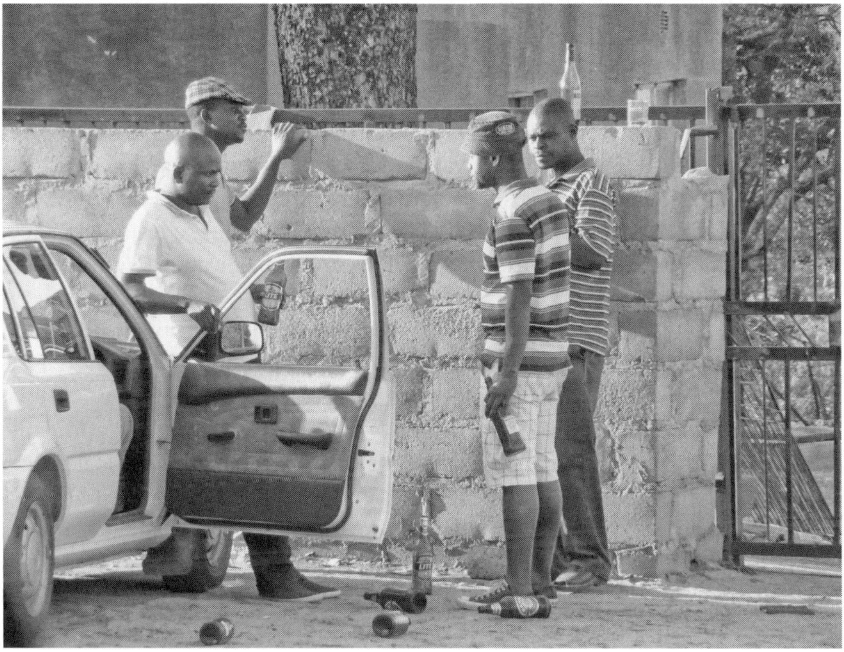

Muchongolo (photograph by Florence Bernault, 2011)

[1] I thank my research assistants, Eliazaar Mohlala and Eric Thobela, for their help during fieldwork. Many of my ideas were shaped in ongoing conversation with Nicole Angotti, Florence Bernault, Fraser McNeil, and Jonathan Stadler. Hansjorg Dilger provided extremely helpful comment on an earlier draft of this chapter.

SINCE THE 1990S, THE GLOBALISATION PARADIGM, advocated by scholars such as Hannerz (1996) and Appadurai (1996), has had deep impact on anthropological theory and practice. This paradigm has been shown to be particularly appropriate to the study of AIDS, a global pandemic, characterised by various transnational flows and assemblages (Nguyen 2005). The rapid diffusion of HIV was accompanied by the distribution of resources and techniques to fight AIDS. These include finance, technologies, drugs, and medical personnel, but also more immaterial goods such as moral agendas, geographies of blame, and blueprints for prevention and intervention. Moreover, HIV/AIDS has brought about new transnational identities and forms of therapeutic citizenship, based on common plight and mutual obligations (Nguyen 2005).

Among these flows, Nguyen (2009, 2010) highlights the transplantation of 'confessional technologies' as one means of confronting the pandemic. These technologies have an exceedingly long history in Europe. Born in Catholic ritual, they were redeployed with the rise of psychotherapy in the early twentieth century (Foucault 1972). The notion of the 'talking cure' is also expressed in 'coming out' narratives that emerged among the gay communities within the United States from the 1960s. Liberation and acceptance were to be found in bringing to words one's innermost, authentic, self (Weston 1997). With the emergence of AIDS, ideologies of religious salvation, psychoanalysis, and sexual liberation merged in new confessional technologies. These include undergoing voluntary counselling and testing, 'coming out' with HIV positivity, and providing public testimony about the sickness and transformative effects of antiretroviral medication (Nguyen 2009, 2010).

In South Africa, the country with the highest rates of HIV infection worldwide,[2] 'confessional technologies' are most widely deployed by the urban-based TAC (Treatment Action Campaign). Headed by the well-known activist for gay and civil rights, Zachie Achmat, the Campaign fought for the provision of affordable antiretroviral drugs, confronting pharmaceutical companies and an obstinate South African government in the process (Leclerc-Madlala 2005; Robins 2004). Robins (2006) shows how TAC activists, drawn from among those attending Médicins Sans Frontières (MSF) treatment programmes, conceptualised their journey from 'near death' to 'new life'. They drew on religious, social and medical meanings to forge new identities. The activists transformed the stigma of HIV/AIDS into a 'badge of pride' that they displayed on T-shirts during township funerals, demonstrations and workshops (Robins 2006: 314). Through speech and story-telling, they strove to overcome pathos and subordination (Fassin *et al.* 2008).

This chapter acknowledges the value of perspectives that focus on the transnational diffusion of medical meanings, and recognises the potential liberatory

[2] By 2007 2.1 million South Africans had died of AIDS-related diseases, and another 5.5 million were HIV-positive (Plusnews 2007).

effect of 'confessional technologies'. But, at the same time, the chapter warns against the assumption that global connections assume a linear character that progressively eradicates plurality and difference (Sahlins 1999). Globalisation not only implies disconnections (Ferguson 1999), but also generates 'frictions' and 'zones of awkward engagement' where competing perspectives and interests combine in unpredictable, often messy, misunderstandings (Tsing 2004). With reference to ongoing, intermittent fieldwork in Impalahoek, a large village of the South African lowveld,[3] I point to various hidden forms of resistance (Scott 1990) against the imported cosmopolitan practice of confessing, and I analyse silence as an alternative response to the pandemic.

Until the end of apartheid in 1994, Impalahoek formed part of the Lebowa Bantustan. But since then it has been administered by the newly constituted Bushbuckridge Municipality and Mpumalanga Province. Impalahoek currently has a population of about 24,000 Northern Sotho and Tsonga (Shangaan) speakers, who rely largely upon the remittances of migrant labourers, employed in Gauteng, and upon social welfare payments such as pensions and child maintenance grants (Niehaus 2006). The HIV/AIDS pandemic reached Bushbuckridge fairly late, but then spread very rapidly. A verbal autopsy survey on common symptoms of death shows that until 1995 the predominant causes of death in Bushbuckridge were infectious diseases and malnutrition in children, accidents and violence in adolescents and young adults, and cardiovascular disease in adults and the middle-aged. But between 1995 and 2002 AIDS was the predominant cause of death in all age groups (Tollman *et al.* 2002). Between 1995 and 2005, life expectancy in Bushbuckridge fell by twelve years for women and fourteen years for men (Kahn *et al.* 2007). In 2008 sero-prevalence among pregnant women receiving antenatal care at Tintswalo Hospital in Bushbuckridge stood at 32 per cent (MacPherson *et al.* 2008: 2).

Despite the severity of the pandemic, many residents of Impalahoek have refrained from undergoing voluntary counselling and testing. Those who do test for HIV antibodies tend to do so in the latter stages of infection, and even then, try their best to avoid speaking about their condition, especially in public domains. My observations confirm the findings of previous studies that show silence to be the predominant response to the AIDS pandemic in rural South Africa (Stadler 2003; McNeill 2011). But I do not merely view silence as a means of avoiding the imposition of a stigmatised identity (Campbell *et al.* 2005; Niehaus 2007). Instead, I focus on beliefs about the intrinsic and transformative capacity of words. I suggest that contrary to activists of the TAC who embrace the liberatory potential of speech, residents of Impalahoek fear the potentially dangerous impact of words, such as pronouncements that one is HIV-positive. In local knowledge, such words can be

[3] I use pseudonyms for the village and all personal names. This is done to protect the identity of my informants.

deadly. They crystallise sickness, invoke negative emotions associated with pending death, and thereby worsen suffering. Therapeutic interventions imposed from cosmopolitan centres frequently ignore these local concerns.

'If I test HIV-positive I will die'

Voluntary counselling and testing – sometimes known by the abbreviation VCT – forms the basis of medical interventions in the case of AIDS. Medical propaganda assumes obvious advantages of knowing one's HIV status. Those who test 'negative' can rest assured. Those who test 'positive' can protect their sexual partners and breastfed babies from being infected with a potentially deadly virus and can also protect themselves from re-infection. Since 2005, they can also access HAART (Highly Active Antiretroviral Therapy), which effectively suppresses viral replication, from public health-care facilities. Moreover, an HIV-positive diagnosis is often a prerequisite for securing highly valued social grants.[4] And yet, many residents of Impalahoek have actively shunned counselling and testing. During 2004 and 2005 I asked twenty-five informants, with whom I was acquainted, whether they might undergo a test for HIV antibodies. My informants included men and women, and were mainly in their twenties and thirties. Many had lost family members during the pandemic, and some had personally cared for kin suffering from AIDS. Only two of my informants said they had tested and both claimed that the results were negative. All others were of the opinion that it was better not to know one's status. A woman teacher, who had attended several workshops on AIDS, aptly summarised their feelings: 'People say they will die if they know [their status]. They say prevention is better than cure and for them prevention is not knowing.'

Such resistance is by no means exceptional. Other studies confirm that many South Africans refrain from undertaking tests for HIV antibodies. In 2000 public health researchers offered 2,500 residents in the mining town of Carltonville free and anonymous tests. Not a single person accepted (Ashforth 2002: 1). After a slow start, the South African Health Ministry launched successive campaigns to increase the numbers of people accessing testing (IRIN 2010), and have achieved some success. Official figures for 2009 show that 32 per cent of men and 71 per cent of women had tested (Government of South Africa 2010).[5] But many barriers persist.

[4] South Africans who tested HIV-positive and registered a CD4 count of 200 (now 350) or less were judged incapable of working and were entitled to receive monthly disability grants valued at R780 ($90) in 2005. These grants frequently constituted a significant source of income to poor households (Leclerc-Madlala 2006).

[5] By the 2000s testing levels had improved significantly in South Africa. A National Communications Survey found that in 2006, only 17 per cent of men and 38 per cent of women in South Africa had tested for HIV antibodies (Government of South Africa 2010). A similar trend is apparent in

People at higher risk of HIV infection, such as victims of gender-based violence, were not more likely to get tested (Steven *et al.* 2010; Adams *et al.* 2011). Moreover, testing by itself does not guarantee the anticipated benefits. Vociferous AIDS awareness campaigns at the University of Limpopo led 17 per cent of first year students to test for HIV antibodies. But only 20 per cent of these actually came for their results (Oxlund 2009: 225).

The statements of my informants give insight into the reasons why they were apprehensive of testing. Ace Ubisi, who had been unemployed for nearly a decade, and occasionally worked as my research assistant, claimed that knowledge of a positive status would only hasten one's death:

> 98 per cent of people from here won't go there [to test for HIV antibodies]. Only 2 per cent might go – maybe the educated ones and the Reborn Christians [bazalwane] . . . They trust themselves. The rest of us don't. If I test HIV positive I will die within three days. I might run away into the forest with a firearm [to commit suicide] . . . If I test positive I will think all the time, thinking about dying or surviving.

Justice Kgwedi, a young man who had recently left school, Joseph Nyathi, a motor mechanic, and Peter Manzini, who operated a small tuckshop – known as a spaza store in this part of the world – expressed roughly similar views:

> I hate to be tested. I hate to know that I'm going to die. I hate people telling me that I'm HIV positive. It will be a problem because I would worry too much. When the disease and the worries get together, I will be mourning too much. I will be fighting two battles.

> If someone says you are HIV positive you won't enjoy your wife or your girlfriend. I will only check my body for TB [tuberculosis] and for other diseases – not for HIV. If you know you have HIV you will never feel alright. You will think.

> I am too scared to be tested. I don't want to hear. It is alright if I die tomorrow, but it is not alright to hear I'm going to die. It will make you worry. If you are aware that you are infected you will think too much. You will become mad.

These responses are not indicative of ignorance of biomedical practice. George Bila had once worked as an AIDS educationist at the local LoveLife Youth Centre, where he taught teenagers to live a positive lifestyle in the context of the pandemic. George echoed the views of others:

> I have never heard of a single person going for an HIV test. We blacks, we are taught to believe that death is a terrible tragedy. If they tell you that you are positive you will think of dying. When they tell you, you automatically become a living dead. If you talk about it, it becomes worse. In this way they [possibly nurses and neighbours] put a negative stigma on you. If you know [your status] you will survive one year, if

neighbouring Botswana. During 2001, the government of Botswana launched an extremely comprehensive programme of free testing and treatment. But after two years, only 15,000 people had come forward to utilise these facilities (Steinberg 2008: 1). However, by 2005, about 158,000 tests had been administered (Klaits 2010: 39).

> you don't know it may even be five or ten years. You worry and you worry that you worry. You worry twice. You will think and you will dream of a grave all the time. In your mind you will see death and what happens to your body.

Many informants not only feared hearing medical personnel pronounce that they had been infected. They were petrified that a positive result might lead to neighbours and friends gossiping about their condition. George Bila said that he would be furious if anyone said his brother had AIDS. 'Even if he is correct, I will beat him.' Lissie Mohlala, a woman in her early thirties who worked as a secretary at the local municipality, responded as follows, when I asked her whether she had tested:

> I might go [for testing], but I will definitely not go around here. There are many people here and they gossip, especially the nurses and your friends. They are the ones who gossip the most. The nurses will tell you that you have AIDS and they will tell you what your CD4 count is. But they will also tell your friends, show them the pills and gossip about you. If you know you are HIV positive you will have stress. You will ignore to eat and you will be unable to sleep. You will die. You will always think about death.

Such statements were made in a context of a super-abundance of information about HIV and AIDS. Throughout Bushbuckridge, the public health-care fraternity and several non-governmental organisations (including the Health Systems Development Unit, Reproductive Health Groups Project, Bushbuckridge Social Service Consortium and LoveLife Youth Project) conducted vigorous campaigns to promote AIDS awareness. Health activists regularly addressed different public forums on the subject of sexual hygiene. The activists also trained teachers as sex educators. By focusing on prevention rather than cure, these interventions portrayed AIDS as an invariably fatal condition, and created the impression that nothing could be done to assist those infected with HIV.

Christian discourses were also prominent in framing people's understandings of sickness and death. Throughout Bushbuckridge, church leaders associated the skin lesions of persons living with AIDS, and sometimes AIDS itself, with biblical leprosy. Like biblical leprosy, they portrayed AIDS as a sign of God's wrath and as divine retribution for sin. They located those suffering from AIDS-related diseases, like biblical lepers, in a liminal domain, betwixt-and-between life and death (Niehaus 2009).

These public health and religious discourses emphasised culpability and also contributed to victim-blaming and stigmatisation. In everyday contexts, residents of Impalahoek blamed persons with AIDS for their own sickness; and condemned them for infecting past and present sexual partners with a deadly virus (McNeill and Niehaus 2010: 33–9). They widely referred to persons living with AIDS as 'living corpses' (setopo sa gopela) whose bodies were literally decomposing whilst they were still alive. This is evidence of the overpowering symbolic load of labelling: it immediately tainted the newly infected person with death, denying the very gradual progression from infection to illness and death (Niehaus 2007).

Woefully inadequate treatment options reinforced the association between AIDS and death. A network of three hospitals and twelve medical clinics screened pregnant women for sero-prevalence, provided voluntary counselling and testing on request, and treated the symptoms of AIDS-related diseases. Hospital amenities, particularly in the tuberculosis ward, were spartan. Only in 2003 did Masana Hospital, located 30 kilometres from Impalahoek, begin to supply the antiretroviral drug, Nevirapine (McNeill and Niehaus 2010: 23–5).

But social prejudice and poor treatment options do not fully explain people's reluctance to test. We are still left with many unanswered questions. Why should people who go through great lengths to act morally under normal circumstances risk infecting their sexual partners and breastfed babies, and re-infecting themselves, with HIV? The relationship between testing and stigma is perhaps less direct than one would suppose. People can simply undertake an HIV test elsewhere, as my informant Lissie Mohlala suggests, and conceal their status from kin and neighbours. Refusing to undertake a test is also no guarantee for avoiding discrimination and social ostracism. It is extremely hard to conceal the symptoms of AIDS, which are well known throughout Bushbuckridge. Constant coughing, drastic weight loss, ugly skin lesions and fluffy hair are sufficient, in themselves, to provoke prejudice, and generate the most malicious forms of gossip (Stadler 2003).

Moreover, treatment options have improved drastically, enhancing the chances for HIV-positive persons to live full and productive lives. In 2005, Rixile ('rising sun' in Tsonga) Clinic, located within walking distance, began to supply HAART to patients who had registered a CD4 count of below 200. Within three years, the clinic had enrolled 6,638 patients. Clinical evidence shows reasonable rates of retention, with a mortality rate only slightly higher than reported in urban settings (MacPherson *et al.* 2008). But people's willingness to learn about their HIV status has not matched these changes. Sick persons generally saw testing as a 'last resort' (Mfecane 2010: 33).

Speaking in euphemisms

Something is clearly amiss. A careful re-examination of the statements by interviewees suggests that they do not simply fear knowing that they suffer from an incurable, potentially fatal, condition. My research participants were terrified of hearing medical personnel and others pronounce that they were 'HIV-positive'. This is apparent in the statements by my research participants: 'I hate people telling me that I'm HIV positive'; 'if someone says you are HIV positive'; 'I don't want to hear'; and 'when they tell you'. My informants were less concerned that neighbours might see their sickness than they were about neighbours speaking and gossiping about their condition. Their statements seem to express a belief that speech about HIV itself could be deadly, and that certain words possess intrinsic agency and transformative power (Basso 1969). Words such as 'HIV' and 'AIDS' have the capacity to materialise, bring into consciousness and thought, and ultimately change the status of persons, from merely being to being afflicted with death.

The fear of hearing others pronounce unpleasant words about one's destiny is evident in the tendency to avoid speaking about HIV/AIDS in public domains. In Impalahoek, as indeed elsewhere in South Africa, talk about AIDS was confined to backstage regions of social interaction (Stadler 2003; McNeill and Niehaus 2010: 60–5). But even in these domains people tend to avoid mentioning the words 'HIV' and 'AIDS' directly. As an alternative, villagers deployed a broad, varied and creative range of euphemisms. They would say that an infected person suffered from the 'three letters' (maina a mararo), 'germs' (twatši), 'the painful sickness' (kukuana hloko), or 'the disease of right now' (bolwetši gona bjalo); had purchased 'a single ticket' (in English); was on 'diet' (dayeta); or had 'eaten herbs that make one disappear' (enga moragela kgole). Other euphemisms for AIDS include twalaza (a dance in which dancers look upwards to the sky). I myself soon learnt to refer to HIV/AIDS as 'the dreaded disease' during interviews and fieldwork.[6]

The agency of words: ethnographic observations

The assumption that words possess intrinsic agency was seldom explicitly formulated, but could be inferred from a number of observations during fieldwork, in contexts that initially seemed to me to have little to do with sickness and healing.

On a Saturday in 2005 I took a break from fieldwork and visited the Mount Sheba nature reserve with fieldwork participants from Impalahoek. My friends were struck by the beauty of nature. Ace Ubisi, who was once an active churchgoer, said that he found it incomprehensible that God could have created the mountains, valleys and forests in only six days. 'It took two hundred men two years to build the new police station and jail in Impalahoek, so how could God make all of this in only six days.' Ace's maternal uncle, who was a preacher of the Zion Christian Church (ZCC), tried to eliminate Ace's confusion. God, he said, brought nature into being through the act of divine speech. 'In the Bible we read that God would say "Let there be light!" and the light appeared. He would also say "Let there be mountains and waters!" and the mountains and waters appeared.' Christian cosmology equates the very act of creation with divine speech.

[6] Danger is generally more apparent when words are spoken in the mother tongue. However, the words 'HIV' and 'AIDS' seemed to have special power because they had recently become vernacularised. People were being forced to bring words into their language which they saw as bringing misfortune into society.

A belief in the power of words was also apparent in secular contexts. During 1996 the South African football team, Bafana Bafana, participated in the World Cup in France. I watched the opening game, between South Africa and the host nation, with friends in Impalahoek. I did not entertain high hopes. Bafana Bafana fielded an inexperienced team, which had never come close to beating top opposition. But to my surprise everyone else said they expected Bafana Bafana to win – not merely the game, but also the tournament. Some predicted that the final would be against Nigeria, another popular African team. I was astonished. My friends included football coaches, an accomplished referee, and a former player in South Africa's Premier League – who knew far more about the game than I did. Bafana Bafana lost the opening game 0–3, and were eliminated after the first round of the tournament in a most humiliating manner. Only much later did some of my friends admit that they too expected South Africa to lose, but could not bring themselves to say so. As an avid football fan explained to me: 'If you say South Africa will lose, we will lose. When we played Switzerland all South Africans said we would win and we won.'

Words seem to possess a certain materiality, and were on occasions treated as if they were things. My research assistants and I were eager to learn about a certain episode of witchcraft accusation. We heard that after several instances of misfortune occurred at a local bakery, all employees hired a bus to consult a witch-diviner close to the Swaziland border. The diviner apparently revealed three witches among the bakery employees. We approached a number of potential informants, but they all referred us to the shop-steward, Freddy Malene. Freddy had organised a witch-hunt and, for this reason, his employers suspended him from work. Freddy warmly welcomed us and offered a splendidly detailed account of events at the bakery. We briefly gave Freddy some advice, saying that his employer could not dismiss him without proper warning, and urging him to consult the legal advisers of his trade union. Freddy's mother overheard our conversation and, as we were about to leave, thanked us 'for the words we gave her son'. To express her gratitude, she offered me a beautiful reed mat, which must have taken her a week to manufacture. I left thinking, were words so concrete that they could be reciprocated with gifts?

In Impalahoek one could clearly observe the constructive power of speech during invocations to the ancestors, Christian hymns, prayers and confessions. Whenever a man set off to seek work in Johannesburg, he would call on his paternal aunt (rakgadi), and kneel with her at an isolated spot in the yard. She would then sip a maize drink and spit the liquid in all four directions, proclaiming, 'Fathers. Here is Fundani! He is going to work in Johannesburg! Give him luck! Let him get work!' Migrants invoked the ancestors in a similar manner upon returning from work, and would then thank them for their protection and support.[7]

[7] See McAllister's (2006) discussion of the importance of oratory in beer drinks, held to welcome home migrants by Xhosa-speaking households in the Eastern Cape.

In the numerous Zionist, Apostolic and Pentecostal churches of Impalahoek, prayers were seldom silent.[8] During sermons and funerals, congregants were expected to kneel on the ground and to pray out loudly to God, as if screaming out the words. Their individual voices mingled in a cacophony of sound (Comaroff 1985: 245–7). People widely acknowledged the miraculous power of prayer. Father Silinda, who was a wealthy storeowner and founder of the Nazarene Revival Crusade, reportedly prayed earnestly after thieves stole money and groceries from his store. Within days the thieves came to him to ask forgiveness, and returned all the cash and belongings that they had taken. These churches occasionally deployed confession (ipolela) as a means of managing the social and sexual lives of congregants. I never confessed myself. But I did observe Zionist church members meeting with ministers out of earshot of the congregation. One confessant told me that he had engaged in an extra-marital affair and afterwards suffered remorse (pona molato, literally, 'seeing crime in oneself'). After verbalising what he had done, the minister simply replied, 'This is sin! May God forgive you!' 'Hereafter I immediately felt relief', he told me. Unlike prayer, confessions were strictly private.

Deadly words, unfortunate names and curses

As shown, residents of Impalahoek acknowledged the agency of words, and in certain contexts, ranging from sport to religion, deployed the power of speech in a constructive manner. These meanings might well support 'confessional technologies' as employed by activists of the TAC, as a means of confronting HIV and AIDS (Nguyen 2009; Robins 2006). But there is one crucial difference: fear about the dangerous and destructive potential of words regularly outweighed faith in their therapeutic potential. This too is apparent in numerous everyday contexts.

Gossip and swearing provoked great unease among my informants. Jonsson (2004: 23) writes that young women in Bushbuckridge very seldom discussed sex or private affairs with each other, and when they did talk about these topics, they generally spoke in the third person. Young women distrusted each other, and feared that gossip might spoil their reputations. They told Jonsson that one good thing about having boyfriends was that they could talk with them about intimate matters without provoking envy. People took even greater offence at swearwords, particularly when others insulted their mothers. Men who swore frequently used the Afrikaans words bliksem ('lightning') and moerskont (literally 'mother's vagina'), as if they were acting outside of themselves, and dissociating themselves

[8] At the time of fieldwork there were twenty-seven churches in Impalahoek with a combined total of nearly 6,000 adult baptised members; 75 per cent of the Christians in the village belonged to 'Zionist-type' churches, 16 per cent to Pentecostal-type churches, and only 9 per cent to mission churches (Niehaus, with Mohlala and Shokane 2001: 31–6).

from swearing. Others swore by calling persons animal names. I heard a mother shout 'donkey' (bongolo) and 'witch-familiar' (thuri) at her disobedient daughter, when she was in a state of rage.

Certain words, that were not necessarily swearwords, seemed to have the power to disrupt social hierarchy, create envy and conflict, provoke disgust, and unleash powerful emotions. Rules of respect (hlonipa) dictated that it was morally inappropriate to pronounce them in certain social contexts. For example, younger persons were not allowed to call elders by name. They had to address related elders by kinship terms such as 'maternal uncle' (malome), and unrelated adults by their relation to their peers, such as 'mother of Fundani' (MmaFundani). Neither were they allowed to ask an elder where he or she had been, since the answer might prove embarrassing. They were not allowed to say directly that someone was drunk, but had to use euphemisms – 'he chases goats' (o kgapa diputi) or he 'has eaten maize' (a jele mabele) – instead. Villagers also had to deploy euphemisms when referring to urination or excretion. Instead of saying 'urinate' (rota), villagers had to use phrases such as 'blindfold rats' (fahla magotla) or 'spill water' (ntšha meetse). Instead of 'excrete' (nya), they had to say I'm 'going outside' (go ya ntla), or 'I'm going to send myself' (ke nyaka go te thoma).

Talk about sex and death was strictly proscribed. Elders, particularly parents, were prohibited from speaking directly to younger people about sex, and vice versa. Notable exceptions were the mother's brother and father's younger siblings, who could speak to youngsters about sex in a pedagogical manner. A male teacher told me that he found it exceptionally difficult to teach sex education as part of the curriculum for life orientation. In local practice, he said, it was taboo to refer to sexual organs when addressing children. He thus decided to use the English alternatives instead. 'Had I used the Northern Sotho terms, their parents might even have demanded my resignation.' Only grandparents could joke with grandchildren about sex. But such joking was not reciprocal. One could only speak directly about sex with spouses, lovers, coevals, friends, and also to outsiders such as anthropologists. Moreover, cousins shared a reciprocal joking relationship, in which they frequently shared lewd sexual jokes. In these forms of talk, sex was referred to indirectly, by euphemisms such as 'to share a blanket' (ke lepai re ya apolelana), 'penetrate' (tobetsa), 'taste' (kwa), 'perform' (maka) or 'sleep' (robala).

Similarly, no person could refer directly to death. In many contexts, adults signified death by non-verbal means. For example, an initiation master indicated that a young man had died at a circumcision lodge by breaking a clay pot in front of his mother.[9] Symbolic inversions, such as turning around logs in a fire and placing their thick ends in the centre, also signified death (Berglund 1976: 230–8). Common euphemisms for death were that the deceased had been 'taken by a hyena' (tšerwe

[9] See De Heusch's (1980) analysis of the analogy between birth and the baking and firing of clay pots among Tsonga-speaking people.

ke phiri) or 'gone to the place of the ancestors' (o ile badimong), or that the 'house has fallen' (o wetše ke ntlo), the 'water had dried up' (meetse a pshele), or the 'sun had set' (dikeletswe ke letšatsi).

My informants were also sensitive to dissonance between words and their referents. I often cross-checked the information supplied by research participants and I was surprised how seldom they lied. My research participants sometimes shied away from unpleasant facts through omission, and by distorting minor details in the storyline. But they were usually honest, sometimes brutally so. A former prisoner told me that he was incarcerated for the illegal possession of a firearm. But, he said, the police should actually have arrested him for attempted murder: the firearm belonged to a man who had hired him to kill his wife's lover, and friends of his intended victim overpowered him before he could shoot.

Residents of Impalahoek were anxious about the predictive power of words. There is hardly any local tradition of prophecy. People seem to fear that, as in the case of witchcraft, unpleasant words could bring about unpleasant consequences. Mabetha Monareng recalled that in 1986 lightning struck next to a Zionist church, killing two boys and two cows. Neighbours incorrectly informed Mabetha's mother that he was one of the deceased. When Mabetha arrived at home, she was delighted to see that he was still alive. But she immediately placed ash on Mabetha's forehead to protect him against the destructive power of the pronouncement. Having withstood the flames of fire, ash was a prominent cooling substance, and was frequently used in healing rites (Hammond-Tooke 1981: 154).

The agency of words was apparent in personal names. Individuals had up to six different names. Whereas mothers gave birth to babies, fathers named them and bestowed them with social identity. A baby's first name usually pertained to an incident that occurred at the time of his or her birth. For example, a man named his son 'Soweto', because he was visiting this city at the time of the baby's birth. Children soon earned additional names. Nurses and teachers conferred on them English or Afrikaans names, used when interacting with white employers and government bureaucracies. Such names were often taken from the Bible. The third name was usually that of an ancestor. Elders sometimes perceived a baby's incessant crying as a sign that a forgotten ancestor was plaguing him or her. The crying would stop only once a diviner had identified the responsible ancestor and parents appeased the ancestor by naming the baby after him or her (Mönnig 1988: 102–7). Children also earned nicknames (dikwero) from their playmates and peers. These could include Lepara ('walking stick'), Badzy (a 'cousin' to everyone), Duma (a talkative person), or Dubuka (someone who assists people). Finally, upon returning home from the circumcision lodge, a boy was entitled to give himself his own name. Kelebotse ('I am handsome') is an obvious example.

Names were never simply rhetorical, but closely described a person's dispositions. It was never quite clear whether the dispositions led to the name or vice versa. Naming a person after an ancestor created a special bond between living and deceased persons. One man was named after his maternal great-grandmother, called Ramadimabe ('father of misfortune'). He explained that she was prone to misfortune, but also extremely resilient and able to contain the misfortune she experienced. 'Like her', he said, 'my life has also been a life of long suffering, but I am also resilient and tough.' Other informants told me that they appropriated the dispositions of the ancestors after whom they were named. Mbhekeni said that like his great-grandfather, he was prone to be short-tempered. Kotšo (a mispronunciation of the Northern Sotho word for 'peace', kgotšo) said that like his great-grandfather, he was rude and fortunate in money matters. During rituals a person named after the most senior ancestor was treated as the most senior sibling, even though he or she might not actually be the first-born.

Names which referred to specific events at the time of a person's birth could also shape his or her destiny. A woman named Bareforiye ('we have been calmed') claimed that she was good at resolving disputes. Mohlopeng ('someone who is troubled') told me that as a child he was always restless and cried throughout the night. As he grew older, he was prone to experience bouts of aggression. Lekhudani ('one who is ill') said, 'Even as an adult I have never been well.' Tshikiwane ('to be abandoned') was forsaken by her own parents, and later deserted by her husband. 'I believe you follow your name', she told me. 'What I have lived throughout my life was the same as my name.' In these instances it was deemed impossible to avoid one's destiny. This is captured by the saying, 'tolerate a good name, tolerate a bad name' (Lebitso lelebotse seroma, Lebitso lebe seroma).

The agency of words is also apparent in witchcraft. Observers have noted that whereas Mediterranean people tend to fear the malevolent power of sight, as in the evil eye (Galt 1982), in much of southern Africa people fear the malevolent power of sound. West (2007) argues that Muedans in Mozambique construct sorcery through speech and experience it through threats and accusations. 'People do not speak of sorcery', he writes, 'they actually speak sorcery' (West 2007: 21).[10] My fieldwork in Bushbuckridge, on the other side of the Mozambique/South African border, supports some of these observations. It would be unwise to reduce witchcraft to words, only because these words often have very real material referents, such as concrete episodes of misfortune. But the power of cursing was, nonetheless, obvious. The most well-known curse in Bushbuckridge was the simple expression 'I'll see you!' (Ke tlo go bona). These words were purported to have deadly consequences, particularly if the speaker possessed innate malevolent power.

Two examples attest to the potentially destructive power of cursing. Rexon Khoza once suspected another man of having an extra-marital affair with his wife. Rexon confronted him in public and in a state of severe anger threatened: 'I'll see

[10] A belief in the malevolent power of words is evident in the case of the sahir in Northern Sudan. Here the casting of evil is attributed to utterances in the form of metaphors, rather than to the gaze of one's eye (Ibrahim 1994).

you'. Only two days later an unknown assailant shot dead this man, in what appeared to be an incident of robbery. Onlookers did not regard the murder as coincidental, and henceforth suspected Rexon of harbouring the power of witchcraft.

My second example is of Khazamula Nyathi, a man in his seventies who was the leader of the local muchongolo dance team. At one event his 28-year-old grandson, Maguduza Nyathi, a lawyer, said that he would never dance for the team. A fierce argument erupted. Khazamula apparently shouted at Maguduza, 'You are a Shangaan! Muchongolo is our tradition!', and beat him with a stick. Maguduza retaliated with his fists. Khazamula then reportedly cursed him, saying 'For beating me, you'll die! You think I'm nothing and that you're a lawyer. I'm your grandfather. You can be a lawyer in heaven or in hell.' Only one month later, Maguduza tried to separate two fighting men at a drinking tavern, and was fatally wounded. Onlookers believed that Khazamula's curse brought about his death.

Another practice bordering on witchcraft, which also shows the destructive power of words, is the 'bottling' of football players. Ace Ubisi, a former player of Impalahoek Fast Eleven, recalled that their team manager sometimes brought a bottle containing strong, dark-coloured, potions that smelt like rum, to their camp. Three hours before the game, he would call Ace and ask him to speak into the bottle. Ace recalled that he usually said words such as: 'Givens [the name of his opponent]! I'm Ace! I'm going to play against you. Today I bottle you! You have nowhere to go!' Ace then breathed into the bottle, the manager closed the lid, and buried the bottle in a termite heap, behind the goal box. Bottling, Ace believed, made his opponents useless.

Powerful words were also deployed as vengeance magic (letšwa), and were used to make witchcraft rebound. Loicy Shai suspected that she had been bewitched. She was unable to find work, her fiancé left her for another woman, and she was plagued by the most horrible nightmares. She would, for example, dream that her younger sister, who was still alive, was deceased. A Zionist healer revealed to Loicy that her boyfriend's mother had spoken a curse against her. The healer instructed Loicy to do the following. She had to take a Coca-Cola bottle, speak into the bottle, verbalise her distress and anger, and immediately close the lid. She then had to take the bottle to a crossroads, smash it on a stone, and walk away without looking back. 'This', the healer said, 'would remove your misfortune (bati). It will make those who want you to suffer, suffer.' Within a year after she had performed the ritual, Loicy secured a secretarial position and found a new boyfriend.

HIV/AIDS: concealment, silence and discreet speech

Anxiety about the potentially destructive effects of words underlies people's fear of hearing medical personnel pronounce that they had tested HIV-positive. It also illuminates the tendency to avoid speaking about HIV and AIDS in public domains.

Unlike activists of the urban-based TAC, residents of Impalahoek resisted the practice of confession (Nguyen 2009), and responded to HIV and AIDS by deploying alternative tactics – concealment, silence, and on occasions, also discreet speech.

Klaits's (2010) analysis of speech in an Apostolic church of Botswana illuminates some of the reasons for the prominence of silence in Impalahoek. He observes that church members perceived faith (tumelo) as vital to healing. In cases of sickness, they communicated faith and love from their own bodies to those of persons who were unwell. Church members believed that hymns, prayers and words of compassion mitigated harm and assisted healing. By the same token, they perceived expressions of scorn and of jealousy as morally inappropriate forms of speech that worsened suffering. The church members avoided certain topics. To protect themselves from the power of witchcraft, they refrained from speaking about it, and refused to share in the sentiments of those they suspected of practising it. Apostolic Christians also avoided speaking about AIDS, and never pronounced AIDS as the cause of death at funerals. To call an illness AIDS would amount to a curse that prophesies imminent death. Moreover, announcing AIDS as a cause of death at funerals would cast aspersions on individual character (see also Durham and Klaits 2002). Hence, in matters of witchcraft and of AIDS, silence avoided anger, victim-blaming, and strife.

Silence and concealment were most prominent during the early stages of the pandemic, before the availability of effective antiretroviral medication. As soon as the first symptoms of AIDS became apparent, fellow household members secluded the afflicted person. This was done not only to avoid others polluting him or her, or vice versa, but also to preclude speech about his or her condition. Only a select few people – usually a mother, sibling or a younger relative – nursed, washed and fed the sick person. The carers were expected to comfort and strengthen (phorola) him or her verbally. Even if the situation was gravely serious, it was deemed inappropriate to name the person's disease, speak about any topics that might upset him or her, or worse still, say that he or she was about to die. Carers hardly ever announced the nature of the sickness to neighbours. Instead, a constantly burning fire indicated sickness in a household. Visits to hospital were hedged in secrecy. Joseph Mnisi, the only person to own a van in his village section, told me that his neighbour once came to his home late one evening and begged him to take her critically ill daughter to hospital. He suspected that she might suffer from AIDS-related diseases because they draped a blanket over her head.

Some carers, themselves, were unsure whether their patients suffered from AIDS-related diseases. Jonas Mohlala, who was a medical doctor, asked his nephew, Thabo, and his nephew's wife to take care of his critically ill son. But Jonas did not tell them anything about the nature of his sickness. The couple, nonetheless, assumed these duties with great moral compassion. They gave Thabo's sick cousin medicine, fed him, washed him, and did his laundry, each day. They also invited their church choir to stand outside his room and sing for him. On a few occasions they took Thabo's cousin to hospital, in the hope that doctors might alleviate his suffering. But these visits always happened at night.

My informants condemned those who failed to provide proper care for close kin suffering from AIDS-related illnesses. They also criticised open speech about AIDS. After Roniah Mashile's daughter became critically ill, she confided in neighbours that her daughter's condition was terminal, because she had contracted AIDS. This statement provoked suspicions that Roniah might actually have bewitched her own daughter, and merely invoked AIDS as a means of hiding her own culpability.

In 2005, there was great improvement in the prospects of persons living with AIDS. For many the availability of effective antiretroviral medication brought new hope. Once a terminal illness, AIDS had now become a potentially chronic, manageable condition. Medical researchers monitored 1,353 patients who were initiated onto HAART at Rixile Clinic between October 2005 and September 2007. After twenty-four months, 84 per cent (1,131) of the patients were retained on treatment: 9 per cent (124) had died, 5 per cent (63) had been transferred, and 3 per cent (35) could not be traced (MacPherson *et al.* 2008: 2). Several patients experienced drastic improvement. Within four months the weight of one patient receiving HAART increased from 20 kg to 70 kg.

But HAART has not suddenly generated a spate of confessions. My research participants still perceived AIDS as a potentially life-threatening and stigmatising condition. Fears of hearing medical personnel pronounce that one is HIV-positive have persisted, and residents of Impalahoek delayed testing for HIV antibodies until they were severely ill (Mfecane 2010). Medical personnel at the Rixile Clinic experience late presentation and advanced levels of immuno-suppression as formidable barriers to effective treatment (MacPherson *et al.* 2008: 4).

Those who did present for treatment expected health workers to treat their health status with the utmost confidentiality. Tintswalo Hospital sometimes dispatched volunteers to provide home-based care for sick persons residing in their neighbourhoods. The volunteers washed disabled persons, cooked for them, did their laundry, and cleaned their yards. Nurses issued all volunteer carers with hospital cards, providing a profile of the patient's medical history. But the cards never explicitly indicated whether the patient was HIV-positive. As one volunteer observed:

> Sometimes, on the corner of the card, there would be a picture of a book. This tells us that the person has AIDS. You must never say it out loudly. The patients usually conceal this. Even the family members may not know.

People using medication perceived speech acts as a crucial dimension of therapeutic encounters. Whereas the indiscreet pronouncement of dangerous words might impede healing, in certain contexts, appropriate words instilled faith in the therapeutic potential of antiretroviral drugs. This is very evident in the case of

Reggie Ngobeni, a man in his mid-forties. By August 2005, Reggie was in a desperate situation. He had previously resided in Johannesburg, but returned to his mother's home in Impalahoek after he was retrenched from work, and started suffering from excruciating stomach cramps. He spent a month in the tuberculosis ward, and began an apprenticeship to qualify as a diviner. But Reggie's condition grew worse. He had diarrhoea, his nose bled, and he vomited and coughed throughout most nights. Reggie eventually blamed the woman who had trained him in the art of divination for his deteriorating health. She had reportedly warned him that if he did not pay his training fees of R3,000 (£250), AIDS would strike him down. Reggie told me, 'I cried when I heard those painful words. When someone promises you AIDS you will remember it.' This statement suggests that Reggie saw his AIDS-like symptoms as the product of a curse. It was out of desperation that Reggie's brother took him to the Rixile Clinic. Here Reggie tested positive for HIV antibodies and registered a CD4 count of only 94. After being given HAART, Reggie's health improved, and his opportunistic infections disappeared. Reggie also became a baptised member of the Zion Christian Church. Reggie told me that the doctor at Rixile warned him that unless he took his medication as instructed, he would die. This statement prompted him to comply with treatment. 'If I don't take these tablets people would say that AIDS killed me.'

The uncoupling of HIV and death has, in certain contexts, paved the way for supportive and discreet speech. Custom Chiloane relayed to me that his friend, Lucas Malebe, who was seriously ill, had lost all hope of recovery, and refused to go to hospital. Custom was shocked because he had anticipated a more positive response from his friend.

> Lucas told me, 'There is no need for me to go to hospital. I will go there, I will return, and I'll still be sick. No doctor or nurse can help me. The best thing is simply to stay here and die. I was involved with three girls. They all died. People gossiped that it was HIV.'
>
> Lucas lay in bed waiting for death. I think his problem was hope. I went home and came up with a strategy. I decided to lie to Lucas. I told him: 'Lucas the dreaded disease affects everyone. I too am HIV positive. I only look healthy because I am on [antiretroviral] treatment.'

One week later Lucas phoned Custom and told him that he had tested and was now 'taking tablets'. However, Lucas was furious when he discovered that Custom had lied to him, and yelled at Custom on the mobile phone. But Lucas later sent a text message, expressing the wish to continue their friendship. Custom told me, 'HIV needs positive thinking. If you do not think positively it will destroy you.'

Conclusions

This chapter has warned against the assumption that confessional technologies – such as coming out with HIV positivity – provide a universally appropriate means of confronting the AIDS pandemic. Confessional technologies are premised upon the assumption that speech has the capacity to transform persons, combat stigma, and bring new hope in the context of suffering and pain. These assumptions accord with classical anthropological observations that the potency of ritual lies as much in the uttering of words as in the manipulation of objects (Malinowski 1965; Tambiah 1968). For example, Lévi-Strauss (1968) argues that South American shamans utilise speech to heal cases of problematic childbirth. By naming the mother's pains and chaotic sensations, and by placing them in a meaningful symbolic framework, the shamans make them bearable. But, as we have seen, words can also be deadly. They also have the capacity to invoke negative emotions such as jealousy and scorn, and bring about harmful effects.

But words operate in material contexts. Urban-based activists of the TAC have used these technologies as a means of forging social support, accessing medication and attaining the benefits of therapeutic citizenship (Nguyen 2010; Fassin *et al.* 2008). But in insecure rural areas such as Bushbuckridge and Venda concealment and silence have continued to be the predominant response to HIV and AIDS (McNeill and Niehaus 2010). Here anxiety about the destructive capacity of words – as in cursing, swearing, and direct speech about sex and death – was overpowering. The words 'HIV' and 'AIDS' bore a negative symbolic load, foretold death, and enhanced sickness. Being pronounced as – and pronouncing oneself to be – 'HIV-positive' was more likely to provoke stigma than compassion. Prior to 2005, effective medication was out of reach for everyone suffering from AIDS-related illnesses. After this date it was generally available to all. With the availability of medication discreet speech has gradually replaced complete silence. People generally delay testing, and they expect medical personnel to speak in a supportive manner and to maintain confidentiality.

It makes greater sense to treat speech and silence as alternative, perhaps equally appropriate, modes of dealing with disease. It is imperative that health workers learn to deal with silence, maintain confidentiality and speak with discretion.

References

Adams, J., N. Hansen, A. Fox. B. Taylor, M Jansen van Rensburg, R. Mohlahlane and K. Sikhema. 2011. 'Correlates of HIV testing among abused women in South Africa', *Violence against Women*, 4 July.

Appadurai, A. 1996. *Modernity at Large: Cultural Dimensions of Globalisation*. Minneapolis: University of Minnesota Press.

Ashforth, A. 2002. 'An epidemic of witchcraft? Implications of AIDS for the post-Apartheid state', *African Studies* 61(1): 121–44.

Basso, K. 1969. *Western Apache Witchcraft*. Tucson: University of Arizona Press.

Berglund, A.-I. 1976. *Zulu Thought-Patterns and Symbolism*. Uppsala: Swedish Institute of Mission Research.

Campbell, C., Y. Nair and S. Maimane. 2005. *Understanding and Challenging HIV/AIDS Stigma*. Durban: University of KwaZulu/Natal.

Comaroff, J. 1985. *Body of Power, Spirit of Resistance: The Culture and History of a South African People*. Chicago: University of Chicago Press.

De Heusch, L. 1980. 'Heat, physiology, and cosmogony: rites de passage among the Thonga', in I. Karp and C.S. Bird (eds), *Explorations in African Systems of Thought*. Bloomington: Indiana University Press, 53–76.

Durham, D. and F. Klaits. 2002. 'Funerals and the public space of sentiment in Botswana', *Journal of Southern African Studies* 28(4): 777–95.

Fassin, D., F. Le Marcis and T. Lethata. 2008. 'Life and times of Magda A: telling a story of violence in South Africa', *Current Anthropology* 49(2): 225–46.

Ferguson, J. 1999. *Expectations of Modernity: Myths and Meanings of Urban Life on the Zambian Copperbelt*. Berkeley: University of California Press.

Foucault, M. 1972. *The History of Sexuality. Volume One: An Introduction*. New York: Vintage.

Galt, A. 1982. 'The evil eye as synthetic image and its meanings on the island of Pantelleria, Italy', *American Ethnologist* 9(4): 664–81.

Government of South Africa. 2010. *The National Communications Survey of HIV/AIDS, 2009*. www.info.gov.za./issues/hiv/survey_2009.htm#implications (accessed 15 September 2011).

Hammond-Tooke, W.D. 1981. *Boundaries and Belief: The Structure of a Sotho Worldview*. Johannesburg: Witwatersrand University Press.

Hannerz, U. 1996. *Transnational Connections: Culture, People, Places*. London: Routledge.

Ibrahim, A. 1994. *Assaulting with Words: Popular Discourses and the Bridle of Shar'ia*. Evanston, IL: Northwestern University Press.

IRIN. 2010. 'South Africa: national HIV testing campaign disappoints'. World Countries News. http://world-countries.net/archives/74328 (accessed 15 September 2011).

Jonsson, G. 2004. 'The construction of young women's sexuality in a Limpopo village, South Africa'. BA Honours diss., Department of Anthropology and Archaeology, University of Pretoria.

Kahn, K., M. Garenne, M. Collinson and S. Tollman. 2007. 'Mortality rates in the new South Africa: hard to make a fresh start', *Scandinavian Journal of Public Health* 35(69): 29–34.

Klaits, F. 2010. *Death in a Church of Life: Moral Passion during Botswana's Time of AIDS*. Berkeley: University of California Press.

Leclerc-Madlala, S. 2005. 'Popular responses to HIV/AIDS and policy', *Journal of Southern African Studies* 31(4): 845–56.

Leclerc-Madlala, S. 2006. '"We will eat when I get the grant": negotiating AIDS, poverty and antiretroviral treatment in South Africa', *African Journal of AIDS Research* 5(3): 249–56.

Lévi-Strauss, C. 1968. 'The effectiveness of symbols', in *Structural Anthropology*, vol. 1. New York: Basic Books, 186–205.

MacPherson, P., M. Moshabela, N. Martinson and P. Pronyk. 2008. 'Mortality and loss to follow-up among HAART initiators in rural South Africa', *Transactions of the Royal Society for Tropical Medicine and Hygiene* 1: 1–6.

Malinowski, B. 1965. *Coral Gardens and their Magic*, 2 vols. Bloomington: Indiana University Press.

McAllister, P.A. 2006. *Xhosa Beer Drinking Rituals: Power, Practice and Performance in the South African Rural Periphery*. Durham, NC: Carolina Academic Press.

McNeill, F. 2011. *AIDS, Politics and Music in South Africa*. New York: Cambridge University Press.

McNeill, F. and I. Niehaus. 2010. *Magic: AIDS Review 2009*. Pretoria: Centre for the Study of AIDS.

Mfecane, S. 2010. 'Exploring masculinities in the context of ARV use: a study of men living with HIV in a South African village'. Unpublished PhD thesis, WISER, University of the Witwatersrand, Johannesburg.

Mönnig, H.O. 1988. *The Pedi*. Pretoria: L.J. Van Schaik.

Nguyen, V.-K. 2005. 'Antiretroviral globalism: biopolitics, and therapeutic citizenship', in A. Ong and S. Collier (eds), *Global Assemblages: Technology, Politics, and Ethics as Anthropological Problems*. Oxford: Blackwell.

Nguyen, V.-K. 2009. 'Therapeutic evangelism – confessional technologies, antiretrovirals and biospiritual transformation in the fight against AIDS in West Africa', in F. Becker and P.W. Geissler (eds), *AIDS and Religious Practice in Africa*. Leiden: Brill, 359–78.

Nguyen, V.-K. 2010. *The Republic of Therapy: Triage and Sovereignty in West Africa's Time of AIDS*. Durham, NC: Duke University Press.

Niehaus, I. 2006. 'Doing politics in Bushbuckridge: work, welfare and the South African elections of 2004', *Africa* 76(4): 521–48.

Niehaus, I. 2007. 'Death before dying: understanding of AIDS stigma in the South African lowveld', *Journal of Southern African Studies* 33(4): 845–60.

Niehaus, I. 2009. 'Leprosy of a deadlier kind: Christian conceptions of AIDS in the South African lowveld', in F. Becker and W. Geissler (eds), *AIDS and Religious Practice in Africa*. Leiden: Brill, 309–32.

Niehaus, I., with E. Mohlala and K. Shokane. 2001. *Witchcraft, Power and Politics: Exploring the Occult in the South African Lowveld*. London: Pluto.

Oxlund, B. 2009. 'Love in Limpopo: becoming a man in a South African university campus'. PhD-series no. 54, Department of Anthropology, University of Copenhagen.

Plusnews. 2007. 'HIV/AIDS barometer – May 2007', *Mail and Guardian Online*. http://www.mg.co.za/articlePage.aspx?articleid=306829&area+/insight/hiv-aids-barometer (accessed 20 July 2007).

Robins. S. 2004. '"Long live Zackie, long live": AIDS activism, science and citizenship after apartheid', *Journal of Southern African Studies* 30(3): 651–72.

Robins, S. 2006. From "rights" to "ritual": AIDS activism in South Africa', *American Anthropologist* 108(2): 312–23.

Sahlins, M. 1999. 'What is anthropological enlightenment? Some lessons of the twentieth century', *Annual Review of Anthropology* 28: 1–23.

Scott, J.C. 1990. *Domination and the Arts of Resistance: Hidden Transcripts*. New Haven, CT: Yale University Press.

Stadler, J. 2003. 'Rumour, gossip and blame: implications of HIV/AIDS prevention in the South African lowveld', *AIDS Education and Prevention* 15(4): 357–69.

Steinberg, J. 2008. *Three Letter Plague: A Young Man's Journey through a Great Epidemic.* Johannesburg: Jonathan Ball.

Steven, M., A. Cockroft, G. Lamothe and N. Andersson. 2010. 'Equity in HIV testing: evidence from a cross-sectional study in ten South African countries', *International Health and Human Rights* 10(23): 67–89.

Tambiah, S. 1968. 'The magical power of words', *Man* 3(2): 175–208.

Tollman, S., K. Kahn, K. Herbst, M. Garenne and J. Gear. 2002. 'Reversal in mortality trends: evidence from the Agincourt field site, South Africa, 1992 to 1999', *AIDS* 13: 1091–7.

Tsing, A. 2004. *Friction: An Ethnography of Global Connection*. Princeton, NJ: Princeton University Press.

West, H. 2007. *Ethnographic Sorcery*. Chicago: University of Chicago Press.

Weston, K. 1997. *Families We Choose: Lesbians, Gays, Kinship*. New York: Columbia University Press.

Part 3

TRANSNATIONAL IDEAS AND LOCAL DISCOURSES ABOUT SEXUALITY

10

'If You Cannot Control Yourself'

Christian Leaders as HIV Preventers in Malawi

ANAÏS BERTRAND-DANSEREAU

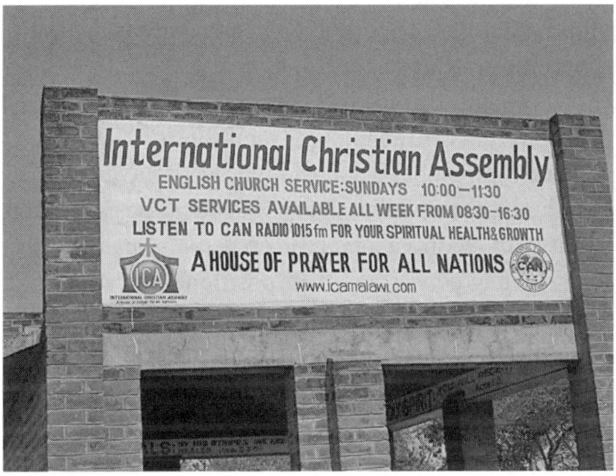
International Christian Assembly
ENGLISH CHURCH SERVICE:SUNDAYS 10:00–11:30
VCT SERVICES AVAILABLE ALL WEEK FROM 0830–16:30
LISTEN TO CAN RADIO 101.5 fm FOR YOUR SPIRITUAL HEALTH& GROWTH
A HOUSE OF PRAYER FOR ALL NATIONS
www.icamalawi.com
ICA
CAN

The International Christian Assembly in Lilongwe, part of the Assemblies of God in Malawi, has an 'HIV Pastoral Counselling and Testing Ministry' that operates as a drop-in centre for voluntary testing and counselling (VCT) (author's photo, 2008).

Introduction

IN 2007, CASSANDRA BALCHIN WROTE THAT 'If you want to get ahead in international development policy today, you've got to use the F-word: faith-based' (Balchin 2007). Balchin's scathing criticism of the 'F-word' was targeting development agencies' discourses and practices related to faith-based organisations (FBOs), but her remarks about the popularity of the term apply to some extent to the scholarly world as well. Indeed, there has been a keen interest in the links between religion and development in recent years (Deneulin and Bano 2009;

Deneulin and Rakodi 2010; Hefferan and Fogarty 2010; Jones and Petersen 2011; Rakodi 2012) and more specifically in the field of HIV/AIDS (Becker and Geissler 2007; Prince *et al.* 2009; Munoz-Laboy *et al.* 2011; Trinitapoli and Weinreb 2012). Part of the interest may stem from scholars of development simply following development agencies, but part of it is also a recognition, following the failure of the secularisation thesis (Deneulin and Bano 2009: 53), that in many parts of the world, religion and religious organisations are meaningful presences in social life (Jones and Petersen 2011: 1292–3).

This was certainly the case in Lilongwe, Malawi, where Christian institutions shape the social life of Lilongwe: the Catholic church runs the best schools, American missionaries run the best hospital and Assemblies run the best gospel shows. When I first went to Malawi to research HIV prevention and sexuality education in 2008, I had no intention of including religion in what I thought was a matter of public health. It soon became apparent however that most people who worked in secular organisations did include religious principles in HIV prevention, but also that religious actors had surprisingly sex-positive and holistic approaches to sex education (Bertrand-Dansereau 2010, 2013).

This chapter offers some examples of the ways in which certain Christian actors and organisations in Malawi are adapting to their role as 'HIV preventers', in a way that is more nuanced than global debates might lead one to expect. It presents an analysis of some Christian discourses about sex education as religious leaders have to adapt to the realities of life in a generalised epidemic, balancing absolute religious values, concern for young people and their position as a crucial node in networks of transnational concern over the suffering caused by HIV and AIDS. I first provide a brief overview of the historical and the policy context in which FBOs operate in Malawi, before examining what we know about their work in the field of HIV and AIDS. I then turn to the words of my respondents to illustrate the ways in which these Christian leaders try to resolve some of the tensions that arise from their engagement with HIV prevention.

Methods

This chapter is based on fieldwork conducted in central and southern Malawi, from August to October 2008, on the topic of HIV prevention for young people. I interviewed eighty-five individuals and I spoke with members of eleven groups (youth groups and village associations) who were involved with HIV prevention activities, be it in the public sector, in non-governmental organisations (NGOs), in community-based organisations, or in FBOs. The latter included twelve individuals who worked for Christian umbrella organisations, for the national headquarters of certain denominations, for ecumenical Christian youth organisations and for specific churches. My informants were Protestant, both from mainline and evangelical/Pentecostal denominations, but many worked for ecumenical or interfaith organisations. Semi-structured interviews were conducted and, in most cases, recorded and transcribed. Notes or transcripts were sent to the respondent for approval and further comments. Such texts were then analysed by themes according to the initial research question in 2009, and re-analysed in 2013 for this chapter. This second analysis was informed, in part, by additional fieldwork conducted in 2011 on the topic of young people's love stories, in the central region of Malawi.

The sampling of Christian actors and organisations was not systematic, since the initial research question did not focus solely on FBOs, who were only a subgroup in the overall sample. A weakness of this research is the absence of representatives from the Catholic Church and from churches preaching the gospel of prosperity and the more flamboyant Pentecostal churches. I also decided not to include Muslim FBOs, because of limited time and resources, and because of the specific social and cultural characteristics of Malawi's Muslim minority. For an account of transnational networks among Malawi's Muslims, see Van Kol (2008).

While I refer to them as 'Christian leaders', the people I interviewed cannot be considered representative of all Christian leadership in Malawi. They are part of Malawi's urban elite, with many of them having post-secondary education, a senior position within their organisation and experience with foreign donors; their work is fundamentally different from that of local clergy. For an examination of the role of religious leaders in rural communities, see the work of the Malawi Religion Project.[1] My goal here is not to paint a representative picture of Christian responses to HIV in Malawi, it is to explore some of the less conventional responses that have been shared with me.

Context: Christianity and HIV in Malawi

Monotheistic faiths came to the shores of Lake Malawi through trade and missions in the nineteenth century (Murray 1922: 10–11; Bone 1982: 127–8). According to the 2008 census, 83 per cent of Malawians are Christian, while the rest are Muslim (13 per cent), or belong to other religions (2 per cent) or no religion (2 per cent) – numbers that have remained constant since the 1998 census (National Statistical Office of Malawi 2000: xv, 2010: 13). Among the country's population, 21 per cent are Catholic, 17 per cent are Presbyterian, 13 per cent are Muslim, 7 per cent belong to the Seventh Day Adventist or to a Baptist denomination, and a whopping 40 per cent of women and 35 per cent of men belong to another Christian denomination

[1] The Malawi Religion Project (MRP) is a sister project of the former Malawi Diffusion and Ideational Change Project (MDICP), now the Malawi Longitudinal Study of Families and Health (MLSFH). More information can be found at http://malawi.pop.upenn.edu/malawi-data-qualitative-religion.

(National Statistical Office of Malawi 2011: 26). This very broad last category seems to point to the large and growing number of evangelical and Pentecostal churches that are not captured in standard survey response categories. In reality, religious affiliation and practice in Malawi is much more complex than any set of fixed categories can capture. Tellingly, the MDICP found that a quarter of its respondents identified as born-again – including 20 per cent of Catholics (Manglos 2010: 410).

Christian organisations have been involved in social services since their arrival in Malawi, in the form of missionary schools and hospitals that provide, to this day, some of the best health and education services in the country. President H.K. Banda, who ruled the country from its independence in 1961 until 1994, encouraged the churches to 'support the government's efforts to improve the world through development, rather than just concentrating on the afterlife' (Forster 1997: 169). The first Christian NGO, the Christian Service Committee, was founded in 1965, but it was really in the 1980s and 1990s that mainline churches established separate organisations dedicated to development work. Those were the decades in which Malawi and other countries in sub-Saharan Africa saw 'the invasion of the acronyms' as AIDS, NGOs and SAPs took front stage (Nugent 2004: 326). Following the political transition in 1994, Malawi saw an explosion of civil society organisations (Morfit 2011: 72), encouraged by the new political opening and by funding from Western development agencies (Makuwira 2011: 619–20). While the first confirmed cases of HIV infections date back to 1985, prevalence soared in the 1990s, peaked in 1997–8 and has since slowly decreased (UNAIDS 2012). The latest epidemiological data show that in 2010, the national prevalence rate stood at 10.6 per cent, down from 12 per cent in 2007 (Malawi Ministry of Health 2008: 26; National Statistical Office of Malawi 2011: 196). Youth prevalence has also decreased in recent years, from 6 per cent in 2004 to 4 per cent in 2010, with a consistent difference between young men and women that reflects the reality of age difference between sexual partners and of young women being infected earlier (National Statistical Office of Malawi 2011: 203).

The disease itself made a severe impact in the country, but the *response* to the epidemic has also shaped contemporary Malawi in significant ways. While official development assistance grew globally in the 2000s decade, the area of HIV/AIDS saw one of the fastest increases in dedicated funding with a 700 per cent growth rate between 2002 and 2009 (Kates *et al.* 2011: 7). Currently, the National AIDS Commission (NAC) is responsible for coordinating the myriad projects and programmes implemented by development partners, and for channelling available funds according to its strategic priorities. One of these is HIV prevention with young people, the main objectives of which are to delay sexual debut and to increase safer sexual practices (National AIDS Commission 2009a: 22). The strategy to achieve this is implemented through behaviour change interventions, especially life skills education (LSE) in schools and in informal settings, as well as through the provision of youth-friendly health services and edutainment (radio drama, youth festivals, magazines, etc.). In 2009, 12 million copies of life skills materials had been printed and distributed across the country (National AIDS Commission 2009b: 16). In 2010, the Ministry of Education made LSE examinable, thus ensuring that it would be taught, even by reluctant teachers; thus, in 2010 and 2011 3.8 million pupils were taught life skills (Government of Malawi 2012: 30).

As part of the initial response to the epidemic, religious organisations were natural partners in caring for 'the infected and the affected', but increasingly they became involved in other aspects of HIV/AIDS programming, including prevention. This was facilitated by USAID's emphasis on partnership with FBOs (Bush 2002) and by the sheer amount of money that was pouring into Malawi (Swidler and Watkins 2009: 1185). This period also corresponds with the involvement of evangelical and Pentecostal churches in social services, something they were less familiar with than their colleagues in mainline churches (Mkandawire 2008). All Christian umbrella bodies[2] now have active HIV programming, as do the major ecumenical Christian youth organisations.[3] In 2003, the Malawi Interfaith AIDS Association (MIAA) was established in order to 'facilitate and coordinate the faith based response to HIV and AIDS using gender sensitive and rights based approaches', with funding from USAID. In 2010, MIAA listed 127 active FBOs in the field of HIV/AIDS, and this does not include the work of the 'mother bodies', and of countless youth groups, prayer circles and parish committees that are active in HIV interventions but are not officially registered with MIAA.

Such a level of activity by FBOs, and funding by international donors, has not escaped the attention of scholars. Malawi's diverse and dynamic religious context has provided the ideal setting to study some links between religion and HIV. Researchers found little significant difference in the HIV prevalence of Malawians belonging to different denominations, which may be explained by Malawians' religious tolerance, and the ensuing lack of bounded sexual networks – people date, marry and sleep with others regardless of their religion (Thornton 2008; Muula *et al.* 2012). What does seem to play an important part in congregants' attitudes towards safer sexual practices is their level of religious involvement (Trinitapoli and Regnerus 2006; Trinitapoli and Weinreb 2012: 44) and the level of knowledge and openness displayed by their religious leaders – pastors, priests, preachers and imams. AIDS-related activities are nearly universal in Malawian religious congregations:

[2] The 'mother bodies' that represent Malawian churches are the Episcopal Conference of Malawi (Catholic), the Malawi Council of Churches (mainline Protestant) and the Evangelical Association of Malawi (evangelical).

[3] These organisations are the Students Christian Organisation of Malawi (active in secondary schools and tertiary institutions) and the Scripture Union (active in primary schools).

> Religious leaders in Malawi use a variety of approaches to address the AIDS problem in their communities: they preach about it, they reinforce biomedical prevention strategies (condoms and [HIV testing and counselling]), and they also directly intervene in the private lives of their members – admonishing sexual indiscretions and encouraging divorce for members who are at risk of being infected by an unfaithful spouse. The AIDS-related activities of religious leaders in rural Malawi are also plentiful, with over 90% of religious leaders reporting involvement in at least one of the six prevention efforts explored here.
>
> (Trinitapoli 2011: 48)

The importance of religiosity, religious leaders and congregations, rather than denomination, corroborates research that found leaders' attitudes to have more influence on women's family planning choices than did denomination (Yeatman and Trinitapoli 2008). In terms of the messages conveyed, it seems that the impact of preaching about HIV is much greater when leaders engage in specific discussions of sexual practices and feelings – something with which most of them feel uncomfortable – rather than advising against 'bad behaviour' in general (Lindgren *et al.* 2013: 9). The fact that nearly half of the leaders who took part in the Malawi Religion Project had attended a workshop about HIV/AIDS is potentially encouraging with regard to the quality of basic information to which they have access, and leaders' ability to discuss sexuality openly (Trinitapoli 2011: 46).

While workshops provide valuable information on biomedical questions, they are not the primary motivation in speaking up and most AIDS-related activities of religious leaders come from the feeling that HIV/AIDS is an important concern for congregants (Trinitapoli 2011: 49). This corresponds largely to religious leaders' roles as brokers and problem-solvers for their congregation – a role heightened by the stiff competition for congregants (Manglos 2011). It is in this role as brokers and problem-solvers, and in this quest to make their church attractive, that religious leaders actively seek and make the most use of their transnational connections, thereby deploying specifically religious forms of extraversion (Englund 2003; Freidus 2010).

Becoming HIV preventers

If local religious leaders in rural Malawi are brokers who solve the problems faced by their congregants, the staff who work at religious headquarters have become Lilongwe brokers, whose professional role is to link foreign organisations with local communities from across the country (Tawfik and Watkins 2007: 1091; Watkins and Swidler 2013). Such brokers are expected to translate flows of ideas and resources that come from Western countries into concrete actions meant to improve the lives of villagers – who have their own ideas about if and how their lives need improving. Lilongwe brokers are often the only Malawians with whom foreigners interact in any depth, and they are expected to explain Malawi to the world. Yet they tend to be urban upper-class men and women, whose knowledge of 'village life' is often tinted with elitism (Englund 2004). The respondents I interviewed hold positions that make them key nodes in transnational networks: they are important opinion leaders, who can make strategic choices about the direction their organisation will take, and who wield considerable power. At the same time, they must handle and reconcile, as much as possible, the pressures of believers, of religious leaders, and of international donors, which makes them vulnerable to everyone's criticisms.

With regard to sexuality, the difference between the discourses of international organisations, brokers and villagers is striking. International donors speak a language of public health, in which sex is *always* a risk factor, although some practices can be made safer. Unsafe behaviours must be changed through interventions inspired by the Health Belief Model (HBM), which 'presumes that individuals will act rationally in order to reduce the risk of infection (or ill-health) once they know about the undesirable health consequences of a given behavior' (Trinitapoli and Weinreb 2012: 50). In this perspective, the problem is that unsafe sex is an individual health risk, and it can be solved by persuading individuals to adopt safer sexual practices – a process known as 'behaviour change'.

At the receiving end of HIV prevention interventions are rural Malawians, many of whom hold 'positive attitudes to sex at all ages', and for whom being sexual is an essential and joyful part of being an adult, granted to them by God (Freeman 2012: 171, 197). As is the case in many other parts of Africa, in rural Malawi communal roles and social norms often take precedence over individual wishes, including with regard to sexuality (Izugbara and Undie 2008: 161). Sexual interactions are thus not just about individuals: they are extremely meaningful forms of social and physiological exchange, in which individuals exchange vital fluids and, through them, the life force that links them to generations and to the wider environment (Thornton 2008: 215–16; Freeman 2012: 80). Sexual relationships are also a major vector of the circulation of wealth and of its redistribution (Poulin 2007; Swidler and Watkins 2007). In rural Malawian communities, sex is a relational, social and material issue, and its health consequences derive as much from social risks and supernatural causes as from pathogens that hospitals can cure.

All HIV prevention work in Malawi involves the attempt to bridge the epistemic differences between these two conceptions of sex. This somewhat acrobatic feat must be done while producing the indicators of success required by monitoring and evaluation officers and pursuing an organisation's own agenda and priorities, whether it is simple organisational survival, women's empowerment or spreading the gospel. HIV preventers are not neutral implementers, and their own worldviews and agendas may be in conflict with those of both the donors and the beneficiaries. The Christian beliefs about sex with which I became familiar in Malawi have in common with villagers' worldview the idea of a joyful God-given sexuality, but restrict this to those sexual practices that occur within the bonds of heterosexual monogamous lifelong marriage. Those Christian beliefs, much like public health, frame sexuality in terms of risks incurred by individuals. This leads to condemnations of both cultural norms that tolerate discreet extra-marital sexual activity, and condoms as a way to make sexual practices safer. Giving advice to congregants about relationships, marriage and sexuality has always been part of the care provided by church leaders, and it is done with sincere concern for the well-being of young congregants. Such advice cannot, however, be dissociated from the not-so-distant fight of Christian missionaries against the 'enduring evils of traditional society', for which the only cure was thought to be 'a deeper extension of Christian morality' in its most Victorian dimensions (Vaughan 1991: 136; Tamale 2013: 273).

It is somewhat misleading to present these conceptions of sexuality separately, when in reality most of us hold conflicting visions of sexuality simultaneously, and draw on one or the other according to circumstances (see for example Hopkins 1980; Prince 2007: 86–7). In Malawi, 'most Christians and Muslims do not hold their religious beliefs to the exclusion of African indigenous cosmology'; indeed Christianity's full engagement with witchcraft seems to be one key reason for its popularity (Forster 1998: 537). Both public health and Christianity, however, demand absolute priority for their sexual prescriptions, making all other considerations secondary to avoiding risks of infection and damnation, respectively. In the case of HIV, there is a considerable overlap between these two sets of prescriptions, both of which include recommendations to avoid sex or to have only one sexual partner at a time. The area of disagreement lies in the issue of condoms, whose use by unmarried partners violates Christian proscription of extra-marital sex while protecting against HIV infection. This is where HIV prevention by Christian organisations becomes a potential minefield; it is also this question that complicates FBO involvement with transnational networks of HIV prevention.

'Now the compassion needed skills': projects, donors and professionalisation

As I mentioned, transnational networks have always been part of Christianity in Malawi, and churches have long been 'used' for purposes other than spiritual. Despite this long experience, the worldwide push to 'leverage religious leaders' for the diffusion of public health messages (Trinitapoli and Weinreb 2012: 78) seems to have significantly altered the reality of religious organisations in Lilongwe. Contrary to many NGOs, which were formed in the 1990s, many churches and ecumenical organisations pre-date both democracy and the wave of HIV/AIDS international funding. Compared with the secular organisations which gave me information on their funding, FBOs tend to generate more income locally, as opposed to depending on foreign donors, something which Leurs also found in Nigeria (Leurs 2012: 716). Indeed, many of my informants saw their involvement with 'development', including HIV prevention, as side projects that would come and go, while the activities related to their main religious mission were continuous.

These side projects, however transient and incidental, did occupy a significant proportion of FBOs' time. In some cases, foreign donors funded projects that had begun as activities of a church, while in other cases donors came to the organisation when they were looking for implementers. Michael, who managed an ecumenical youth organisation, gave me the most details about his relationship to donors. In thirteen years, Michael had dealt with three bilateral donors and four NGOs, mostly working on projects that lasted two or three years. Michael did not express any irritation at these frequent changes; on the contrary he seemed proud of the ability of his organisation to attract donors, and to keep some of them over the long run. When I asked him about conditionality, his answer was equally calm.

> There are moments when we've said no to a prospective donor because of the conditions they want to attach, if they contradict our position on certain issues. We say 'Thank you for your willingness to offer this money, no matter how much it is, but we might not be comfortable' – when we are implementing a programme we have to be natural [. . .] I can give you two examples. One UN organisation wanted us to be distributing condoms to schools. But one it's against our ethics, two it's against the policy of the Ministry of Education. When it comes to youth programmes, we do them among church youth so we can't go to church youth with boxes of condoms. That time, five million kwachas was a lot of money, plus a bus and five landrovers we were about to sign. Without the condoms they couldn't give us the resources, but we had to decline because we have to be principled. Then another secular organisation in the Netherlands also wanted us to distribute condoms, to go with 24 million kwachas. We also refused that.
>
> (Michael, programme director, ecumenical youth organisation, Lilongwe)

Michael is telling the opposite of what has often been said about HIV and condoms in the context of PEPFAR (see for example Gordon and Mwale 2006): instead of a secular organisation ceding to the demands of a funding agency to abandon condom programming, he is presenting a religious organisation resisting a funding agency's requirement to include condom programming. James, who also headed an ecumenical youth organisation, reported that 'there have been times when donors refuse to give us funding because of our position, especially because we refuse to distribute condoms'. Hence, when donors' demands were in conflict with the organisation's core values, the African organisation refused Western funding.[4] Contrary to certain secular NGOs, which are willing to adjust their focus from HIV to human rights and now to climate change (Bertrand-Dansereau 2013: 165),

[4] Other conditions, such as a thematic focus (e.g. orphans), a geographical district or heavy administrative requirements, were seen as acceptable conditionality.

FBOs do not easily change their core mission. FBO leaders felt that like-minded Christian donors could be found, and that even without the support of foreign donors, their organisational survival was not threatened. For some of them, the Christian aspiration to a life of poverty may also make it easier to refuse large sums of money that come with cars and electronic equipment.

Aside from international donors, respondents reported working with the government of Malawi on various occasions. Gloria's organisation provides a good example of the links between a church, the government and foreign donors. As part of their charitable work, some members of the church had decided to spend some time caring for sick people in the hospital.

> After the training the volunteers were treated as professionals, not as church people but as HTC counsellors. As the work increased we discovered that we needed financial support, because all that time it was for free, it was voluntary. But now with the HTC they needed to be there at a certain time, almost all the time. So we started looking for funding and we got some from a certain NGO, which was attached to a bilateral donor. Through that donor, they gave us funding and started building our capacity. We started the work without good capacity, without the skills of counselling, it was just an act of compassion but now the compassion needed skills. [. . .] At first it was two people, from what I can remember, and the numbers increased to reach four counsellors at the first hospital as of now. But our work expanded to another government hospital, and closer to here in a community hospital, where we also have four counsellors. So we have three testing sites within government institutions.
>
> (Gloria)

Gloria's narrative highlights the ways in which public institutions, international donors and FBOs come together in the response to the HIV epidemic. Church members who were engaged in conventional charity work, caring for the sick, were asked to become counsellors by the government hospital, who had received foreign funding to expand HTC (HIV testing and counselling). The volunteer work thus became increasingly professional, and importantly it started falling into the neat acronyms of HIV/AIDS work: the church started providing HTC, which was soon followed by home-based care (HBC), then work with orphans and vulnerable children (OVCs) and finally some life skills education (LSE) for the youth. Work that fits into an acronym can usually be funded; providing personal hygiene and praying with patients in a hospital ward was charity; HIV testing and counselling, which has an acronym, became 'development'.

Discourses of adaptation

The Christian leaders with whom I spoke thus find themselves involved with very different conceptions of sexuality, having to maintain a delicate balance between various demands and imperatives. Their primary mission as members of churches and Christian organisations remains to take care of the spiritual needs of believers, and in some cases to bring non-believers to Christ. Despite the world's interest in the epidemic, and the funding that some of them received to conduct HIV prevention activities, what mattered most to these Christian leaders remained salvation.

> For the Christian young person, the fear of the Lord is very important; it will help them. If young people fear infection, then it's easy to go for other preventive measures; but if they fear God – for example, Joseph in the Bible, his fear was not of the consequences, but of sinning against God. Whether there are any physical consequences or not, it is not the issue.
>
> (James, programme director, ecumenical youth organisation, Lilongwe)

Despite his assertion that the physical consequences of pre-marital sexual activity are 'not the issue', James and the other respondents are living and working in a society that has been deeply affected by HIV and AIDS over the past three decades. The solution to the tension between their beliefs and the demands of donors seemed straightforward: drop the funding if it comes with unacceptable conditions, and concentrate on the organisation's true calling. There is, however, no easy solution to the tensions between their belief in the promotion of a Christian sexuality, and their concern for young people who are coming of age in a dangerous time. I conclude this chapter with descriptions of three responses to this dilemma, each of which was refreshingly different from popular beliefs about conservative Christians in Africa.

Michael: not happily, but painfully

When we spoke, Michael had been working for his ecumenical youth organisation for a number of years. He has since started working for another youth-oriented FBO, still in Malawi. Michael described himself as a committed Christian, and like many of my other informants, his opinions about pre-marital sex were informed by his own experience of having married as a virgin. He shared some of his thoughts about sexuality education and the promotion of abstinence.

> To us, the biggest challenge is we know that young people cannot 100 per cent abstain, some will succumb to pressure and maybe the percentage will be higher than those who will abstain. However, we find it difficult to say 'You are not married, if you cannot control yourself, use a condom.' Because in a sense, in the spirit of that statement, I'm saying that if you cannot control yourself, you can still go and have sex, and that contradicts my faith. What I see, personally, is that as we are talking about condoms, no matter how much different our opinion might be from the secular world, we should not give a condemning kind of attitude to our young people. We should still passionately speak to them, to say if you want to be 100 per cent sure, then abstain [. . .]
>
> The problem is not the substance [the condom itself], the problem is the action outside marriage. It's painful. I don't think there is a Christian who says no to condoms for

> young people happily, but painfully because we know, we understand that young people, some of them, most of them, are still going to try it. That's when we say, in our case, it's no to sex outside marriage. We cannot compromise on that. But then we say, on issues of condoms you can go to these organisations, who will encourage the use of condoms outside marriage [. . .]
>
> Truthfully speaking, and I cannot lie to people, it's a struggle because I see, I know, I hear, I feel, I understand that mostly unmarried people are not as faithful as we want them to become. But I don't think that is licence to us. The way to Heaven is now. It's hard, it's very hard, even for us Christians it's very, very hard.
>
> (Michael, programme director, ecumenical youth FBO)

Michael articulates the tensions between his religious principles and his awareness of young people's realities, and the very way in which he speaks constantly oscillates between the two. On the one hand, Michael knows that most young Christians are sexually active, and he is aware of the potential consequences of unprotected sexual activity. There is a certain weariness in his words when he says 'I see, I know, I hear, I feel, I understand that mostly unmarried people are not as faithful as we want them to become' – as if responding to secular accusations that Christians are not aware of young people's realities. Yet he feels that he 'cannot compromise' on the question of sex outside of marriage: his faith makes it morally impossible for him to recommend condoms, but does not give him the comfort of feeling righteous. In lieu of the gung-ho abstinence promotion that one might expect from a committed Christian, we find someone who is careful not to have a 'condemning attitude' towards young people who are sexually active, and who says that it is 'painfully' that he does not promote condoms.

There are two strategies that Michael uses to ease the permanent moral discomfort in which he lives. On the one hand, he borrows from public health by saying that abstinence is '100 per cent sure', a favourite argument of conservative American evangelicals. Such an affirmation makes a good catchphrase, but has been discredited as inaccurate (Santelli *et al.* 2006). Nevertheless, it appears to make intuitive sense, and may reconcile him by affirming that the prevention message he favours on spiritual grounds, that of pre-marital abstinence, is compatible with the elimination of health risks.

The second 'way out' is to tell the young people 'you can go to these organisations', referring to other groups that do distribute condoms, a strategy that he is not alone in using. Many FBOs, and many secular organisations for that matter, rely on medical personnel to impart facts about physiology and 'changes in the body' that arrive with puberty. It is often these medical people who, with the authority of their white coat, give information about condoms. This information thus becomes an objective fact of prevention, part of the respected body of expert medical knowledge with which one cannot tamper, and not a condoning of immoral behaviours.

Gloria: 'It's OK to have sexual feelings!'

Michael claims to have been a virgin when he married, and this gives him the authority to say that everyone should be able to abstain. Others with a similar experience use their own narratives of abstinence, on the contrary, to explain that abstinence is a struggle. Gloria works for a Pentecostal church in Lilongwe, where she mentors young people according to the Augustinian principle of hating the sin but loving the sinner. She was the best example I heard of someone using the moral authority conferred by her religious affiliation to break taboos. Her approach manages to be at once extremely sex-positive, and unflinchingly conservative in her condemnation of pre-marital sexual activity.

> When I'm talking to young people, I ask them 'How many of you ever have sexual feelings?' You should look at their faces! Almost all of them will look down. If I say raise up your hands they'll barely lift it up, while looking at who is doing what. I say 'It's OK to have sexual feelings! If you have them you are a normal person. If you don't have them you have a problem, I must pray for you.' It's like you take them out of their shell and they begin to realise it's normal. So we have to bring them to a level when they know it is normal to have sexual feelings, that's how God created us.
>
> Now the challenge is, how do we bring them to manage those sexual feelings? And for me as a person, that's where I find that it's a big tragedy across the world. We have quickly said 'OK, because you have sexual feelings, then the solution is to sleep with a person and here is a condom so that you don't get HIV.' OK, fine. But do you know what we are doing? We are creating a generation that is sexually irresponsible. They are responsible in terms of exercising safe sex. But what kind of generation are we creating? We are moving humanity from being a human being who is able to control these sexual feelings, to an animal like a dog. [. . .] As a church, our promotion is abstinence for the young people, which can be quite controversial when you deal with other stakeholders.
>
> (Gloria)

On the one hand, Gloria is very articulate about topics that are usually avoided in HIV prevention. She names sexual desire, and she gets young women to talk about it – which is no small feat in a setting where female sexual agency is too often repressed and punished. On the other hand, she sees as doomed a society that does not punish pre-marital sexual activity, whose members will assuredly turn into wild animals. Moreover, she presents the promotion of abstinence, in which the whole country is engaging, as a controversial position that 'other stakeholders' do not appreciate.

Gloria's discourse is infused with her own experience of having remained sexually abstinent until her marriage – and the pride that she derives from this comes as much from respecting the divine rules as from the fact that it was so hard to wait all that time.

> It was hard. It was not easy and I never ever went to his house alone. Usually I would have a friend. If we wanted to have a private talk, we'd take each other to a restaurant, buy a bottle of Fanta, sit and talk, or go to somebody's yard and sit on a *chitenje*. You talk, you are outside, people are seeing you. Those four years [of courtship] were not easy. [. . .] We wanted to kiss, but in this relationship we will not kiss because we are afraid of the results. We made an agreement. There were moments where we felt we should just do it, but because we had talked about it we refrained.
>
> That's what I tell young people: abstinence is not easy but it's worth the sacrifice. The moment you tell them that, when the going gets tough they know! But when we just say 'Abstain! Pray to God to help you.' I pray so much, but it's not enough to tell a young person to pray, there's certain measures they need to put in place for abstinence to work. Yes I fear God, I prayed throughout the courtship and said 'God, I want to abstain'. There were moments, even sometimes in meetings, when we were just so sexually aroused and you go home and you say 'God, how long am I going to wait?' And those moments, maybe you put on a spiritual music, you get over it. When I talk to young people I'm so real, I tell them how I felt, what I went through so when they're going through it they know. That's the problem with others, they're not honest.
>
> (Gloria)

Gloria is, indeed, 'so real' about her own struggles with abstinence. This honesty was not reserved to our conversation; it infused all of her interactions with people, young and old. Over the course of the research, it was not unusual for respondents from churches and FBOs to tell me about their personal experiences, but nobody went into as much detail as Gloria.

Gloria's discourse goes against two ideas that are deeply ingrained in discourses of HIV prevention in Malawi: the naturalness of abstinence for young people, and the asexuality of young women. Gloria acknowledges that 'when the going gets tough', prayer and moral righteousness are not sufficient, and that she needed concrete measures to make sure she did not have sex with her boyfriend. In a way, she is admitting that if she had been alone with him during those four years of courtship, it is likely that they would have indeed 'failed to abstain', regardless of her intentions and of her moral positions. By saying this, Gloria acknowledges the difficulty of abstaining until one's mid-twenties, which is the age at which university graduates are expected to marry. She describes in some detail the difficulties she faced, the greatest of which was not 'peer pressure' or poverty, but her own desire.

Gloria's position as a respected church leader allows her to have honest conversations with the young women she mentors about female desire, about being aroused and suffering from not having sex – topics that would quickly lead to accusations of promiscuity coming from someone less morally conservative. Instead of the passive, asexual young women typical of life skills education books, she portrays young women as sexual beings who are struggling as much as boys to remain abstinent – and not just because of the material enticements of sexual relations with older men.

> With girls it's just at the beginning that they're shy. Once you break that ice, they even want to hear more, listen more, talk more. With the girls there's a lot of things on their body that will make them sexually aroused – their breasts, their backs, they easily get sexually aroused. We need to help them. [. . .] Sometimes girls all they want is someone to talk to, not even sleeping with a boy, they just want to be touched. When they talk I like to put my hand around their shoulder and reassure them that it's normal, that it's not time yet. Talking, talking, talking. By the time that girl leaves you, she has changed. She just needed somebody to talk to. [. . .] What I've noticed is that when you are available as an adult, they can tell you everything. They know I'm a Christian, they know my standards, that I wouldn't promote sex, they know. But when they've done it they will come. And that has given me a lot of delight. They don't fear, which is what they feel towards their parents.
>
> (Gloria)

By becoming 'somebody to talk to', Gloria is taking on a role akin to that of the aunt who was traditionally responsible for sex education in much of eastern and southern Africa (see for example Parikh 2005; Glynn *et al.* 2010; Tamale 2013). In doing this, she respects the distaste for parent–child communication about sex, which is common across all cultural groups in Malawi – despite the fact that a public health approach often aims to foster communication between parents and children about sex (World Health Organization 2007). Her discourse also resonates with the therapeutic ethos, which values verbal intimacy and reflexivity (Illouz 1997), and which the African upper classes are increasingly adopting (Spronk 2009). Gloria offers such intimacy to the young women she mentors in the context of a non-sexual relationship, and says that this intimacy is a large part of what they want in a romantic relationship. According to her, by simply 'talking, talking, talking' she solves many of their problems.

Gloria's discourse is a breath of fresh air amid stale repetition by HIV workers that young people should just abstain. It is also, I believe, a very good strategy for giving young people Christian spiritual guidance on sex and relationships and associating this kind of openness and sex-positive discourse with Christianity.

George: give young people choices

When we spoke, George had been working for a Christian denomination for over ten years. He told me about his organisation's approach to peer education in rural areas. In each geographical area, they train a number of young people as peer educators through a two-week training on sexual and reproductive health and HIV. So far, everything seemed very similar to the peer approach taken by all organisations in Malawi. Then came a surprise.

> We even train them on issues of condoms, but we make sure the church leaders don't see us do that. What we are saying is, give young people choices. We train them, we don't encourage them to use condoms because we feel abstinence is the issue and we promote abstinence. But at the same time, I think we'd be silly and . . . and not helpful

> to our young people if we don't train them, if we don't teach them about condoms. They need to know and it's up to them to choose. But we tell them 'this is not the solution'. The way we do it is very smart. We tell them 'Look here, the church doesn't support this, but the world out there, secular NGOs, this is what they teach. We teach them what the secular world teaches' [. . .].
>
> [How do young people react to this message?] Actually young people are very open, they want to hear more about it, because it affects them. They want to know. But somehow in their own churches they don't teach them. However we need to be very smart as an organisation. We need also to know our members. Our members don't like that. But we need to thread very carefully to make sure that we convince our members of what is necessary for them to be taught.
>
> (George, pastor and administrator, Christian denomination, Lilongwe)

While Michael was telling me about his inner struggle over conflicts between public health and Christian teachings, George seems to be mostly concerned with 'keeping face', a common concern for Christian organisations faced with the pandemic (Eriksson *et al.* 2009: 108). Like Michael, George knows that the young members of his denomination are sexually active before marriage, something he does not want to encourage. Unlike Michael, he has settled this dilemma by deferring to the moral agency of the young people themselves. He believes that his role is to 'give young people choices' by giving them full information about prevention, including condoms, and spiritual guidance to inform their choices.

He is aware, however, that this will not sit well with other congregants, as well as with the public image of the church. The dilemma, in this case, is thus not a matter of inner moral struggle over body or soul, as much as an operation in public relations with parents and church leaders. The first solution that George describes is the strategic omission on the part of his organisation, who 'make sure the church leaders don't see us' include information about condoms as part of the peer education training. I was surprised at this subterfuge, and even more surprised that George would tell me about this the first time we met. I had heard of lower-level youth workers including more information about condoms than was allowed by their hierarchy (see for example Bartelink and Meinema, Chapter 8, this volume), but not the other way round. It did, however, resonate with a certain class prejudice of educated, urban Malawians, who often told me they did not think rural people could understand nuanced policies. Later on, George told me:

> Most of our pastors they may not be very independent, they rely a lot on others who are more informed than them. Either their own leadership, or congregations that are being headed by people who are seen to be much more informed and influential. [. . .] Their ability to articulate some issues is limited, some issues are just above their capacity to engage in a conversation. I'm able to engage with you because of your education and your exposure. But if you were a Malawian pastor coming from a rural area, with a Standard 5 education, you may not be able to engage with me at

> that level. So issues like condoms, it's a bit of a problem for them to engage constructively and expect them to be able to contribute meaningfully to that.
> (George, pastor and administrator, Christian denomination, Lilongwe)

It was thus fairly clear that George felt that his own position on condoms was best kept discreet not because it was compromising his Christian morals, but because misinformed, uneducated people might mistakenly think so. Having heard from Malawian leaders and from other evangelicals that condoms are always wrong, they would not understand that he also thought they were wrong, even if he was giving out information about them. Interestingly, young people are spared this harsh judgement of their intellectual capacities, and George seems to trust them more than he trusts their parents – an unusual position in Malawi.

The second solution to the dilemma lies in the strategic engagement with the secular world: George says that churches must speak up about condoms because young people already hear about them from 'the world out there', so the organisation must make sure that they hear the *correct* things about condoms. Later on, he talked about a project in which donors favoured condom demonstration for young adults, and he explained how he convinced his colleague that it was acceptable.

> I said 'Look here, allow them. What you do is simple: the boys should be taught on their own, and the girls on their own. It'll be less embarrassing for the two. But allow them. We cannot cheat ourselves that – as churches sometimes we live in a false world. Those boys we're talking about might have already seen those things, somehow somewhere the secular world has already reached them. There's nothing that you are teaching them they don't already know. At the same time, let's trust the donor.' And he said 'OK, now that you've said to go ahead.'
> (George)

Thus, George has solved the condom conundrum: teaching condoms does no harm to young people who already know about them, while it works to the organisation's advantage by keeping its foreign partners happy. From his previous comments, we know that he thinks young people should be able to make their own decisions, even if he would like them to choose abstinence. He knows that young people want to have complete information, including about condoms, but he also knows that their elders do not want to be associated with condom programming. He navigates these conflicting views by strategically omitting certain information when talking to elders, and by invoking the influence of the secular world and of donors to justify his own actions.

Conclusion

Providing social services and maintaining transnational networks of resources and ideas is not new for Malawian Christians; indeed, they have been doing just that since the establishment of the first missions in the nineteenth century. Since the

1990s, however, Malawian society has been transformed by the AIDS epidemic, as well as by the international response to this epidemic, which brought funds, experts and health promotion messages to the country. As part of these changes, activities that used to belong to the realm of family obligations and charitable deeds became development activities, complete with their acronyms, donors, best practices and UN recommendations; thus 'caring for the sick' became HBC, 'taking in a nephew' qualified as OVC work, and pastoral work with youth was incorporated under LSE. Such redefinition of social and relational work came with funds, but also with strings attached according to donor conditionality.

Christian leaders working with young people took on this role gracefully, in part out of sincere concern for young people, but also in part in response to the high demand on the part of foreign donors for implementers of youth programming. The materials presented here show, however, that they adopt this role as 'HIV preventers' only as far as it does not conflict with their core mission, which remains evangelism and discipleship. In many cases, the limit is condom promotion, which leads them to find various arrangements to reconcile young people's need for complete information and their own Christian duty to promote abstinence. FBOs are not unique in accepting the HIV agenda within limits set by their own pre-existing priorities. They may, however, be firmer and more vocal than others about which lines they will not cross, insistent that their particular limits are based in revealed scriptures.

The discourses of my informants highlight the limits of Christian HIV prevention that focuses on abstinence, but they also point to the creative strategies that are used to reconcile different moral imperatives: some talk about their own experiences, others hide their condom programming from certain members of their organisation. They also highlight the complementarity of the Christian approach with other programming, especially those that emphasise condom promotion, whose presence in the Malawian landscape is implicit in my informants' discourses.

Some of the most important limitations of this chapter include the fact that it is based on interviews alone, and that these were conducted with leaders in Lilongwe and Blantyre (i.e. urban centres) only. Further research could build on this and the work of others by engaging with Christian organisations and leaders in smaller towns and in villages to establish how discourses become actual life skills classes and training sessions for peer educators; and by detailing the political economy of faith-based funding for HIV/AIDS work in Malawi. This chapter does, however, illustrate some of the ways in which Christian leaders are reconciling different conceptions of sexuality, and helping young people come of age in a dangerous time.

Acknowledgements

This chapter is based on research that was funded in part by a master's scholarship from the *Fonds québécois de recherche sur la société et la culture* (FQRSC). Many thanks to Alessandro Gusman, Susan Watkins and Jenny Trinitapoli for their comments and their encouragement.

References

Balchin, Cassandra. 2007. 'The F-word and the S-word – too much of one and not enough of the other', *Development in Practice* 17(4): 532–8.

Becker, Felicitas and P. Wenzel Geissler. 2007. 'Introduction: searching for pathways in a landscape of death: religion and AIDS in East Africa', *Journal of Religion in Africa* 37(1): 1–15.

Bertrand-Dansereau, Anaïs. 2010. 'La prévention du VIH auprès des jeunes au Malawi: paralysie et potentiels de l'éducation sexuelle', Département de Sociologie, UQÀM, Montréal.

Bertrand-Dansereau, Anaïs. 2013. 'Sex is a gift from God: paralysis and potential in sex education in Malawi', in S. Jolly, A. Cornwall and K. Hawkins (eds), *Women, Sexuality and the Political Power of Pleasure*. London: Zed Books.

Bone, David S. 1982. 'Islam in Malawi', *Journal of Religion in Africa* 13(2): 126–38.

Bush, George W. 2002. *Executive Order 13280. Responsibilities of the Department of Agriculture and the Agency for International Development with Respect to Faith-Based and Community Initiatives*. Ed. White House. Washington: American Government.

Deneulin, Séverine and Masooda Bano. 2009. *Religion in Development: Rewriting the Secular Script*. London: Zed Books.

Deneulin, Séverine and Carole Rakodi. 2010. 'Revisiting religion: development studies thirty years on', *World Development* 39(1): 45–54.

Englund, Harri. 2003. 'Christian independency and global membership: Pentecostal extraversions in Malawi', *Journal of Religion in Africa* 33(1): 83–111.

Englund, Harri. 2004. *Transnational Governance and the Pacification of Youth: The Contribution of Civic Education to Disempowerment in Malawi*. Durban: Centre for Civil Society, University of KwaZulu-Natal.

Eriksson, Elisabet, Gunilla Lindmark, Pia Axemo, Beverley Haddad and Beth Maina Ahlberg. 2009. 'Ambivalence, silence and gender differences in church leaders' HIV-prevention messages to young people in KwaZulu-Natal, South Africa', *Culture, Health and Sexuality* 12(1): 103–14.

Forster, Peter G. 1997. 'Religion and the State in Tanzania and Malawi', *Journal of Asian and African Studies* 32(3–4): 163–84.

Forster, Peter Glover. 1998. 'Religion, magic, witchcraft, and AIDS in Malawi', *Anthropos* 93(4/6): 537–45.

Freeman, Emily. 2012. 'Older adults' experiences of ageing, sex and HIV infection in rural Malawi', Department of Social Policy, London School of Economics and Political Science.

Freidus, Andrea. 2010. '"Saving" Malawi: faithful responses to orphans and vulnerable children', *NAPA Bulletin* 33(1): 50–67.

Glynn, Judith R., Ndoliwe Kayuni, Sian Floyd, Emmanuel Banda, Monica Francis-Chizororo, Clare Tanton, Anna Molesworth, Joanne Hemmings, Amelia C. Crampin and Neil French. 2010. 'Age at menarche, schooling, and sexual debut in northern Malawi', *PLOS ONE* 5(12): e15334.

Gordon, Gill and Vincent Mwale. 2006. 'Preventing HIV with young people: a case study from Zambia', *Reproductive Health Matters* 14(28): 68–79.

Government of Malawi. 2012. *2012 Global AIDS Response Progress Report: Malawi Country Report for 2010 and 2011*. Lilongwe: Government of Malawi. http://www.unaids.org/en/dataanalysis/knowyourresponse/countryprogressreports/2012countries/ce_MW_Narrative_Report[1].pdf.

Hefferan, Tara and Tim Fogarty. 2010. 'The anthropology of faith and development: an introduction', *NAPA Bulletin* 33(1): 1–11.

Hopkins, Joseph Martin. 1980. 'Theological students and witchcraft beliefs', *Journal of Religion in Africa* 11(1): 56–66.

Illouz, Eva. 1997. *Consuming the Romantic Utopia: Love and the Cultural Contradictions of Capitalism*. Berkeley: University of California Press.

Izugbara, Chimaraoke O. and Chi-Chi Undie. 2008. 'Who owns the body? Indigenous African discourses of the body and contemporary sexual rights rhetoric', *Reproductive Health Matters* 16(31): 159–67.

Jones, Ben and Marie Juul Petersen. 2011. 'Instrumental, narrow, normative? Reviewing recent work on religion and development', *Third World Quarterly* 32(7): 1291–306.

Kates, Jennifer, Adam Wexler and Allison Valentine. 2011. 'Donor funding for health in low- and middle-income countries 2002–2009', in *US Global Health Policy*. Menlo Park, CA: Kaiser Family Foundation.

Leurs, Robert. 2012. 'Are faith-based organisations distinctive? Comparing religious and secular NGOs in Nigeria', *Development in Practice* 22(5–6): 704–20.

Lindgren, Teri, Ellen Schell, Sally Rankin, Joel Phiri, Rachel Fiedler and Joseph Chakanza. 2013. 'A response to Edzi (AIDS): Malawi faith-based organizations' impact on HIV prevention and care', *Journal of the Association of Nurses in AIDS Care* 24(3): 227–41.

Makuwira, Jonathan. 2011. 'Civil society organizations (CSOs) and the changing nature of African politics: the case of the CSO–government relationship in Malawi', *Journal of Asian and African Studies* 46(6): 615–28.

Malawi Ministry of Health. 2008. *HIV and Syphilis Sero – Survey and National HIV Prevalence and AIDS Estimates Report for 2007*. Lilongwe: Malawi Ministry of Health.

Manglos, Nicolette D. 2010. 'Born again in Balaka: Pentecostal versus Catholic narratives of religious transformation in rural Malawi', *Sociology of Religion* 71(4): 409–31.

Manglos, Nicolette. 2011. 'Brokerage in the sacred sphere: religious leaders as community problem solvers in rural Malawi', *Sociological Forum* 26(2): 334–55.

Mkandawire, Rev. Francis. 2008. 'Roles of churches in a world living with HIV/AIDS', *Global HIV Consultation: Churches Living with HIV*. http://www.micahnetwork.org/sites/default/files/doc/library/09_roles_of_churches_francism.pdf.

Morfit, N. Simon. 2011. '"AIDS is money": how donor preferences reconfigure local realities', *World Development* 39(1): 64–76.

Munoz-Laboy, Miguel, Jonathan Garcia, Joyce Moon-Howard, Patrick A. Wilson and Richard Parker. 2011. 'Religious responses to HIV and AIDS: understanding the role of religious cultures and institutions in confronting the epidemic', *Global Public Health* 6(suppl. 2): S127–31.

Murray, S.S. 1922. *A Handbook of Nyasaland*. London: Published for the government of Nyasaland by the crown agents for the colonies.

Muula, Adamson S., James C. Thomas, Audrey E. Pettifor, Ronald P. Strauss, Chirayath M. Suchindran and Steven R. Meshnick. 2012. 'Religion is not associated with HIV infection among women in Malawi', *International Journal on Disability and Human Development* 11(2): 121–31.

National AIDS Commission. 2009a. *Malawi HIV and AIDS Extended National Action Framework (NAF), 2010–2012, Draft*. Lilongwe: Government of Malawi.

National AIDS Commission. 2009b. *National HIV Prevention Strategy 2009–2013*. Lilongwe: Government of Malawi.

National Statistical Office of Malawi. 2000. *1998 Population and Housing Census Analytical Report*. Zomba: Government of Malawi.

National Statistical Office of Malawi. 2010. *Population and Housing Census. Main Report*. Zomba: Government of Malawi.

National Statistical Office of Malawi. 2011. *Demographic and Health Survey 2010*. Zomba: Government of Malawi.

Nugent, Paul. 2004. *Africa since Independence: A Comparative History*. New York: Palgrave Macmillan.

Parikh, Shanti A. 2005. 'From auntie to disco: the bifurcation of risk and pleasure in sex education in Uganda', in S.L. Pigg and V. Adams (eds), *Sex in Development: Science, Sexuality and Morality in Global Perspective*. Durham, NC: Duke University Press.

Poulin, Michelle. 2007. 'Sex, money, and premarital partnerships in southern Malawi', *Social Science and Medicine* 65(11): 2383–93.

Prince, Ruth. 2007. 'Salvation and tradition: configurations of faith in a time of death', *Journal of Religion in Africa* 37(1): 84–115.

Prince, Ruth, Philippe Denis and Rijk van Dijk. 2009. 'Introduction to Special Issue: Engaging Christianities: negotiating HIV/AIDS, health, and social relations in East and Southern Africa', *Africa Today* 56(1): v–xviii.

Rakodi, Carole. 2012. 'Religion and development: subjecting religious perceptions and organisations to scrutiny', *Development in Practice* 22(5–6): 621–33.

Santelli, John, Mary A. Ott, Maureen Lyon, Jennifer Rogers, Daniel Summers and Rebecca Schleifer. 2006. 'Abstinence and abstinence-only education: a review of U.S. policies and programs', *Journal of Adolescent Health* 38(1): 72–81.

Spronk, Rachel. 2009. 'Media and the ethos of romantic love in middle-class Nairobi', in J. Cole and L.M. Thomas (eds), *Love in Africa*. Chicago: University of Chicago Press.

Swidler, Ann and Susan A. Watkins. 2007. 'Ties of dependence: AIDS and transactional sex in rural Malawi', *Studies in Family Planning* 38(3): 147–62.

Swidler, Ann and Susan Cotts Watkins. 2009. '"Teach a man to fish": the sustainability doctrine and its social consequences', *World Development* 37(7): 1182–96.

Tamale, Sylvia. 2013. 'Eroticism, sensuality and "women's secrets" among the Baganda', in S. Jolly, A. Cornwall and K. Hawkins (eds), *Women, Sexuality and the Political Power of Pleasure*. London: Zed Books.

Tawfik, Linda and Susan Cotts Watkins. 2007. 'Sex in Geneva, sex in Lilongwe, and sex in Balaka', *Social Science and Medicine* 64(5): 1090–101.

Thornton, Robert J. 2008. *Unimagined Community: Sex, Networks and AIDS in Uganda and South Africa*. Berkeley: University of California Press.

Trinitapoli, Jenny. 2011. 'The AIDS-related activities of religious leaders in Malawi', *Global Public Health* 6(1): 41–55.

Trinitapoli, Jenny and Mark D. Regnerus. 2006. 'Religion and HIV risk behaviors among married men: initial results from a study in rural sub-Saharan Africa', *Journal for the Scientific Study of Religion* 45(4): 505–28.

Trinitapoli, Jenny and Alexander Weinreb. 2012. *Religion and AIDS in Africa*. Oxford: Oxford University Press.

UNAIDS. 2012. 'Country page: Malawi'. http://www.unaids.org/en/regionscountries/countries/malawi/.

Van Kol, Willemijn. 2008. 'Ummah in Zomba: transnational influences on reformist Muslims in Malawi', *Journal of Muslim Minority Affairs* 28(3): 435–52.

Vaughan, Megan. 1991. *Curing Their Ills: Colonial Power and African Illness*. Palo Alto, CA: Stanford University Press.

Watkins, Susan Cotts and Ann Swidler. 2013. 'Working misunderstandings: donors, brokers, and villagers in Africa's AIDS industry', *Population and Development Review* 38(suppl. 1): 197–218.

World Health Organization. 2007. *Helping Parents in Developing Countries Improve Adolescents' Health*. Geneva: World Health Organization.

Yeatman, Sarah E. and Jenny Trinitapoli. 2008. 'Beyond denomination: the relationship between religion and family planning in rural Malawi', *Demographic Research* 19(55): 1851–82.

11

Let's Talk about Sex

Islam and Sexuality in Positive Muslims' 'Theology of Compassion'

JONAS SVENSSON

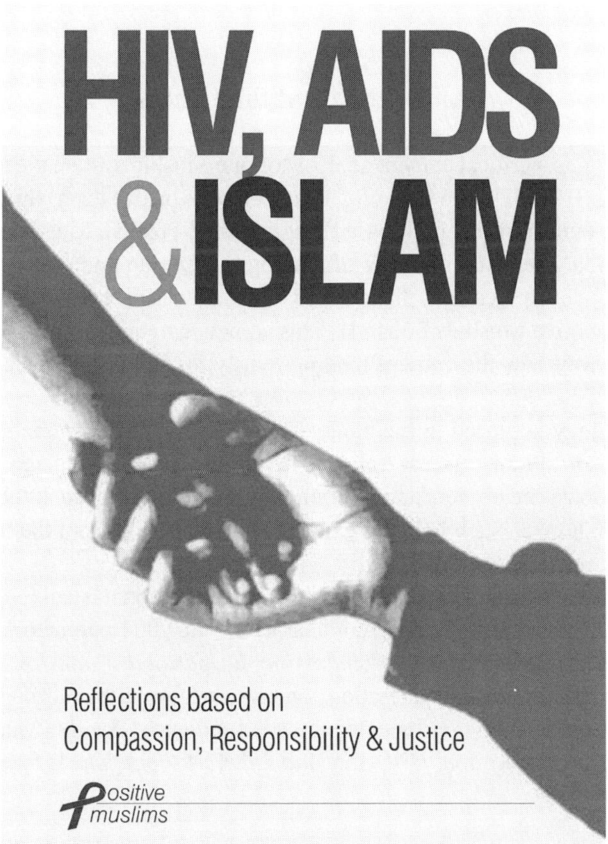

Front cover of the pamphlet in which Positive Muslims outlines the 'theology of compassion'

Proceedings of the British Academy **194**, *219–243*. © The British Academy 2014.

Introduction

IN THE ACADEMIC AND ACTIVIST LITERATURE on Islam and HIV/AIDS, one focal point has been religious beliefs, practices and institutions as obstacles to successful prevention work and as contributing to the stigmatisation of people living with HIV/AIDS (PLWHA), mainly through a 'moralising' discourse on divine punishment (Kelley and Eberstadt 2005; Obermeyer 2006; Atighetchi 2007: 199–234). Another focus has been on Islam as a potential resource in 'faith-based' activism to provide preventive work with a culturally acceptable veneer (Lagarde *et al.* 2000; UNICEF 2003; Hasnain 2005). In these discourses, however, Islam is more often than not taken as a given entity. In contrast to such a view, this chapter will turn the issue around. Instead of asking questions about the actual or potential role of Islam for HIV/AIDS activism, it will give a particular example of how the topic of HIV/AIDS has been used in religious rethinking and reformulation of religious 'authenticity'.[1]

Aim, scope and limitations

The following is a critical content analysis of one Muslim systematic theological[2] reflection on HIV/AIDS and sexuality. It concentrates on two texts which both form part of the South African 'faith-based' organisation Positive Muslims' 'theology of compassion', defined as 'a way of reading the Qur'an and understanding the Sunnah (prophetic precedent) that focuses on Allah who cares deeply about all the creation' (Positive Muslims 2004: 4). This somewhat non-informative definition does not convey how the 'way of reading' partly involves quite radical religious rethinking.

The theology is placed in the context of transnationalism, understood as the 'economic, social and political linkages between people, places and institutions crossing nation-state borders and spanning the world' (Vertovec 2009: 1), posing the question: how do such linkages explain particular features of the 'theology of compassion' relating to sexuality?

The texts are in English, the *lingua franca* of transnational Islam (Nielsen 2002: 22), and they are of slightly different character. The 2004 publication, *HIV Aids and Islam: Reflections Based on Compassion, Responsibility and Justice*, outlines aims and hermeneutical considerations and has local religious leaders, teachers, activists and organisations as its stated intended audience (Positive Muslims 2004: 8–9). The 2007 publication, *HIV, Aids and Islam: A Workshop Manual Based on*

[1] This chapter was written within the framework of a grant provided by Riksbankens jubileumsfond.
[2] 'Theology' is here used in a wide sense to denote any 'discourse on God', i.e. any *reflective* public representation of divine agency and intentionality, more or less elaborated.

Compassion, Responsibility and Justice, contains instructions for the planning and management of workshop sessions. It is directed at those working with Muslims in the context of raising awareness (Positive Muslims 2007: vii). Both texts, at least with regard to their theological content, are in practice mainly the work of Farid Esack, a founding member of Positive Muslims and an internationally well-known Muslim religious intellectual. He is currently a professor of Islamic Studies at the University of Johannesburg. Despite the fact that Esack is responsible for most of the content, his authorship is understated. For that reason I will in the following refer to Positive Muslims as the 'author'.

The texts form part of a larger 'theology of compassion' project. This also includes a third text, which for the most part will not be addressed, since it does not constitute a clear-cut outline or application of the theology as such. Neither was it intended for direct use in local activism. It does, however, testify to the transnational context of the theology. *Islam and AIDS: Between Scorn, Pity and Justice* (Esack and Chiddy 2009) contains academically oriented articles on HIV/AIDS and Islam and is a result of a seminar course held, not in South Africa, but at Harvard Divinity School in 2007 (where Farid Esack held a post as visiting professor until 2008).

As a content analysis of two theological texts, this chapter approaches the issue of HIV/AIDS, sexuality and Islam in Africa in a manner that differs from much previous research in the field, for example ethnographic accounts (see Becker 2009), attempts to provide more comprehensive overviews of local discourses in a particular geographic area (see Beckmann 2009) or particular institutional settings (see Svensson 2009). It also differs from surveys on attitudes towards HIV/AIDS among Muslims in Africa (see Ansari and Gaestel 2010; Maulana *et al.* 2009). It does not address the issue of reception or the actual use of the texts in local activism, and hence does not contribute with any particular on-the-ground insight into HIV/AIDS and Islam in South Africa. Its relevance lies elsewhere.

I am in agreement with Felicitas Becker when she states that we 'need to look further than Islamic scriptures and law in order to understand Muslims' responses to AIDS' (Becker 2009: 183). One could add public reflective theology to her list. The usefulness of religious scriptures, legal tradition or reflective theology in predicting actual beliefs and behaviour in any real-life settings is indeed limited, if any. This does not discount, however, that reflective theology, as one form of religious behaviour, may be a relevant object of study *in itself*. In a reflection on the 'anthropology of Islam' from a Mali context, Benjamin Soares (2000) claims that analysing Islam in African contexts as local and idiosyncratic forms of religious belief and practice risks missing out on an important field of study: the processes where Islamic scriptures, law and theological concepts belonging to a larger 'discursive tradition' are interacted with, referred to, used, criticised, reformulated and interpreted. Such activities constitute 'Islamic discourses and practices at the intersection of the local, the supralocal and the translocal' (Soares 2000: 283). It is in this context, and as a particular case study of such processes, that the following analysis should be placed.

Theoretical considerations

Any particular representation of Islam at any given time and in any given context is a cultural product, a result of human, socially situated responses to and reflections on established beliefs, practices and institutions that have been passed on from earlier generations and social, economic, political and ecological realities. Taking this into account, 'Islam' is not a unitary phenomenon. However, amidst the diversity of religious expressions there is a sense in which it is relevant to theoretically refer to 'Islam' as a 'discursive tradition' (Asad 1986).

Dale Eickelman and James Piscatori use the concept of 'Muslim politics' to denote an ongoing intra-Muslim discursive negotiation of social change and continuity. This discourse relates to a 'widely shared [. . .] tradition of ideas and practices' recognised *by participants themselves* as 'Islamic' (Eickelman and Piscatori 2004: 4). The outcomes of such negotiations, characterised by conflict and competition, are nevertheless diverse.

Growing transnational contacts and movement and the spread of easily accessible information on 'Islamic issues', combined with increased potential for processing such information among a general public, has in modern times prompted discourses on Islam that transcend local settings and relate to an imagined transnational community of a global *umma*. While the notion of such a transnational community is well established as an ideal in classical Islamic thought, it has gained everyday salience among increasingly wider sections of a Muslim public worldwide, particularly in the last century (Mandaville 2011). New actors have also emerged, challenging the interpretational monopoly of formally trained religious scholars, *'ulama*, and claiming to 'speak for Islam' (Mandaville 2007: 302–31). Rapidly expanding possibilities for transnational communication have provided new means for diverse actors within Muslim politics to establish transnational networks and platforms for the dissemination of their particular versions of the 'authentic' religious tradition worldwide.

The effects of the transnational character of contemporary Islam on sub-Saharan Africa have been highlighted in research, for example in the critical academic discussion on the distinction between 'African Islam' and 'Islam in Africa'. This distinction is emphasised in the edited volume *Islam in Africa and African Islam* (Westerlund and Rosander 1997). 'African Islam' is here used to denote 'home-grown' local versions of Islam, characterised as popular, inclusivist, open, flexible, engulfed in the local and with strong connections to Sufism. In contrast, 'Islam in Africa' signifies a reformist Islam 'imported' from outside: scholarly, scripturalist, exclusivist, detached, anti-Sufi, puritanist and rigid. The latter is associated with foreign involvement, mainly state actors such as Saudi Arabia, and transnational missionary (*da'wa*) organisations (Rosander 1997).

Although it is possible to read rather too much rigidity into this distinction, relevant critique has been raised. Rüdiger Seesemann, René Otayek and Benjamin Soares all note how it tends to reproduce colonial and orientalist discourses of a 'pure' Islam and local deviations. Furthermore, they all identify how, possibly as a result of an anthropological bias, some forms of religious beliefs and practices observed in local settings are treated as uniquely 'African', not noting that these are in fact widespread around the Muslim world (Seesemann 2006: 231–9; Otayek and Soares 2007: 3–4). Apart from this, one can also, as Seesemann has done, take a historical perspective and argue that whatever can be viewed as 'African Islam' in a particular setting at a particular point in time might at another point in time just as well be seen as 'Islam in Africa'. There are no clear boundaries between the two (Seesemann 2006: 239–42). Above all, the critique points out how religious change in contemporary or historical Africa cannot be construed as a result of unidirectional flows. The notion of a 'foreign' Islam imported or superimposed on Africa obscures the actual processes involved. The vessels for change are, and have been for a long time, manifold, without a shared agenda and not least indigenous. They involve Sufi orders with transnational networks, Islamic NGOs, transnational or local, state parties and notably individuals, travelling inside or outside the continent, or increasingly producing local religious rethinking based on inspiration through the diverse channels of modern-day communications (Otayek and Soares 2007: 4, 8–9).[3]

Apart from the fact that the agents of transnationalism are varied, contemporary transnational processes of change also affect the Muslim publics with whom these agents interact. An important aspect of religious change due to modernity is what Eickelman and Piscatori, and others after them, have termed the 'objectification of Islam' (Eickelman and Piscatori 2004: 37–45; Roy 2004: 21–2). Increased awareness amongst believing Muslims around the world that there exists a multitude of often competing representations of Islam has resulted in decentralised reflections on religious authenticity. Islam has increasingly become less of a 'natural', integrated and embedded part of everyday life, and more of a delimited object, a 'religion', possible to relate to and reflect upon in relation to other 'religions' and other social and cultural phenomena.

The 'theology of compassion' should be seen as part of a discursive negotiation within the framework of Muslim politics characterised by the 'objectification of Islam'. 'Islam' is not an independent variable that casually *affects* the particulars

[3] There is quite a lot of research on the diversity of agents of transnationalism having religious importance in an African context besides state actors, including transnational piety movements such as Tabligh Jama'at (see Vahed 2003), networks of Sufi orders with roots in African contexts (see Babou 2011; Hill 2012), and Islamic Aid organisations (see Kaag 2011; Petersen 2012).

in this theology, but rather emerges as a *result* of it. The 'theology of compassion' is hence an instance of 'doing Islam' (Varisco 2005: 149). Highlighting this constructive process means paying attention to how Positive Muslims on the level of reflective thought, and with the purpose of convincing others, cite and utilise elements from within a religious 'pool of resources' (Eickelman and Piscatori 2004: 29), e.g. sacred scriptures, narratives, rituals, previous theological elaboration and particular elements in a 'sacred terminology' that carry a positive or negative emotive charge.

Positive Muslims and the transnational context of the 'theology of compassion'

Positive Muslims was founded in 2000 in Western Cape province and formally dissolved in late 2011. All its assets were transferred to the larger 'non-faith-based' NGO Treatment Action Campaign with which Positive Muslims had had a close cooperation throughout (Positive Muslims 2004: 8; Bangstad 2007: 159). According to Farid Esack, they 'had run out of steam and could not find a competent director' (personal communication, 8 May 2012). During its heyday, it was nevertheless internationally noted for its work to reformulate Islam in order to facilitate prevention work and combat stigmatisation of PLWHA (see Francesca 2002: 391–2; Bangstad 2007: 158; Obermeyer 2006: 852).

There are a few scholarly works that provide information about Positive Muslims. One of the organisation's founding members, Abdul Kayum Ahmed, gives a comprehensive overview of its early development and origins in his master's thesis 'Positive Muslims: a critical analysis of Muslim AIDS activism in relation to women living with HIV/AIDS in Cape Town' (2003). In a 2008 paper, Kate Willson provides a vivid presentation based on fieldwork in 2007, including reports from workshops using the above-mentioned manual (Willson 2008: 50–8). In a master's thesis from 2007, Om Lekhraj Lala writes about the diverse activities of Positive Muslims (although the organisation is not mentioned by name), comparing it with corresponding Christian and Hindu 'faith-based' organisations in South Africa (Lala 2007: 57–66). Sindre Bangstad, in his 2007 thesis on Muslims in Cape Town, also devotes a section in a chapter on HIV/AIDS to Positive Muslims, mainly contrasting its religious vision of HIV/AIDS with what he generically refers to as the more conservative and moralising view of the local *'ulama* (Bangstad 2007: 157–9). All these sources provide the impression of a strong core of individual activists, with affiliated volunteers, pursuing a diverse agenda including research, counselling, support, awareness raising and in particular theological rethinking. All allocate particular attention to the 'theology of compassion', but limit themselves to descriptive overviews.

The transnational context of Positive Muslims involves several levels. During its active period, Positive Muslims cooperated with several transnational aid organisations: state, interstate and non-state. The Dutch non-governmental organisation Oxfam Novib, USAID and UNAIDS all contributed with funds in the formulation of the 'theology of compassion' (Positive Muslims 2004: i, 2007: v). Ahmed states that the support from Oxfam Novib in particular provided the economic means for the organisation's expansion in 2002 (Ahmed 2003: 85–6).

In 2007 Positive Muslims co-arranged a large conference in South Africa on HIV/AIDS and Islam with the international NGO Islamic Relief, founded in the UK in 1984. It also cooperated with the NAZ project, which offers information on sexual and reproductive health to South Asian, Middle Eastern, North African and Latino minority communities in the UK. Other activities also indicate an anticipated context for the 'theology of compassion' that extends beyond South Africa. In 2008 a delegation of three prominent members of Positive Muslims, Farid Esack, Fatima Noordien and Faghmeda Miller, travelled to Amsterdam at the invitation of the Dutch organisation SOAAIDS. The explicit purpose was to export the 'theology of compassion', with suitable modifications, to be used in awareness campaigns among Muslim immigrants in the Netherlands (Tempert 2009). The anticipation of a transnational relevance is also clear in the texts under analysis:

> At a broader (beyond South Africa) *ummah* (community) level, we want to let other Muslims living with HIV&AIDS know that they are not alone and we want to alert Muslims to the fact that there are, indeed, Islamically rooted responses beyond knee-jerk prejudice and bigotry.
>
> (Positive Muslims 2004: 8)

In the 2007 manual it is stated that:

> Although this project has developed from Positive Muslims' experience in South Africa, and [*sic*] interactions with Muslims in other parts of the world who are working in this area have reiterated the need for a manual which has a broad appeal and which may be adapted for use elsewhere.
>
> (Positive Muslims 2007: vii)

Another aspect of transnationalism relates to the 'theology of compassion' as a *reaction* to otherwise dominant intra-Muslim religious discourses on HIV/AIDS. Ahmed provides a short characterisation of AIDS activism in South Africa before the establishment of Positive Muslims. He highlights the activities of the national Islamic Medical Association (IMA), affiliated with similar organisations in other parts of the Muslim world within an international Federation of Islamic Medical Associations. Ahmed portrays the IMA as strongly influenced by a 'Malik Badri approach' (Ahmed 2003: 58–65). Malik Badri is a Sudanese-born professor of psychology at the Malaysian Islamic University. His book *The AIDS Crisis* (1997) has been highly influential in the contemporary intra-Muslim discourse on Islam and HIV/AIDS (Bangstad 2009: 43–4). Badri construes HIV/AIDS as a collective divine punishment for (mainly sexual) transgressions of Islamic moral boundaries, ultimately traceable to a worldwide influence of a 'Western' sexual revolution, and in particular its acceptance of male homosexuality (Badri 1997: 35–71). The only way to prevent a further spread of the pandemic is to promote 'true' Islamic sexual morals in society, by force if necessary. Islam, Badri argues, is the solution, even a 'cure' for the AIDS epidemic (Badri 1997: 189–227). Ahmed is clear in stating that the establishment of Positive Muslims was motivated by a wish to construct an alternative to the 'Malik Badri approach' (Ahmed 2003: 62–3), which I believe is better understood as a generic designation of larger moralising discourses on Islam and HIV/AIDS.[4]

Another transnational context in which to place the 'theology of compassion' is particularly important in explaining its particularities *qua* theology. Positive Muslims uses the word 'progressive' as a self-description (Positive Muslims 2004: 59, 2007: vii). This is more than just a positioning against 'conservative' or 'traditional' approaches. Ahmed clearly identifies Positive Muslims as part of a 'Progressive Muslim Network' specified as 'a group of academics and activists from various parts of the world, including Cape Town, who communicate primarily via their web site and Internet discussion forum' (Ahmed 2003: 20). The website and forum, traces of which at the time of writing (October 2012) could still be found on the internet (see, for example, progressivemuslims.tripod.com/index2.html), were established in 1998 and involved an international network of individual scholar-activists calling for a radical reinterpretation of Islam on the basis of human rights, social justice and democracy. In 2003, as a consequence of the 9/11 events in New York, members of the network, several of whom occupied influential positions at higher educational institutions in the US, published the volume *Progressive Muslims* (Safi 2003). It featured contributions from several internationally well-known Muslim scholar-activists such as Omid Safi, Ebrahim Moosa, Amina Wadud, Scott Siraj Kugle and Kecia Ali, and not least Positive Muslims' own Farid Esack.

'Progressive Islam' has received some academic interest, both as a relatively identifiable network and more loosely understood as a tendency or a movement (Duderija 2008, 2010; Frisina 2010: 568; Shannahan 2010). The more formal organisation Progressive Muslim Union of North America (PMU) was launched in New York in 2004, dissolved after internal conflicts in 2006, and succeeded by the likewise North America-focused Muslims for Progressive Values, which is still active.[5] When the term 'progressive Islam' is used in the following, however, it

[4] For an introduction to such discourses, see for example Francesca (2002), and in the South African and Cape Town context, see Bangstad (2007: 153–7), which also mentions Badri's book as influential.
[5] The subsequent development of the concept of 'progressive Islam' within a North American context, and how it became a topic for discussion, polarisation and conflict, is not an issue pursued here.

refers to the suggestions for reinterpretation of Islam outlined in *Progressive Muslims*. There is a connection with the later organisations in the sense that some of the contributors to the volume were also engaged in the early activities of the PMU and participated in its advisory board, but the main individual important hereinafter declined to do so – Farid Esack.

While the contributors to the 2003 volume *Progressive Muslims* address different topics, they share certain basic views which could be summarised as follows: a general critique of essentialist constructions of Islam as a monolithic unity and an acknowledgement of intra-Muslim religious diversity; a stress on the *validity* of a multiplicity of understandings of the religious tradition; a call for a socially contextual, historically conscious reinterpretation of Islam that focuses less on interpreting the scriptures to the letter, and more on what the authors identify as basic religio-ethical principles contained mainly in the Qur'anic revelation.[6]

The distinctiveness of progressive Islam in contemporary Muslim politics becomes clear only when considering two strong alternative interpretational tendencies against which its proponents position themselves, more or less explicitly: apologetic modernism and salafism (at times termed neo-fundamentalism or wahhabism). Both share the notion of *one* single, ahistorical and decontextualised 'authentic' Islam, although the methods for discerning this and the conclusions reached on particular topics differ. Salafism can be roughly characterised as the tendency to restrict authentic Islam to the *literal* reading of the religious scriptures, the rejection of both traditional scholarship throughout the ages and the employment of human reasoning in a process of interpretation. The rising prominence of this tendency among Muslims around the world has received a great deal of attention during the last decade.[7] Apologetic modernism, on the other hand, has been a prominent trend for a longer period, at least since the late nineteenth century. As in salafism, there is a rejection of classical scholarship in favour of approaching the scriptures directly. However, here the use of human reasoning is pivotal. A characteristic feature is the ambition to accommodate authentic Islam with concepts and values associated with modernity. Hence, the scriptures, correctly interpreted (often with great effort and detail) and freed from the constraints of traditional Islamic scholarship, contain 'Islamic' and therefore 'superior' versions or alternatives of, for example, human rights, democracy or gender equality. The tone is often idealistic, distinguishing between what Muslims do (bad) and what Islam 'really' says (good) and claims, as in the case of salafism, that the majority of what can be observed within the diversity of 'Muslim' beliefs and practices around the world and in history, particularly those that in one way or the other conflict with modern sensibilities, is really not 'Islamic'.

[6] For a presentation of these shared views, based on an analysis of the 2003 volume and other texts, see Duderija (2010).

[7] The best overview to date of the phenomenon of salafism, and current research in the field, is the 2009 edited volume *Global Salafism: Islam's New Religious Movement* (Meijer 2009).

Mention has already been made several times of the chief architect behind the 'theology of compassion', Farid Esack. Although there is no tendency in the texts under analysis to stress or even point out any prominent position for him, all secondary sources are univocal in this respect. Esack is the main personal link between the 'theology of compassion' and progressive Islam. As one of the contributors to the 2003 volume *Progressive Muslims*, it is his chapter that most clearly outlines a programme for the proposed movement (Esack 2003).

Esack's personal history also reads as a prime example of an 'individual' agent of transnationalism in Africa: born in a Cape Town suburb, he was involved at an early age in the transnational piety movement *Tabligh Jama'a*, and travelled to Pakistan for *madrasa* studies and earned a degree as a religious scholar; later on in life he pursued theological and philosophical studies in Great Britain and Germany and gained secular university degrees. He has held academic posts as a widely acknowledged theologian and scholar in the study of religions in South Africa, Germany, the UK, the Netherlands and the US. Firmly rooted in a South African context of anti-apartheid and gender activism, he has been an inspiration to other Muslims who have striven to apply the religious tradition to social issues. His book *Qur'an, Liberation and Pluralism* (1997) is an attempt to formulate a Muslim version of liberation theology.

This section has outlined the multi-faceted transnational context of Positive Muslims and the 'theology of compassion'. The remainder of this chapter will connect these varied aspects of transnationalism to the particular *content* of the theology in the field of sexuality.

Islam, sexuality and the 'theology of compassion'

Justifying prevention: Islam, condom use and sex education

Positive Muslims provides a commonplace overview of sexually transmitted infections and prevention methods, with facts on both male and female condoms and arguments for their effectiveness with reference to scientific studies (Positive Muslims 2004: 42, 2007: 8, 54, 56). Reluctance among believing Muslims against the large-scale promotion of condoms, based on the view that such endorsement would encourage promiscuity, is recognised. Still, Positive Muslims counters such disinclination first by pointing out condom use within 'legitimate' sexual relations where one partner is infected as religiously unproblematic (Positive Muslims 2004: 41, 2007: 59), and second by referring to a well-established ethical principle in Islamic thought – the choice between a 'greater' and a 'lesser' evil. The latter takes on a prominent position in the argumentation and constitutes the sub-heading for the section on condoms in the 2007 workshop manual: 'The lesser of two harms' (Positive Muslims 2007: 55). In Muslim ethical tradition, this principle is based on an analogy with 'necessity', *darura*, and the Qur'anic verse 6:145 concerning forbidden meat that becomes legitimate in case of need (Atighetchi 2007: 34). It has frequently been used in the contemporary intra-Muslim discourse on Islam, HIV/AIDS and condoms as a (last resort) method of prevention, both in theological outlines on Islam and HIV/AIDS, such as for example in the above-mentioned Malik Badri's book (Badri 1997: 248–50), and in everyday discourses on prevention and in activism (see Beckmann 2009: 140; Svensson 2009: 206–7). Positive Muslims also explicitly cites Badri (Positive Muslims 2004: 42) as well as giving references to Malaysian state policies based on the same ethical considerations (Positive Muslims 2007: 58).

Thus, in the case of promoting condom use, Positive Muslims provides a theological response that is fairly commonplace. This is also the case concerning sex education, particularly sex education for youth. In response to critical voices that claim sex education is tantamount to encouraging promiscuity, the organisation quotes UNAIDS' studies. These show 'scientifically' that sexual health education delays sexual activity in young people, and reduces both the frequency of sex and the number of sexual partners. The main point is that rejecting these facts is basically 'un-Islamic': 'Since the Qur'an emphasizes knowledge, it compels people to consider evidence produced by scholars and scientists, even if they are uncomfortable with that evidence' (Positive Muslims 2007: 50). Here, there is an implicit reference to widely held notions in contemporary Muslim politics of a scriptural dictum to 'search for knowledge' as a religious duty, and a contemporary view that 'true' knowledge, including knowledge from modern science, is fully compatible with religious 'truths'.[8]

On the positive side of theologically *promoting* and not merely justifying sex education, Positive Muslims urges Muslims to break the silence and talk openly about sexual issues. Also in this case direct references to scripture are utilised, as is the principle 'search for knowledge'. As a more direct reference, 'historical' information concerning attitudes among the first Muslims, Muhammad and his companions, is invoked. They had no problems discussing intimate matters, including sexuality (Positive Muslims 2004: 21). Hence, modern-day sex education is provided with a religious coating through a standard modernist reference to the normative example of the 'pious forefathers', *al-salaf al-salih*, due to their spatial and temporal proximity to the initial divine revelation.

The manner in which both condom use and sex education are approached within the 'theology of compassion' thus displays a familiar way in which a shared 'pool of resources' – the Qur'an, early Islam and established ethical principles – is applied in contemporary Muslim politics. The scriptures are construed as carriers of clear,

[8] For a thorough analysis of contemporary Muslim discourses on Islam and science, and the way in which scriptures, as in the case of Positive Muslims here, feature as discursive resources, see Stenberg (1996).

easily accessible information directly relevant for and applicable to contemporary concerns. However, when moving into other topics in the field of sexuality, the radical character of the 'theology of compassion' in terms of hermeneutics becomes more conspicuous.

Redrawing sexual boundaries

Positive Muslims rejects an 'apologetic approach' (Atighetchi 2007: 200) that is otherwise common in contemporary Muslim discourses on HIV/AIDS, which claims that Islam, contrary to 'Western culture' and due to high standards of sexual morality, provides protection against HIV. There is an emphasis that Muslims are not, by virtue of their religious affiliation, in any way protected against HIV/AIDS. On the contrary, such an attitude may have disastrous effects on HIV/AIDS prevention (Positive Muslims 2004: 12–13). An idealised view that 'true' Muslims *should* not engage in sexual activities outside of religiously prescribed boundaries must not obscure the fact that many do: 'The Qur'an [. . .] contains clear injunctions on sex outside the permissible boundaries, but the reality of Muslims' lives does not always conform to this' (Positive Muslims 2007: 13).

The quotation could give the impression that Positive Muslims affirms the existence of an 'Islamic' sexual morality that can be easily deduced from the scriptures. Likewise, in a passage on prevention strategies it is stated that 'Islam teaches that sexual activities outside the permissible boundaries of the Qur'an are wrong. An Islamic approach to HIV prevention must include this message' (Positive Muslims 2007: 12). However, as it turns out, the concept of Qur'anic *boundaries* present in both these quotations becomes an object for theological redefinition.

In classical Islamic legal tradition, illicit sexual activity is generically termed *zina*, one of the crimes against divinely set 'boundaries', *hudud.* These crimes (which are usually considered to be five in number) are not social crimes, but crimes against God. They are mentioned in, or directly deduced from, the words of the Qur'an and merit harsh punishments – in the case of *zina*, corporal or capital punishment (depending on the marital status of the offender) (Peters 2012). Homosexuality, or rather male homosexual penetrative sex, often referred to as *liwat*, is at times counted as *zina* and as a *hudud* crime, but has also come to occupy a particular position in the legal tradition as a crime in its own right, likewise meriting death (Bearman *et al.* 2012).

However, classical Islamic law concerning *zina* and *liwat* has little bearing on the sexual boundaries that Positive Muslims outlines:

> Our bodies are a sacred trust from Allah that must be returned, and Allah will ask us about how we treated these bodies. We cannot cheapen our bodies by having sex with just anybody, thus exposing ourselves to all sorts of risks [. . .] Abstaining from casual sex is not just about being prudish – it is about self-respect and the awareness that one is accountable to Allah. A good Muslim understands that 'no soul carries

> the burden of another' (Qur'an 6:164), and will not succumb to peer pressure to have casual sex.
>
> (Positive Muslims 2004: 35)

Here, irresponsible sexuality replaces illegitimate sexuality. The reference to a sacred trust, *amana*, exemplifies a utilisation of a 'sacred terminology'. It is a Qur'anic term that, when it occurs in verse 33:72, is usually associated with a particular view of human nature and destiny, and a particular relationship or covenant with God. In classical exegesis, *amana*, as it stands in the Qur'an, is something offered by God and accepted by human beings. Strong candidates for what the term actually denotes are reason or free will (see Sherif 1995: 58). However, in the quotation above, the use corresponds more to how *amana* recurs within a contemporary religious bio-ethical discourse, where it is connected to *the human body* as ultimately the property of God, but entrusted to individuals (Atighetchi 2007: 35). This interpretational principle of what can be termed 'conceptual hermeneutics' is a recurring feature in the texts. An emotionally charged, Qur'anic key term is chosen as fundamental to the overall message. It is invested with meaning so that it becomes relevant to the issue at hand and is then used to contest established interpretations. Other such terms used in a similar manner include 'compassion' (*rahma*) and 'justice' (*'adl*).

However, replacing a *legal* notion of illegitimate sex with the *ethical* notion of religiously 'irresponsible' sex is not the only way in which the 'theology of compassion' questions established notions of Islam and sexuality. Sex is presented as a basic, legitimate and divinely created human need, just like hunger. 'In the same way that all of us have the right to enjoy our food, so too do we have the right to sexual enjoyment' (Positive Muslims 2004: 38). This comparison is elaborated with reference to intra-Muslim diversity and historical change. In the case of food, Positive Muslims argues, historical records testify to Muslim diversity on what qualifies as *halal* (allowed) and *haram* (forbidden). The organisation notes a lack of consensus among the different schools of law, *madhahib*, and claims that Islamic legal thought always mirrors historical change and cultural differences (Positive Muslims 2004: 38). The notion of historical change is then transferred to sexuality in the following manner: Muslims today are convinced that the only form of legitimate sex is between husband and wife within the framework of marriage. All other forms of sexual encounters constitute *zina*. This view, however, is not that of the Qur'an, nor of the classical legal tradition. Here, a man may also have legitimate sexual relations with his female slaves. Still, Positive Muslims argues, Muslims today find concubinage repulsive, reject slavery as an institution and claim that neither the Prophet nor the Qur'an, *from a basic ethical point of view*, condones the tradition. Instead the scriptures encourage its abolition. The narrow understanding of legitimate sexuality as being confined to heterosexual marriage, dominant in contemporary Muslim politics, is thus put forward as a novel 'modern' perception, as is the negative moral evaluation of slavery (Positive

Muslims 2004: 38–40). Changes in perception in the latter case show how 'Islam has been able to adjust eternal principles to changing times' (Positive Muslims 2004: 38). Hence:

> The insistence on marriage between male and female as the only other legitimate basis for sexual fulfilment is approached as if it is timeless and as if all other forms of sexual fulfilment between two persons are regarded as adultery. Clearly though, from the example of slavery, Islamic scholarship is capable of responding to new understandings of what it means to be human and to respond humanely to impulses around us without dismissing these as mere Western-induced promiscuity or as anti-Islamic.
>
> (Positive Muslims 2004: 39–40)

Challenging contemporary understandings of what constitutes an 'eternal' or 'authentic' religious norm in the context of sexuality through invoking scriptures, legal tradition and historical changes becomes a starting point for religious rethinking. The consequences in the field of sexuality are only implied. The 2007 manual instructs the facilitators at a workshop session with the title 'Shari'ah Muslim society and gender' to ask participants to rate the three phenomena 'slavery', 'sex outside marriage' and 'interest or usury' on a scale from 1 to 5 of approval/disapproval. After that, the information on sex, marriage and concubinage, as above, should be given. Participants should then be asked to reflect on whether slavery can be justified in Islam and if 'it is proper to do so'. They are also asked to morally compare a man having sex outside marriage with a slave to consensual sex with a prostitute, with a casual partner, and, last but not least, 'with a girlfriend' (Positive Muslims 2007: 46–7).

The explicit reference to *diversity* in Islamic legal tradition in the example above should be noted. It is a recurring feature in the texts (see Positive Muslims 2004: 40, 51, 2007: 51–2), but becomes most prominent in the section of the workshop manual mentioned in the previous paragraph. The text provides a very short overview of Islamic law, pointing out differences between schools, and basic principles employed by legal scholars and historical changes. The stress is on inherent and above all legitimate flexibility (Positive Muslims 2007: 44–8).

The theological strategy employed in these examples of redrawing sexual boundaries is one of simultaneously challenging perceived dominant views on what constitutes legitimate and illegitimate sex, and providing a proposal for an *ethically* valid alternative. This is a qualification of the above-cited adherence to a clear 'Islamic' teaching on sexuality, and the need to heed that teaching in activism. The method echoes what feminist scholar (and contributor to the 2003 volume *Progressive Muslims*) Kecia Ali has proposed as one strategy for religious reform in sexual ethics in her book *Sexual Ethics and Islam* (2006). Pointing out the discrepancy between actual norms and the literal content of the scriptures – as well as the diversity in Islamic law throughout the ages – can be used to challenge dominant contemporary views on 'Islamic sexuality' (Ali 2006: 156). The similarity is not a coincidence. Ali's contributions to the 'theology of compassion' are clearly acknowledged in the 2004 publication (Positive Muslims 2004: 9).

Homosexuality is not mentioned very often in the two texts. This can be interpreted as a strategic choice, since the association between HIV/AIDS and homosexuality, as the ultimate form of sexual transgression, is strong both in the contemporary intra-Muslim discourse in general (Francesca 2002), and in the local South African context (Bangstad 2007: 132, 156–7), and could easily overshadow other important themes. The 2007 manual mentions 'male–male intercourse' in a discussion of a particular *hadith*, i.e. a saying from the Prophet Muhammad, often cited in the contemporary discourse as 'proof' that HIV/AIDS is a divine punishment. Positive Muslims translates the *hadith* as follows: 'If unlawful *fahishah* (bad deeds or speech) become common in any group or nation, Allah will punish them with epidemics and diseases which were not known to their forefathers and earlier generations' (Positive Muslims 2007: 21). The term *fahisha* can be found in the Qur'an (e.g. verses 7:28, 27:54, 29:28) and is often translated as 'abomination', 'lewdness', 'sexual indecency' and similar terms. It is also frequently used to denote homosexuality (Siddiquee 2009; Rowson 2012). Malik Badri, in his paraphrasing of the *hadith*, translates it as 'fornication and all kinds of sinful sexual intercourse' (Badri 1997: 210). Positive Muslims challenges this in its choice of wording and the subsequent discussion. The *hadith*, taken as a whole, enumerates several 'bad deeds' not related to sexuality, and in Islamic tradition *fahisha* has been taken to mean a wide range of transgressions. Ultimately, Positive Muslims poses the rhetorical question 'who decides what a word should mean?' (2007: 22).[9] The 2004 publication mentions homosexuality four times, noting the connection often made to HIV/AIDS and acknowledging it in the local South African context (Positive Muslims 2004: 8, 22). Nevertheless, the topic is approached in a more implicit manner in both publications. This is done by including sexual diversity in a more general discussion on divinely instituted human diversity and a basic notion of a common, sacred humanity transcending this diversity (Positive Muslims 2004: 37, 2007: 34).

Positive Muslims' redefinition of sexual boundaries can be summarised as follows: widespread notions among Muslims on eternal norms of legitimate and illegitimate sexuality are wrong, as evidenced by historical facts showing a continuing process of change and redefinition. From this, a general strategy for religious reform can be deduced: identify the *basic* unchanging ethical foundations of the divine message and construct new norms from them. This becomes a challenge to both contemporary and historical formulations of 'authenticity'. While the topic at hand is HIV/AIDS and sexuality, the suggestions for reform, and in particular its methodology, have much wider aspirations and go much deeper in

[9] For a thorough discussion on the *hadith*, its use, and an interpretation of its meaning in line with that suggested by Positive Muslims, see Siddiquee (2009).

questioning widely held premises of contemporary Muslim politics. This becomes even more evident when context and diversity – still applied to the issue of sexuality – are used not only to challenge interpretations of Islam throughout history in the contemporary world, but also to challenge the very content of the scriptures themselves.

The individual sexual subject and power structures

When Positive Muslims, in the quotation above, claims that the demand not to transgress sexual boundaries should not obscure the fact that many do, it is not primarily a statement about individuals' moral shortcomings. Rather, sexuality is placed within a larger intersectional context of gender, social justice and unequal power structures; a reality posed against idealistic constructions of Islamic authenticity regarding sex. Such constructions abound in contemporary Muslim politics. In widely distributed, contemporary pamphlet literature on sex, 'Islam', in a reified manner, is often attributed with a positive view on sex and sexual pleasure, as long as it is confined within the boundaries of the *shari'a.* This view is often apologetically contrasted with both a perceived 'Christian' denouncement of sex as a 'necessary evil' and a 'Western' perverted, destructive and exploitative sexual morality. 'Islam', it is claimed, holds sex as a divine gift, and the securement of the mutual sexual gratification of spouses, and particularly women's sexual pleasure, is construed as a religious obligation.[10]

In contrast to such idealistic and apologetic constructions of 'Islamic' sexuality, Positive Muslims clearly states that sexual intercourse is far from always a matter of individuals' free rational choice. This is particularly relevant for women whose capacities for sexual negation are often circumscribed. A prevention strategy that preaches that Muslims should heed Islamic sexual morals is not enough: 'In addition to teaching people to say no to sexual advances, it is important to work towards a world wherein people have the freedom to do so' (Positive Muslims 2007: 13). An indication that sex as a matter of individual free choice is regarded as problematic is the way in which the 2007 manual, when summarising the measures needed to be taken in an effective 'Islamic' prevention policy, does not mention sexual abstinence, although the B (be faithful) and C (condoms) of the ABC are included. Instead of abstinence, focus is directed at the need for reform in gender structures and actions against other forms of social inequality (Positive Muslims 2007: 54).

In the theological elaboration on social inequality and sexuality, there is a prominent perspective that questions important foundations in contemporary Muslim politics. The beginning of the Qur'anic verse 2:223 reads, in Yusuf Ali's

[10] For a prototypical example, see Waris Maqsood (2000).

translation: 'Your wives are as a tilth unto you; so approach your tilth when or how ye will.' The verse has been interpreted as establishing a religious obligation for married women to always accept the sexual advances of their husbands, unless they are in a state of ritual impurity (Ali 2006: 129–31). While not quoting the verse outright, Positive Muslims nevertheless addresses the conjugal duty of sexual availability, again referring to the concept of *amana.* Marriage should not be construed as a contract providing husbands with unlimited access to their wives' bodies, since this would be sexual exploitation. It deprives women of the possibility to perform their religious duty to safeguard their bodies as sacred trusts. Just as in the context of responsible sexuality, the body is not owned by the individual or any other human being. Hence, according to Positive Muslims, it is 'Islamic' to strive against such exploitation, and against the power relations upon which it rests. This involves not only a struggle against gender inequality, but also against a whole, intersected system of inequalities. When doing this, the individual is fulfilling her or his God-given role, specified in the Qur'an, as His vicegerent, *khalifa*, on earth (Positive Muslims 2004: 35–6).

Thus, a particular scriptural reference – and not only an interpretation of scripture – is directly questioned with reference to basic ethical principles *and* social reality, utilising an emotionally charged 'sacred terminology'. This way of reasoning mirrors that of Muslim feminist Amina Wadud, mentioned above as a contributor to the 2003 volume *Progressive Muslims*. She caused an uproar with her paper 'Vulnerabilities: HIV and AIDS', during an HIV/AIDS conference of 'Muslim leaders' in Malaysia in 2003. The paper was eventually withdrawn. The incident is recounted by Farid Esack, who was present at the conference, in an appendix to his UNAIDS report on Muslim attitudes to HIV/AIDS (Esack 2007: 232–41), but it was also noted in the international news flow (Singh 2003). In June 2003 Wadud published the paper on the blog MuslimWakeup, closely affiliated with the Progressive Muslim Union of North America referred to above. She later published it again in her book *Inside the Gender Jihad* (2006).

Wadud's text criticises the notion that abstinence from *zina* is the main way to combat HIV/AIDS. The stress on abstinence obscures the existence of religiously legitimised gender-based inequalities that impede women's control over their sexuality. The important – and controversial – claim was that such inequalities are not just a matter of deficient interpretations or human shortcomings in understanding the sacred texts. On the contrary, the texts in themselves are part of the problem. Androcentrism is integral in the Qur'an. According to Wadud, the majority of Muslim women who become infected with HIV are monogamous and heed Islamic sexual morals. The problem is that their husbands do not. Due to the conjugal duty of intercourse as expressed in 2:223, women are in a difficult position. For this reason, Wadud argues, any feasible strategy to combat HIV/AIDS among Muslims must entail a radical rethinking of the religious heritage, with reforms that go beyond reinterpreting sacred texts and challenge the very word of the scripture. A literalist approach characteristic of much contemporary Islamic discourse must be replaced by a wider search for a 'divine intent' in face of current social realities (Wadud 2006: 233–44). Given Positive Muslims' approach to verse 2:223, the 'theology of compassion' would appear to be one such feasible strategy. The *meaning* of the verse is not challenged through an alternative interpretation other than the long-established one – an interpretation that would render it less objectionable. The verse is taken at face value, but its normative force is questioned with reference to a 'divine intent' that in practice overrides it.

Relativism and authenticity

It has been shown above how Positive Muslims utilises the fact of religious diversity and the role of interpretation in questioning established 'truths' about sexuality in contemporary Muslim politics. Islam is diverse and understandings change. This is followed through in many instances in the texts, and in a noteworthy manner. In the critique of gender inequality, Positive Muslims takes a relativistic stand on interpretation. The organisation does not reject as *incorrect* understandings that condone male authority over women. Such interpretations of the scriptures may very well be true. Similar reluctance to make definitive claims to religious truth is found elsewhere in the texts. Hence, there is no claim that the 'theology of compassion' is *the* 'true' and 'authentic' interpretation of Islam. Indeed, the definition as quoted above describes it as '*a* way' of reading the scriptures, not '*the* way'. Likewise, in the discussion on *fahisha* mentioned previously, the claim is not that translations such as 'abomination' or similar, or even 'homosexuality', are necessarily incorrect. The reference is rather to a more general questioning of 'Who speaks for Islam?'

The relativist stance on religious 'truth' and 'authenticity' and its theological implications become particularly evident in the way the organisation handles the widespread notion of HIV/AIDS as a divine punishment for sexual transgressions, either as an individual punishment for those affected, or as a punishment on a social level for a more general deviance in society. This is a central theme in the contemporary intra-Muslim discourse, well testified in ethnographic studies as well as local and regional surveys (Charnley 2007; Beckmann 2009; Maulana *et al.* 2009; Svensson 2009).[11] Positive Muslims takes an explicitly 'agnostic' position on whether or not such an interpretation of HIV/AIDS is correct. On the one hand, it is clearly stated that HIV/AIDS is 'an illness among other illnesses; in other words, it is not a peculiar disease for which a particular group has been singled out by Allah or by nature' (Positive Muslims 2004: 4). On the other hand, there is a

[11] For a more detailed study of this aspect of the discourse on HIV/AIDS, and suggestions as to why the notion is so widespread, see Svensson (forthcoming).

concession that narratives in both the Qur'an and the *hadith* literature testify to the 'fact' that God also punishes human beings in this world (Positive Muslims 2004: 22, 2007: 20). In conclusion, the organisation asserts that 'Since we are not able to tell apart which [events] are simply natural occurrences and [which are] signs of Allah's displeasure we must suspend our judgement in this matter.' The Qur'anic verse 17:36 is cited, with the advice not to speak about things of which one does not have knowledge (Positive Muslims 2007: 38). However, regardless of the ultimate cause of HIV/AIDS, the duty for Muslims to show compassion, *rahma*, to those affected is absolute (Positive Muslims 2004: 22).

Therefore, the multiplicity of Muslim claims to religious authenticity and the impossibility in practice to determine which one is correct become part of the 'theology of compassion'. This means that any claim to authenticity based on a particular reading of the scriptures is in practice a matter of meaning invested into that text by the interpreter, firmly rooted in a particular context. This has consequences for constructive theology. In the introduction to the section on 'Shariah, Muslim society and gender' in the 2007 manual, it is stated that:

> This section does not seek to address any specific question about women in Islam but suggests that alternative interpretations which value men and women as equal partners must be found in a world where women's already difficult lives are made worse by illness and disease.
>
> (Positive Muslims 2007: 43)

The very existence of HIV/AIDS becomes a contextual factor that influences which interpretation, among the multiple variations available, should be *chosen* as 'authentically Islamic'.

Conclusions

Positive Muslims' 'theology of compassion' is more than merely a locally produced and motivated pragmatic religious coating of HIV/AIDS activism. True, there are many instances in the texts, some of which have been highlighted above, where religious legitimacy for particular standpoints or suggestions for action are justified by reference to a selection of verses in the Qur'an or prophetic *hadith*. As shown above, this is exemplified mainly on issues of condom use and sex education. Both belong to prevention strategies endorsed by a multitude of actors in the field and both have been identified as problematic in a Muslim context. In the texts, they are provided with backing from scripture and religious ethics in a way that reflects a 'culturally sensitive' approach to prevention (Hasnain 2005). But the 'theology of compassion' exhibits wider ambitions. It also promotes a particular vision of Islam, and of what Islam ought to be in the contemporary world.

The question posed in the introduction concerned how transnational linkages can explain particular features of the 'theology of compassion'. From the analysis above, it becomes clear that if the transnational context is not taken into account a full understanding of the theology and its features cannot be reached.

One obvious aspect of the impact of transnationalism concerns resources. Producing reflective theology, publishing and distributing it in an appealing manner requires financing. It was noted above that Positive Muslims' 'theology of compassion' was developed with the help of financial resources provided by transnationally active state, interstate and non-state agencies involved in HIV/AIDS prevention, and presumably with a positive attitude to 'faith-based' initiatives. By providing financial backing to the development and distribution of the theology, these international donors become active participants in contemporary Muslim politics. Whether or not the financing has also had an influence on the theological content is difficult to ascertain, but it is highly unlikely that donors' presumed or explicit views as to what may constitute central areas of prevention work will be neglected by the producers of the theological material. As noted above, the topics of condoms and sex education are dealt with in a straightforward manner, with clear references to the scriptures. Here, the relativist view on interpretation is rather toned down. One reason may be that the niceties of post-modern theology would not be appreciated if applied to these issues.

Transnationalism is also a matter of the ambitions tied to the texts themselves. These are clearly addressed to *Muslims* and not only South African Muslims. While produced locally in South Africa, the content of the theology and the stated ambitions are not limited to that context but are stated as being at least possibly relevant to Muslims elsewhere, and the *umma* as a whole. Activities arranged and the institutional connections forged transnationally further indicate such ambitions, which are recognised by other agents. This also affects the way in which the theology is presented: examples of Muslim diversity, contemporary and historical, that are provided in the texts are in no way limited to South Africa. When Islamic law is outlined, the perspective is on *all* schools of law, not merely the dominant tradition of the Shafi'i school in South Africa. Cases used to illustrate the difficult situation of Muslim PLWHA are selected from a wide range of geographical locations around the world. In a sense, there is little in the content of the texts that necessarily and exclusively ties the 'theology of compassion' to a South African or even African context.

Still, of course, the very production of the texts and the 'theology of compassion' are tied to a local situation where HIV/AIDS is an issue of immediate social concern. The motivation to produce a 'theology of compassion' in the first place must be understood against the background of a local situation involving a combination of high HIV prevalence *and* stigmatisation and denial among Muslims in South Africa. But even here there are relevant transnational linkages to consider. Ahmed cites the prominence of a 'Malik Badri approach' to HIV/AIDS among Muslims in South Africa as the motivating factor behind the 'theology of compassion'. The published work of a Pakistani-born, Malaysia-based activist, distributed through a transnational network of Islamic Medical Associations provides important input in the production of the 'theology of compassion' *because of its local impact*. This impact is also dependent on the actual South African situation. For Positive Muslims, it affects the themes addressed in the 'theology of compassion', the attitudes anticipated and the theological positions attacked. Apart from unequivocal statements to this effect, there are several instances in the 'theology of compassion' where a stance against Badri's position and similar positions in a transnational discourse of HIV/AIDS is clear: Badri's view that 'Islam is the solution' is qualified by questions as to 'which Islam'; his statements on HIV/AIDS as punishment and his 'apologetic approach' to HIV/AIDS are both opposed or, at least, relativised. In general, the relativistic position on religious 'truth' that is detectable in the texts analysed does stand in stark contrast to a much less modest approach characterising many other Muslim religious responses to the disease.

The 'theology of compassion', and the way in which it addresses sexuality, is a result of two intersecting transnational currents within Muslim politics. First, a reaction to an initial wave of 'moralising' discourses which sets the scene, motivates action and, in a sense, defines the topics; and second, as a response to this, an employment of a particular alternative to the theological reasoning underlying these discourses, i.e. that associated with progressive Islam. The analysis of the 'theology of compassion' has shown how prime themes within a progressive Muslim agenda recur in the texts. There is an opposition to both literalist and apologetic modernist ways of approaching the sacred texts. Ahistorical, essentialist and non-contextual formulations of Islam and sexuality are rejected and there is stress on the need to rethink Islam, focusing on basic and eternal values of the religious message, and the actual context and position from which the interpretation is executed. Without taking this connection with a particular position in transnational Muslim politics and how it relates to other positions into account, what makes the 'theology of compassion' *qua* theology unique as a local response to HIV/AIDS is lost.

In a way, progressive Islam, also as it occurs in the 'theology of compassion', is in itself shaped by academic reflections on a transnational level of contemporary Islam. The way in which essentialist, ahistorical and literalist interpretations are challenged, and posed against a diversity of beliefs and behaviour worldwide, resulting in a relativist position in relation to religious 'truth', is identical to views widely held in the academic study of Islam (including the views of the present author). Most of the proponents of progressive Islam mentioned above, including Farid Esack, are also academics within the field of the secular study of religion. In a sense, the *theological* agenda they champion constitutes a second level of the 'objectification of Islam'. Objectification on the first level denotes how 'Islam', in the minds of believing Muslims and as a result not least of experiences of religious diversity, becomes an object for reflection and delimitation, and motivates a search for and a struggle over religious 'authenticity' transcending local contexts. Objectification on the secondary level takes the resulting diversity of multiple 'authenticities' as the object of reflection and the starting point for a *constructive* theology. The 'theology of compassion' mirrors this. The references to contemporary and historical intra-Muslim religious diversity in views on sexuality rest upon an expectation that the audience will be familiar with, understand and, in some ways, accept the fact of such diversity.

The 'theology of compassion' constitutes an on-the-ground, local application of progressive Islam. Does this mean that it can be seen as an example of 'Islam in Africa', as imported and essentially alien? I believe not. On the contrary, the 'theology of compassion' rather exemplifies how the dichotomy of 'Islam in Africa' and 'African Islam' becomes problematic when actual examples are closely examined. Although progressive Islam has received particular attention in North America, possibly as a result of the events on 11 September 2001, it emerged prior to this time as a *transnational* initiative. In this, South African Muslim activists, shaped not least by the anti-apartheid struggle and the role of religion in that context, most notably Farid Esack, had key roles. Esack himself, as a result of transnational linkages, has a set of competences and experiences that makes him particularly suitable for contributing to the progressive Muslim agenda, especially dual competence in traditional Muslim scholarship and the secular academic study of religion, and a long engagement in activism. Hence, if the 'theology of compassion' is to be seen as a local application of 'imported' 'Islam in Africa', it is just as reasonable to see progressive Islam, with its rather radical suggestions for Islamic reform on a transnational scale, as – at least partly – an 'exported' 'African Islam', shaped by both local and transnational experiences.

References

Ahmed, Abdul Kayum. 2003. 'Positive Muslims: a critical analysis of Muslim AIDS activism in relation to women living with HIV/AIDS in Cape Town'. Master's thesis, Department of Anthropology and Sociology, University of Western Cape.

Ali, A. Yusuf (trans.) 1983. *The Holy Qur'an: Text, Translation and Commentary*. Brentwood, MD: Amana Corp.

Ali, Kecia. 2006. *Sexual Ethics and Islam: Feminist Reflections on Qur'an, Hadith, and Jurisprudence*. Oxford: Oneworld.

Ansari, David A. and Allyn Gaestel. 2010. 'Senegalese religious leaders' perceptions of HIV/AIDS and implications for challenging stigma and discrimination', *Culture, Health and Sexuality* 12(6): 633–48.

Asad, Talal. 1986. *The Idea of an Anthropology of Islam*. Georgetown, Washington, DC: Center for Contemporary Arab Studies.

Atighetchi, Dariusch. 2007. *Islamic Bioethics: Problems and Perspectives*. Dordrecht: Springer.

Babou, Cheikh A. 2011. 'A West African Sufi master on the global stage: Cheikh Abdoulaye Dieye and the Khidmatul Khadim International Sufi School in France and the United States', *African Diaspora* 4(1): 27–49.

Badri, Malik. 1997. *The AIDS Crisis: An Islamic Socio-Cultural Perspective*. Kuala Lumpur: International Institute of Islamic Thought and Civilization.
Badri, Malik. 2009. 'The AIDS crisis: an Islamic perspective', in F. Esack and S. Chiddy (eds), *Islam and AIDS: Between Scorn, Pity and Justice*. Oxford: Oneworld, 29–42.
Bangstad, Sindre. 2007. *Global Flows, Local Appropriations: Facets of Secularisation and Re-Islamization among Contemporary Cape Muslims*. Leiden: ISIM.
Bangstad, Sindre. 2009. 'AIDS and the "Wrath of God"', in F. Esack and S. Chiddy (eds), *Islam and AIDS: Between Scorn, Pity and Justice*. Oxford: Oneworld, 43–58.
Bearman, P.J., T. Bianquis, *et al.* (eds) 2012 [1983]. 'Liwat', in *Encyclopaedia of Islam*, 2nd edn. Leiden: Brill Online.
Becker, Felicitas. 2009. 'Competing explanations and treatment choices: Muslims, AIDS and ARVs in Tanzania', in F. Becker and W. Geissler (eds), *AIDS and Religious Practice in Africa*. Leiden: Brill, 155–88.
Beckmann, Nadine. 2009. 'AIDS and the power of God: narratives of decline and coping strategies in Zanzibar', in F. Becker and W. Geissler (eds), *AIDS and Religious Practice in Africa*. Leiden: Brill, 119–54.
Charnley, Simone. 2007. *Speaking up: Muslim Views on HIV and AIDS*. Bangkok: Asian Muslim Action Network.
Duderija, Adis. 2008. 'The interpretational implications of Progressive Muslims' Qur'an and Sunna Manhaj in relation to their formulation of a normative Muslima construct', *Islam and Christian-Muslim Relations* 19: 411–29.
Duderija, Adis. 2010. 'Progressive Muslims: defining and delineating identities and ways of being a Muslim', *Journal of Muslim Minority Affairs* 30(1): 127–36.
Eickelman, Dale F. and James P. Piscatori. 2004. *Muslim Politics*. Princeton, NJ: Princeton University Press.
Esack, Farid. 1997. *Qur'an, Liberation and Pluralism*. Oxford: Oneworld.
Esack, Farid. 2003. 'In search of progressive Islam beyond 9/11', in O. Safi (ed.), *Progressive Muslims: On Justice, Gender and Pluralism*. Oxford: Oneworld, 78–97.
Esack, Farid. 2007. *Muslims Responding to AIDS: Mapping Muslim Organizational and Religious Responses*. Observatory, South Africa: Positive Muslims.
Esack, F. and S. Chiddy (eds), *Islam and AIDS: Between Scorn, Pity and Justice*. Oxford: Oneworld.
Francesca, Ersilia. 2002. 'AIDS in contemporary Islamic ethical literature', *Medicine and Law* 21: 381–94.
Frisina, Annalisa. 2010. 'Young Muslims' everyday tactics and strategies: resisting Islamophobia, negotiating Italianness, becoming citizens', *Journal of Intercultural Studies* 31(5): 557–72.
Hasnain, Memoona. 2005. 'Cultural approach to HIV/AIDS harms reduction in Muslim countries', *Harm Reduction Journal* 2(23). http://www.biomedcentral.com/content/pdf/1477-7517-2-23.pdf.
Hill, Joseph. 2012. 'The cosmopolitan Sahara: building a global Islamic village in Mauritania', *City and Society* 24(1): 62–83.
Kaag, Mayke. 2011. 'Connecting to the umma through Islamic relief: transnational Islamic NGOs in Chad', *International Development Planning Review* 33(4): 463–74.
Kelley, Laura M. and Nicholas Eberstadt. 2005. *Behind the Veil of a Public Health Crisis: HIV/AIDS in the Muslim World*. Seattle: National Bureau of Asian Research.

Lagarde, Emmanuel, Catherine Enel, *et al.* 2000. 'Religion and protective behaviours towards AIDS in rural Senegal', *AIDS* 14(13): 2027–33.

Lala, Lekhraj. 2007. 'The role of faith-based organisations mitigating HIV/AIDS-related stigma in religious communities: examining religiously-based anti-stigma messages in three South African faith-based organisations'. Master's thesis, University of Cambridge, Institute of Public Health.

Mandaville, Peter G. 2007. *Global Political Islam*. London: Routledge.

Mandaville, Peter G. 2011. 'Transnational Muslim solidarities and everyday life', *Nations and Nationalism* 17(1): 7–24.

Maulana, Aisha Omar, Anja Krumeich, *et al.* 2009. 'Emerging discourse: Islamic teaching in HIV prevention in Kenya – Short Report', *Culture, Health and Sexuality* 11(5): 559–69.

Meijer, Roel (ed.) 2009. *Global Salafism: Islam's New Religious Movement*. New York: Columbia University Press.

Nielsen, Jorgen S. 2002. 'Transnational Islam and the integration of Islam in Europe', in S. Allievi and J.S. Nielsen (eds), *Muslim Networks and Transnational Communities in and Across Europe*. Leiden: Brill, 28–51.

Obermeyer, Carla Makhlouf. 2006. 'HIV in the Middle East', *British Medical Journal* 333(7573): 851–4.

Otayek, René and Benjamin F. Soares. 2007. 'Introduction: Islam and Muslim politics in Africa', in B.F. Soares and R. Otayek (eds), *Islam and Muslim Politics in Africa*. New York: Macmillan, 1–26.

Peters, Rudolph. 2012 [2002]. 'Zina', in P.J. Bearman, T. Bianquis, *et al.* (eds), *Encyclopaedia of Islam*, 2nd edn. Leiden: Brill Online.

Petersen, Marie J. 2012. 'Islamizing aid: transnational Muslim NGOs after 9/11', *Voluntas: International Journal of Voluntary and Nonprofit Organizations* 23(1): 126–55.

Positive Muslims. 2004. *HIV, AIDS and Islam: Reflections Based on Compassion, Responsibility and Justice*. Observatory, South Africa: Positive Muslims.

Positive Muslims. 2007. *HIV, AIDS and Islam: A Workshop Manual Based on Compassion, Responsibility and Justice*. Cape Town: Positive Muslims.

Rosander, Eva Evers. 1997. 'Introduction: the Islamization of "tradition" and "modernity"', in D. Westerlund and E.E. Rosander (eds), *African Islam and Islam in Africa: Encounters between Sufis and Islamists*. Athens, OH: Ohio University Press, 1–27.

Rowson, Everett K. 2012. 'Homosexuality', in J.D. McAuliffe (ed.), *Encyclopaedia of the Qur'an*. Washington, DC: Brill Online.

Roy, Olivier. 2004. *Globalized Islam: The Search for a New Ummah*. New York: Columbia University Press.

Safi, Omid (ed.) 2003. *Progressive Muslims: On Justice, Gender and Pluralism*. Oxford: Oneworld.

Seesemann, Rüdiger. 2006. 'African Islam or Islam in Africa? Evidence from Kenya', in R. Loimeier and R. Seesemann (eds), *The Global Worlds of the Swahili: Interfaces of Islam, Identity and Space in 19th and 20th Century East Africa*, Berlin: Lit, 229–50.

Shannahan, Dervla Sara. 2010. 'Some queer questions from a Muslim faith perspective', *Sexualities* 13(6): 671–84.

Sherif, Faruq. 1995. *A Guide to the Contents of the Qur'an*. Reading: Garnet Publishing.

Siddiquee, Nabilah. 2009. 'When fahishah becomes widespread – AIDS and the Ibn Maja hadith', in F. Esack and S. Chiddy (eds), *Islam and AIDS: Between Scorn, Pity and Justice*. Oxford: Oneworld, 59–75.

Singh, Jasbant. 2003. 'Malaysia: American academic causes uproar at conference on AIDS and Islam'. Associated Press, 21 May.

Soares, Benjamin F. 2000. 'Notes on the anthropological study of Islam and Muslim societies in Africa', *Culture and Religion* 1(2): 277–85.

Stenberg, Leif. 1996. *The Islamization of Science: Four Muslim Positions Developing an Islamic Modernity*. Stockholm: Almqvist & Wiksell International.

Svensson, Jonas. 2009. '"Muslims have instructions": HIV/AIDS, modernity and Islamic religious education in Kisumu, Kenya', in F. Becker and W. Geissler (eds), *AIDS and Religious Practice in Africa*. Leiden: Brill, 189–219.

Svensson, Jonas. forthcoming. 'God's rage – Muslim representations of HIV/AIDS as a divine punishment from the perspective of the cognitive science of religion', *Numen*.

Tempert, Bertus. 2009. 'Positive Muslims experience', *Life2Live* 5: 1–4.

UNICEF. 2003. *What Religious Leaders Can Do about HIV/AIDS: Action for Children and Young People*. New York: UNICEF.

Vahed, Ghoolam. 2003. 'Contesting "orthodoxy": the Tablighi-Sunni conflict among South African Muslims in the 1970s and 1980s', *Journal of Muslim Minority Affairs* 23(2): 313–34.

Varisco, Daniel Martin. 2005. *Islam Obscured: The Rhetoric of Anthropological Representation*. New York: Palgrave Macmillan.

Vertovec, Steven. 2009. *Transnationalism*. London: Routledge.

Wadud, Amina. 2006. *Inside the Gender Jihad: Women's Reform in Islam*. Oxford: Oneworld.

Waris Maqsood, Ruqayya. 2000. *The Muslim Marriage Guide*. Beltsville, MD: Amana Publications.

Westerlund, David and Eva Evers Rosander (eds) 1997. *African Islam and Islam in Africa: Encounters between Sufis and Islamists*. Athens, OH: Ohio University Press.

Willson, Katherine Davila. 2008. 'Breaking the silence: South African Muslim responses to HIV/AIDS and a theology of compassion. A case study of religio-cultural approaches to HIV/AIDS'. Bachelor's thesis, The College of William and Mary, VA.

12

The Choice of Health

Christian Family Planning among Cosmopolitan Educated Professionals in Time of HIV/AIDS in Botswana

ASTRID BOCHOW

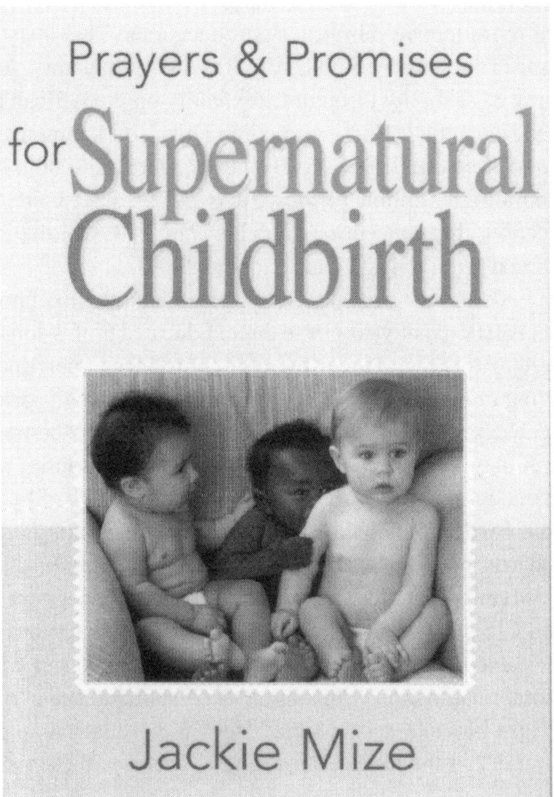

'God wants you to be faithful' – Pentecostal messages provide hope to conceive by the strength of faith. (Photograph used by permission of the book's publisher: Harrison House Publishers, Tulsa, OK 74153, www.harrisonhouse.com)

Proceedings of the British Academy **194**, *245–267*.

Introduction

PATRICIA IS 45 YEARS OLD and suffers from a condition that, in biomedical terms, is labelled 'infertility'. She works in a managing position in a bank and is a member of a leading Pentecostal-charismatic church.[1] She was 30 years of age when she entered into her first marriage, still childless. Her marriage turned sour and she did not feel secure having children with her husband: 'We never sat together and planned to have a baby', Patricia indicated. After little more than one year of marriage, she divorced. Although she remarried, she has not had any children, yet (interview, 3 October 2010).

Tswana people – one of the main ethnic groups in Botswana – have been described as valuing motherhood and childbirth (Upton 2001; Mogobe 2005). How is it then that educated and financially independent women in Botswana do not pursue having children in their marriages? This is the starting question of this chapter. In what follows, I explore the impact of elite lifestyles, HIV/AIDS, and Christianity on reproductive moralities and decisions. This question is a rather unexplored angle in the study of both HIV/AIDS and Christianity. Anthropologists study the shaping of sexuality through Christianity on the African continent (Ojo 1997, 2007; Sadgrove 2007; Bochow and van Dijk 2012), ranging from religious involvement to matters of HIV/AIDS (Becker and Geissler 2009; Nguyen 2009). From an epidemiological point of view, it is not only sexuality that becomes potentially infectious, but conception (Wilcher *et al.* 2009), birth (Chapman 2010) and breastfeeding as well (Blystad and Moland 2009).

In a context with an HIV prevalence of 30 per cent, the likelihood that one or the other partner is HIV-positive is one in three. Educated professionals in Botswana are highly aware of this fact. Under these circumstances, reproduction bears the risk of contracting or passing on an HIV infection, unless both partners cooperate and seek medical help; and confronts women and men with a dilemma: if they want to have children they must have unprotected sexual intercourse, and yet having unprotected sexual intercourse would expose them to the risk of being infected. In my contribution, I will problematise women's decision-making or non-decision-making on child bearing, which is tied into general reflections on decision-making in the context of family planning in relation to female life courses. This relates to the literature on Christianity and subject formation in this region: Comaroff and Comaroff (1997: 365–6) pointed to the psychological power of Christianity that introduces a moral imagination with a sense of personhood and a 'modernist self', which is the 'right bearing, responsible "free" individual' among the Tswana-speaking community in the nineteenth century. Thereby, these new conceptions

[1] To ensure the anonymity of my informants, I not only use pseudonyms but also disguise other markers of their origin and identity. Therefore, I will not name the churches, places, or professions of those I interviewed.

of personhood travelled via English nonconformist Methodist missionaries into local Tswana culture. The choice of health versus having children appears to be influenced by if and how Christianity enables individuals to make decisions in twenty-first-century Botswana. The transnational elements, which will be discussed in this contribution, are the travelling ethics of health, the body and personhood, and how these are implemented in single individuals' reproductive life courses.

Personal tragedy and social change in individual biographies: notes on concepts and methodology

My analysis of the changing reproductive dynamics among Christian urban professionals in Botswana is based on biographical interviews with about seventy urban women and fifteen men that I conducted during several visits to the country in the years 2009 to 2011. These interviews were conducted alongside fieldwork and participant observation in urban households and at the University of Botswana. I will analyse the biographical interviews of three women in particular, who have remained childless in their marriages, partly because they have been protecting themselves from HIV/AIDS. I call them Patricia, Ruth, and Tsholo (interviews, 3 October 2010; 1 March 2011; 16 November 2010).

People who remain childless are exceptions in Botswana as well as in most other societies, even though people in Gaborone have perceived infertility to be a common problem. Their situation is particular and appears to be a personal problem rather than a social one. Anthropologists working on infertility have pointed out that infertility is likely to appear in women's life courses, if 'something goes wrong', and have coined the term 'reproductive disruption' for these cases (see Sundby and Larsen 2006; Inhorn 1996, 2002; Feldman-Savelsberg 1999). Infertility often results from unusual circumstances in a person's life, and these circumstances may be attributed to social dynamics. Poor health care for women who had an abortion might be an example (Hörbst and Schuster 2006). Other circumstances described in the literature include education that postpones childbirth in women's life courses and therefore heightens the risk of remaining without children (cf. Caldwell 1982). I argue that these life courses I encountered during my fieldwork in Botswana reflect reproductive dynamics; they speak about new gender roles, new approaches to the body, new spiritualities, and alternative ways into reproduction. Looking into biographical circumstances, I propose, allows understanding of some of the factors that have shaped gender relations, reproductive moralities, and reproductive decisions (compare also Leonard 2002).

The second conceptual question that arises out of my research on reproduction among elites in Botswana is how to understand reproductive agency and how it is influenced or directed by culture, gender, and health and family politics, transporting new ideas of the body, health, and technologies. Demographers hypothesise that demographic transitions are motivated by larger social processes, as for instance the introduction of schooling on a national level or the enhancement of medical care (Caldwell 1982). Others attribute people's striving for fertility to specific family and household structures (Caldwell and Caldwell 1987; Lesthaeghe 1989). These studies do not question individuals' motivation to reproduce. In contrast, person-centred approaches, as they have been put forward by anthropologists like Andrea Cornwall (2007), Jane Guyer (1994) and Liv Haram (2004), discuss single persons' agency in reproductive decisions, showing how individuals use their reproductive capacities in order to achieve other social goals or how these decisions are embedded in wider processes of producing meaning and moral contestations of family planning practices. In my study, I pursue such a person-centred approach.

Thirdly, I wish to comment on the methodology of the biographic interviews and the context in which these interviews took place. For interviews, I met women (as well as men) mostly in public spaces, cafés, or restaurants. The interviews, lasting between forty-five minutes and two hours, resembled the kind of intimate chats that urban women are used to. My interactions with men outside the context of my research were limited, so I do not know how men usually speak about these issues outside the interview situation. Chatting with me gave women the opportunity to talk about some of their troubling conditions, such as HIV infection or infertility. Narrating their lives, they engaged in meaning making so that the interviews can be read as reflecting reproductive ethics, and how these enter the subjectivities of people. They give evidence of how to evaluate individual agency. In talking about their lives I also refer to 'life events', a term that is often used in psychology (compare also Langness and Frank 1981). Like birth, remaining childless is a life event of significant effect in women's lives.

During the conversation, I took notes, and later I finalised 'memory minutes' based on these notes and my memory.[2] Twenty-five of the women sought medical assistance in order to conceive; only nine women had not given birth to any child so far. Their ages, and therefore also their chances of conceiving, varied considerably, from 28 to 55. Of this sample, five women showed, like Patricia, that they were strongly influenced by Christian and in particular Pentecostal values (see below). The reproductive histories of these five women were visibly impacted by their Christian/Pentecostal background, and two others suffered a similar fate to Patricia: their reproductive wishes had represented a danger for their health and well-being in their short-lived marriages, and they also did not conceive later on.[3] This will become clear in the discussion of their life courses below.

Lastly, I will comment on the religious affiliation of my respondents. As I will show in the following paragraph, the formation of a group of educated professionals

[2] Most respondents did not feel comfortable when I recorded.

[3] Two other childless women, who are now beyond child-bearing age, suffered abusive relationships and finally divorced. However, their inability to conceive was (at least partially) attributed to medical problems.

is deeply rooted in the history of mission churches in African societies. The southern African region is best known for its involvement with the so-called African Independent movements of churches, which put a high emphasis on healing and prophecy (Fernandez 1978; Klaits 2010). Presently, the church with the highest membership is the Zion Christian Church, an African Independent church. However, the Christian landscape is very diverse and fragmented: long-established mission churches, African Independent churches and Pentecostal churches exist alongside one another. Several of my respondents worshipped in one of the biggest Pentecostal churches, and by and large I could recognise that some elements of the Pentecostal paradigm, healing practices and sexual morals, were relevant also for those who were of other denominations. I will write about Pentecostal couples and Pentecostal family planning, and in particular about the life courses of Pentecostal women who had, like Patricia, remained childless or had lower levels of childbirth. The person-centred approach, however, reveals that *several* Christian influences possibly *merge* in a single person's striving for fertility, their bodily practices, and hopes. Women who are members of Pentecostal churches might call upon elements of other forms of Christianity, and non-Pentecostal women might draw upon Pentecostal ideas in their narratives.

In what follows, I will first locate these women in a social-historical context of educated elites in Botswana by illuminating how Christianity permeates the building of elites. I will then discuss the Christian moral sphere of family planning and sexuality that impacts these women's decisions; and finally I will discuss their childlessness in the light of paradoxical reproductive moralities in twenty-first-century Botswana.

Elites: Christianity and cosmopolitanism

The building of a local educated elite is closely related to the arrival of Christianity. Christianity itself has been described as a transnational religion (Adogame 2005; Nieswand 2005; Krause and Hüwelmeier 2010) that not only brought new ideas of sin, soul, and salvation into the receiving societies but also new knowledge, new modes of consumption, new forms of governance and administration, and new medicines (Comaroff and Comaroff 1991; Vaughan 1991). In Botswana, as in many other African countries, mission churches, such as the nonconformist evangelists of the London Missionary Society described by Comaroff and Comaroff, contributed considerably to the evolution of these elites, as their institutions such as hospitals and schools offered possibilities to gain social prestige outside local hierarchies. Thus, at the beginning of the 1900s, 'Christian marriage' with lavish wedding celebrations became popular among elites (Comaroff and Comaroff 1991: 385).

Economic diversification took place in Betchuanaland (today southeastern Botswana and northeastern South Africa) from the first half of the twentieth century onwards with men migrating to the mines. These first elites retained their commitment to farming; most men were still raising cattle, the main source and sign of wealth, and most women continued to farm. Even though the local administrators distinguished themselves by the houses they lived in (cemented and roofed) and the vehicles they drove (cars instead of donkey wagons), those who are in their sixties to eighties today displayed modesty concerning their family backgrounds, pointing at the farming activities of their parents. In contrast to South Africa, where educated professionals had a specific function in the colonial administration and later on in the national state of South Africa under Apartheid, in Botswana educated professionals do not focus on their distinctiveness from, but rather emphasise belonging to, these rural communities.

By the time of independence, there were only a handful of graduates, and yet women had belonged to the educated elites since the beginning of the twentieth century (Werbner 2004). These first elite women stood out from their peers and even from their (male and female) siblings. They pursued education, unlike their age mates who usually dropped out at standard five in order to go to South Africa to work or because they became pregnant. These early-educated professionals found themselves well educated and specialised enough to take on responsibilities when the country experienced economic growth and diversification. Reproductive relations and ethics had begun to change from the beginning of the twentieth century onwards, and not only among elites. Schapera (1933) reported that a new childbearing pattern had emerged in rural Tswana communities according to which women bore children before they married.[4] In a restudy, Comaroff and Roberts (1977) confirmed this trend. In their analysis, Comaroff and Roberts attribute the detachment of reproduction from the institution of marriage to the decline of polygamy. This, in turn, they attribute to the increasing influence of Christianity. The early elite women of my sample pursued their education, mostly at Lesotho International College, and gave birth later in life when their education was completed. By that time, most of them were in their mid-twenties. They married, however, earlier than most of their peers, as they believed in the Christian ideal of marriage according to which childbirth and sexuality should fall within marriage and not outside marriage. Therefore, the transnational religion of Christianity contributed considerably to the reshaping of the moralities of local communities in the first half of the twentieth century.

After independence and during the time when Botswana's economy boomed, Christian ethics were enriched by transnational ethics of spiritual healing, new models of monogamous marriage, marital love and sexuality, and from

[4] Not all women in this study are Tswana, but in the process of nation-building Tswana became a lead culture among educated professionals (Werbner 2004). Especially among urban educated professionals elements of Tswana became popularised. I therefore use the historical reports on these groups as a background against which I understand and analyse contemporary developments in this group.

the 1990s onwards also by HIV/AIDS prevention campaigns. During the years of economic growth, the government needed highly qualified people to manage the state apparatus and the growing infrastructure. This enabled social mobility for many through education, which was freely provided by the government. By that time, educated professionals increasingly acquired their education not only in South Africa but also in the UK, the US and Australia, where they went to study. Most of them retained their strong Christian orientation. During their travels, they were inspired by global popular culture, which influenced their sense of fashion as well as their views on relationships. Therefore, transnational travels were and are important for the educational histories of these elite groups. Education acquired abroad guaranteed their social mobility. In addition, this outward orientation serves as an identifier so that these educated middle-class and elite groups exhibit a strong cosmopolitan orientation. One example was a divorced woman in whose household I stayed during my first visit to Botswana. She had received part of her education in the UK and the US. As a devoted Christian she had been campaigning to include HIV/AIDS in Christian teaching. In addition, she was an advocate of equal rights for women, on which she was very outspoken in her professional environment as well as in her private life. I met several Christian educated professionals like her during my stay in Botswana. They often play a pivotal role in their Christian communities. Not only do these educated professionals inform themselves on matters of love, life, and health, but they also bring these new ethics on relationships, reproduction, and health into their Christian communities.

Independently of their Christian affiliation, educated professionals are also beneficiaries of private biomedical services that provide fertility care in Botswana. Assisted reproductive technologies are only available in South Africa, which adds to the transnational orientation of some of the educated professionals' biographies discussed here.

In the following sections I will explore these ethics of Christian family planning as they transpire through the life courses of educated elites.

The travelling moralities of family planning: controlling reproduction

Patricia felt that her marriage did not provide the space for her to take care of her fertility. 'We never sat down together and discussed things', she repeatedly stated. Her statement indicates a strong sense that matters of reproduction need communication, consent-seeking and finally cooperation, which she felt was not possible with her ex-husband. From the perspective of this educated professional Christian woman, reproduction (within marriage) does not happen 'naturally' but rather needs planning and is subject to a decision.

This section will analyse how Christian, and in particular Pentecostal, elite women adhere to ethics of planning reproduction. Herein, Pentecostal reproductive moralities link up with other globally travelling health ethics of family planning and HIV prevention programmes, offering a pool of globally circulating ethics on marriage, sexuality, and health. With their emphasis on the controllability of the body, these ethics differ from historically recorded and culturally important reproductive ethics that emphasise fertility (Schapera 1966). I discuss Pentecostalism in relation to these questions as women's life courses appear to be impacted by this doctrine in a specific way, although only two of the three mentioned women actually belong to a Pentecostal church (the third exhibits certain elements of Pentecostal-spiritual healing paradigms). This means that all women who appeared to have lower levels of childbirth or who remained without children were members of Pentecostal churches. Again, I would like to point at the messiness of how religious beliefs, practices, and belonging transpire through an individual's life course. Studying these life courses has a strong heuristical value but statistically relevant claims cannot be made about whether or not elite women have lower levels of childbirth.

Elites striving for fertility exhibit a great need and believe in planning their reproduction. A standardised reproductive life course starts at the age of 20, the average age of first childbirth in Botswana. At that age, women are generally not married yet, as the average age at first marriage was recorded to be 26.4 for women and 30.9 for men (United Nations 2013). The high cost of a wedding and the *lobola* – these are payments to the wife's family when a couple marry – postponed the average age of marriage throughout the twentieth century. Women present first pregnancies mostly as 'accidents' and as a result of 'broken condoms'. Sometimes women state in a confessional manner that they had loved their first child's father, who had also wanted the child and had promised to marry them. Yet, when they had become pregnant the relationship ended. The second child should follow ideally within their marriage in their late twenties or early thirties. This child is then planned and sometimes women face difficulties becoming pregnant again (five of my sample). Women often wish to have a last child in their late thirties or early forties just before menopause.[5]

Elite women (and men) in their thirties *plan* their reproductive life. Women at that age often indicated that they wanted to 'try' to have a baby and pointed out a specific time when they wanted to have it. This demonstrates that, in their view, having children is a volitional act that they influence with their own decision. 'Trying' thereby could imply different things: it could mean to intensify sexual contacts or, when couples were not living and working in the same city, to

[5] While in rural settings these last born children are also those who will stay on the farm and take care of their parents in old age and inherit the farm from them, elite women's reasons for having a last child are expressed on the basis of emotions: they want this child 'before the house becomes empty'.

synchronise their visits with the fertile days of the woman's cycle. Their need to plan their reproduction also derived from educated professionals' time constraints as working mothers and their concerns over the costs of raising children, especially school fees for private education. They feel the burden of combining their job responsibilities with the emotional task of mothering and they are concerned about the rising costs of education, holidays, and other activities they want their children to enjoy.

Educated professionals' planning also demonstrates their knowledge about reproduction and how to possibly control it, thus showing a sense of their right to monitor their reproductive lives, continuing a process that Comaroff and Roberts had already observed in 1950s Botswana. As many of my interviews have revealed, elites have incorporated the messages of family planning and fertility medicine that regard the procreative body as controllable. If they face reproductive challenges they would first consult a specialist, understand that they need to undergo a lot of tests, and expect that the doctor would be able to help them. Gynaecologists even complain about women's instrumentalist attitude towards biomedicine and towards the possibilities of manipulating their bodies: women would expect to get a pill that would solve their problem, not understanding that fertility treatments are often time-consuming processes. In this sense, elite women might be labelled as being the prototypical 'pragmatic woman' as described by Lock and Kaufert – women who 'use whatever biomedicine can provide in pursuit of their own goals' (1998: 7). The preferred method of contraception is condom use in combination with the calendar method. In this societal group, especially male partners (husbands) favour the use of condoms. The contraceptive pill is widely regarded as having negative effects on women's child-bearing capacities.

Furthermore, in their quest for conception, educated professionals enjoy privileged access to private fertility care. Many women feel that the fertility care offered by the comparatively well-functioning public health-care system does not meet the need for advanced fertility care. This comprises diagnostics and treatment of fertility problems but also cancer screenings and other more pressing needs. The public health-care system provides these services; however women have to wait up to six months for an appointment. Educated professionals, and in fact any woman who can afford to, therefore consult private specialists, who offer a broader spectrum of diagnostics, treatment, and care. Taking care of one's fertility to such a high standard reflects the material condition of the elites' fertility practices concerning the controllable and manipulable procreative body.

Elites' striving for controlled fertility may be informed by various sources that provide information on fertility control as well as knowledge about available technologies and fertility services and biomedical ideas about the controllability of the body. Family planning programmes propagate powerful paradigms in matters of reproduction all over the continent. These programmes travel from the desks of international organisations to the desks of national politicians and from there on to health facilities, schoolbooks, and the minds of the people in Africa. By propagating biomedical ideas of procreation, family planning programmes introduce new ethics of well-being into the domain of reproduction (Paxson 2005: 105) and import Western concerns of 'overpopulation' to African countries (for a critique, see Hunt 2005). Botswana has always been a sparsely populated country, with only two million inhabitants in a country the size of France. Nevertheless, the government has been integrating family planning into the national maternal care and child health programme since 1973. Thereby, the number of outlets for contraceptives increased from 50 in 1973 to 350 in 1984 (Way *et al.* 1987: 8), and Botswana is noted for being a country with well-organised distribution of contraceptives, in rural areas more than in urban ones (ibid.). The biomedical idea of controlling and manipulating procreation, if not invented by family planning programmes – Schapera (1966) reported on the method of withdrawal as a common technique to control reproductive outcomes – has been enforced by these programmes. Family planning programmes suggest a specific idea about fertility, namely one that is restricted by biological age but also located in a body comprised of single, functioning, reparable parts and certain medical practices (Woliver 2002: 39).[6] With school education teaching the 'biological facts' of reproduction and pointing at the possibility and importance of controlling fertility with biomedical measures, educated professionals were and are willing recipients of the biomedical concept of controllable conception.

Controlling conception: Pentecostal reproductive moralities and biomedicine

Churches, and Pentecostal churches in particular, meet educated professionals' need to plan reproduction and even encourage them to pursue family planning within marriage. They even organise weekends with courses on family planning methods. Family planning and sex education also takes place in pre-marital counselling sessions. It was in one of those sessions that a teacher (his wife had a good position in the civil service) had learned about the practical and technical sides of prevention methods, such as how to hold and roll a condom (interview, 27 August 2011). Pentecostal linkages with the biomedical rationale supporting the manipulation of reproduction are not unique to Botswana: for instance, authors have described Pentecostals' adoption of global knowledge of biomedicine,

[6] Feminist-inspired literature has claimed women's rights to their bodies. It has criticised biomedical advancement as a way of subjecting women to biomedical regimens and authorities (that are mostly male) and therefore fostering women's dependency on these technologies, which leads to women's alienation from their bodies.

especially in the domain of (assisted) reproduction, in Nigeria and Ghana (Pearce 1995, 1999; Asamoah-Gyadu 2007). Some of these churches foster an approach to women's reproduction that supports the biological manipulation of fertility.

Similar to Patricia, many other church members indicated this idea of postponing childbirth, even within marriage, so as to create the ideal emotional and financial conditions for the start of the new family. While her church does not prescribe a specific reproductive timeline as ideal, many members feel that they would like to take some time after marriage before they have their first child (Pastor Seithamo, 27 August 2011). With lavish wedding feasts becoming an indicator of successful participation in Botswana's economic growth (van Dijk 2010) most couples face huge debts after their wedding (focus group discussion, Molepolole, 2009), or they might want to finish some building project (focus group discussion, Molepolole, 2010). The psychological reason given is that the child shifts the attention of the couple, which might endanger their relationship if it is not well established. Planning in the context of Pentecostal churches makes biological fertility control relevant for pursuing a specific lifestyle, in which having a family with many children is not an indication of wealth and well-being but rather adds costs to the establishment of a lifestyle of prosperity with houses, cars, and private education for the children.

Alongside incorporating family planning paradigms of fertility control, Pentecostalism also provides a strong notion of God's almighty healing power that is stronger than the biomedical healing paradigm of cause and effect. The women inspired by Pentecostalism, like other charismatic and prophetic Christians (cf. van Dijk 1997; Csordas 1997), believe that health is a gift from God, which his children are eligible to receive and which they can acquire through prayer and blessing. Prof. F., one of the founding members of Patricia's church, said that as a student he had witnessed prayer sessions that had cured blind and crippled people whom he personally knew. He later acquired the gift of healing through the Holy Spirit himself and passed it on to other church members. In Pentecostal circles and beyond, a book called *You Shall Not Be Barren*, by David Oyedepo, the bishop of the Winner's Chapel, a Nigerian Pentecostal church, is quite popular. Bishop Oyedepo (1998) assures his readership that 'God wants you to be fruitful'. It is possible to conceive if one's faith is strong enough. To support his claim he quotes examples from the Bible of seemingly barren women who conceived at a late age, such as Ruth or Hannah, mother of Samuel. He further works with the technique of affirmation by addressing his audience: 'I can see the child in your womb. The child is there. You will conceive!'

In my conversation with Ruth, aged 47, married, divorced, and remarried without children, I could sense that she was under the influence of this Pentecostal healing paradigm. She was keen to keep the picture I let her draw to understand her conceptualisation of the process of procreation (it sketched which substances would go from the woman into the new baby and which from the man). Maybe she felt by drawing this picture she helped her child to materialise. Also the name Ruth, under which she wanted to appear in this study and which she had chosen for herself, suggested that the above-described Pentecostal imagination was a source of hope for her. Ruth is now seeking to conceive using IVF. In addition, she uses the Pentecostal technique of visualisation in order to conceive (interview, 1 March 2011).

Christianity, and Pentecostalism in particular, enters into strong alliances with the biomedical paradigm and practices, while it also provides the healing paradigm of the 'all is possible for those who believe'. Building on historical grounds, the alliances of Christianity and biomedical knowledge and practices are well established. Along with its new theologies of sin and salvation, Christianity brought new medicines and medical practices to the African continent that appeared to be efficient cures for many afflictions of the African population. Alongside healing and preaching, Christians created a new language and imaginary of thinking about oneself and the body (Landau 1996: 283). In twenty-first-century Botswana, these new conceptions of the self and the body build on the biomedical paradigm of fertility that reduces the concept of fertility to a bodily biological capability of conceiving children, which can and ought to be controlled and manipulated. If 'magic' is, as Frazer has argued, 'a technique, a way of humans trying to shape the world to their will – if only by mistaken techniques' (Graeber 2005: 22), both the educated professionals' use of biomedical technologies (embodied by their gynaecologists) and their use of the omnipotent power of faith to invoke conception exhibit – from an ethical point of view – magic elements of Christian thinking. Contrary to what the debate on 'rational science' and 'irrational religion' has suggested, throughout the first half of the twentieth century these two practices appear not all that different from one another. Evangelical Christian approaches towards reproduction resemble what Pamela Klassen (2011: xiv) has described as the 'robust supernaturalism' of liberal Protestantism in North America that fostered engagement with the public health-care system by the end of the last century and allows for 'yoga under the cross' and laying on hands in the twenty-first century. Klassen terms both developments in flirtation with Weber as 'spirits' of 'medicalized, enchanted, cosmopolitan and local rhetoric of love and human universality' (2011: xiv). Understood through the lens of life courses of educated professionals, Christian approaches to reproduction comply well with family planning messages of replaceable fertility and introduce an understanding of a controllable fertility by means of both faith and biomedicine.

Protestantism, sexuality, and infectious reproduction

This section discusses how Pentecostal moralities on sexuality shape the elites' reproductive life courses. These moralities are, on the one hand, informed by the Pentecostal doctrine on pre-marital sexual intercourse and, on the other, by the biomedical preventive paradigm that enters educated professionals' discourses on sexuality.

Christian teachings, and the Pentecostal doctrine of sexual abstinence before marriage in particular, have been noted not just for introducing strong sexual moralities into societies that reportedly did not moralise sexuality as such but rather judged people on their sexual behaviour according to their reproductive outcomes: whether children arrived inside or outside wedlock or at all (Schapera 1966; Delius and Glaser 2005). While in the first half of the twentieth century, Christianity's influence on destroying polygamy had the adverse effect of the detachment of marriage and reproduction, more recent Christian influences on educated professionals' family planning stem from Pentecostal churches. They propagate sexual abstinence before marriage. This has implications for the age at childbirth, especially in a context in which a woman's age at first childbirth is 20 while the average age at marriage is 30.

Following the doctrine of her church, Patricia had not yet borne any children when she married at the age of 30. Other women in my sample, though not all women worshipping in Pentecostal churches, had followed a similar pattern, for instance Tsholo, who married at the age of 28 while still childless. She believed in her church's doctrine of pre-marital abstinence as a means to achieve greater spiritual clarity and greater closeness to God. Consequently, she courted according to the standards of her church, meaning she insisted on not having sexual intercourse with her future husband. When she did not conceive in the first four years of her marriage, her anxieties about remaining childless grew. Considering her age, she was worried about her biological ability to bear children and sought help from gynaecologists.

Taken together the Pentecostal doctrine puts forward new ideas and moralities of family planning and reproduction and introduces a factor into educated professionals' reproductive lives: time and the experience of having one's fertility restricted by one's diminishing biological fertility. Timing and planning reproductive life courses is an approach that not only appears in the context of Pentecostal churches. The Pentecostal doctrine of abstinence before marriage accelerates a process of increasing the emphasis on controlling reproduction and finding the right time for having children, which is indicative for educated professionals' lives in Gaborone. Restricting childbirth was already a concern of educated professionals in the 1990s, especially among single working mothers (Mannathoko 1999). This raises the question of how to understand 'time' and 'timing' better in educated professionals' lives: if and how elite women are timing their reproduction and the moralities that inform their decisions.

As mentioned above, in the context of a high HIV/AIDS infection rate, reproduction becomes potentially infectious, as it would, if unmonitored by biomedical supervision, 'naturally' require unprotected sexual intercourse. Educated professionals are aware of this: 'Throw a stone and you hit three out of ten', commented Reneilwe when we discussed 'making babies' in Botswana (interview,

16 March 2011). For about twenty years, Botswana's HIV/AIDS infection rate has been one of the highest in the world, the most visible effects being a decade-long experience of death and dying and a radical demographic decomposition of the society. This, in conjunction with various HIV/AIDS-related public campaigns and health interventions, has accelerated the public's knowledge on HIV/AIDS-related matters. Education and surveillance campaigns had been launched already in 1988, as well as an ARV programme in 2001, which gave each citizen in need access to free ARVs, and routine testing among pregnant women (Heald 2006). Social marketing campaigns, public testing centres (Steen *et al.* 2007), and condom distribution were also part of such campaigns. The biomedical preventive paradigm promotes an idea of sexuality as potentially infectious; it thus mediatises sexuality and also dissociates matters of sexuality from matters of reproduction (Beckmann *et al.*, Chapter 1, this volume; Adam and Pigg 2005).

Like many other elite women, Christian educated professionals are aware that unprotected sexual intercourse is potentially infectious, and revolt against the patriarchal rights of husbands to extra-marital sexual intercourse. Feminist-Christian discourses attribute the spread of HIV/AIDS (among other diseases) to these rights and claim that men should be discouraged from engaging in casual sexual intercourse with multiple partners (Dube 2002). In elite women's discourses on marriage in Gaborone, they commonly accuse men of 'cheating', thus indirectly accusing them of bringing them the virus. The female discourses thus inverse a commonplace in patriarchal discourses, which traditionally deems women's sexuality as polluting. The Pentecostal teaching introduces a morality directed towards the sexual act itself – and not only towards the question of whether children are born within marriage (Schapera 1966; Delius and Glaser 2005) – and provides the moral framework for women's rejection of (their husband's) extra-marital sexuality. Even though Pentecostal churches do not explicitly encourage women to use condoms within their marriage for preventive purposes, being a (Pentecostal) Christian strengthens women in their rejection of having unprotected sexual intercourse within their marriage.

The interview with Patricia also reflects this attitude: the experience of emotional abuse was a central topic in the ninety-minute conversation I had with her during our meeting at Wimpy's, a fashionable fast-food chain restaurant in Gaborone. Her husband was a policeman, and the relationship had turned sour when she was promoted in her job. He started drinking and began cheating on her. She reported that she repeatedly had dreams and visions from God who told her about her husband's mischievous behaviour. One day, she woke up hearing God's voice: wake up and call your husband to check where he is! When she did, another woman answered the phone and Patricia discovered that her husband was on a trip with her outside the country.

Talking about visions and God's voice that led her to discover her husband's cheating, Patricia refers to a source of female power that women of charismatic circles frequently draw upon (see also Klaits 2010). As prophecy is the core element of the widespread African Independent churches, they use an idiom of power and resistance with a long history in this area (Comaroff and Comaroff 1991). Women's visions were mostly concerned with their close family members' well-being and contained prospective sickness, accidents, or, as in Patricia's case, the cheating of a partner. Thus, this rhetoric indicates Patricia's will to take her life into her own hands as well as her will to protect herself from being infected. In the Pentecostal sphere the widespread practice of having extra-marital sexual partners is transformed into the moral concept of 'cheating'. In the context of HIV/AIDS, this concept gains urgency as it is related to the medical discourse of HIV/AIDS prevention. Elite women understand that their husbands' extra-marital relationships are a real danger to their lives, and they feel they have the right to protect themselves against it. Other, non-elite women I talked to exhibited a similar sense of danger originating from their husband. Women from lower economic backgrounds tend to reject marriage or relationships so as not to risk their health but also not to threaten their freedom and financial situation, as they fear that a partner might use their income for his drinking and womanising. One solution that some women propagate is to remain single.

In this Christian context, women expressed that their fear of being infected overshadowed the fear of remaining childless and they insisted on *not* engaging in unprotected sexual intercourse with their husband.

Ruth, aged 47, had remained childless in her first marriage. She married at the age of 27. When I asked her whether she had already sought medical assistance in order to conceive during her marriage she stated shyly: 'We had used contraception.' And added after a pause: 'Condoms. The marriage wasn't . . .' Leaving the sentence open suggested that she did not feel secure having intercourse with this man without protection against HIV/AIDS.

Tsholo's anxieties about childlessness gained another dimension when she came to talk about her sexual relationship with her husband. Tsholo courted according to the rules of her church, practising abstinence before marriage. She and her husband met mostly at weekends in restaurants and spent some time chatting. The pastor of her husband's church presented him as a devout Christian, thus confirming his moral integrity. It was only after the wedding that she discovered her husband's habit of extra-marital affairs. Her growing anxieties about not conceiving also related to her growing ever more uncomfortable about having unprotected sexual intercourse with her husband. After she had her child she decided to file for a divorce (interview, 16 November 2010).

Ruth had never imagined that her insistence on condom use could have such drastic consequences for her life. Towards the end of the conversation, just before we left the table, she commented in a low voice: 'I never thought I would never have children.' This indicates that she had perceived her will to protect herself as a measure to save her own life and had not thought about the consequences for her reproductive life. Christianity supports a specific imaginary of the procreative body according to which the procreative body becomes controllable through biomedicine and faith. Carried by these beliefs, some educated professionals, like Patricia and Ruth, prioritise their health over their fertility.

At the time of the interview, Ruth had married again, just like Patricia. While Patricia's husband brought children into the marriage, Ruth's husband did not. The couple had found it difficult to communicate about the fact that they were unable to have children and Ruth was too shy to ask him whether he had any children from other relationships. Nevertheless, both women were grateful for their second marriage and described their new husbands as supportive and kind. These second husbands also supported them in the fulfilment of their desire for children, accompanying their wives to gynaecologist appointments and agreeing to take the necessary tests (sperm screening) to identify possible causes for the couple's childlessness. In sum, while the first marriages were marked by experiences of abuse, fights, and cheating, these second marriages are havens of respect and support.

Both women found hope in the prospect of successful conception via in vitro fertilisation (IVF), a treatment that can only be sought in South Africa. The cost of one IVF cycle ranges between 4,000 and 6,000 euros, excluding travelling costs – something that only wealthy people can afford. Patricia had sought IVF twice already, so far without success. During the last course of treatment no more eggs could be extracted. Ruth was planning to undergo IVF at the time of the interview. For both women their second marriage represents a financially and emotionally secure place to seek conception, and both hope for the late realisation of their desire for children.

Perspective on fertility of elite women in contemporary Botswana

Patricia had everything that many Batswana dream of: a good job, a house, a big car, and she had re-married, to a man with two children who was supportive and understanding. Yet, Patricia suffered a lot from her childlessness. While elite women are supported by Pentecostal teachings to plan their reproductive lives and postpone childbirth to their late twenties, childlessness as a solution to reduce the risk of HIV infection is not approved by (Pentecostal) pastors and church members. In fact, it was in one of the Pentecostal churches that I met very harsh comments on my own situation in being single and childless, when I approached people for interviews. However, I did not find any indication that pastors themselves would condemn these women for being childless, and I doubt that they were knowledgeable of the factors that led to their childlessness. Infertility tends to be regarded as a 'private matter', as pastors of all denominations explained to me. They would only interfere if church members asked them for assistance.

In Patricia and Tsholo's environment such child-bearing behaviour is met with scorn and disapproval. There are 'comments' from people at work, church members, and 'even my own sibling', Patricia exclaimed at a certain point in the interview. Tsholo reported that she was asked in a tone full of pretended sympathy: 'Is it difficult to get pregnant?' Others were more upfront: 'Next time when I see you I want to see you pregnant!' Especially nagging was the hostility from her in-laws: 'Do you want people to think that our son is infertile?' Among the comments that both women received was the accusing question 'what are you waiting for?' as well as the put-down 'they have waited too long'. While professional women have practised birth control for decades in Botswana, the practice is still met with suspicion. Especially when children were not arriving at the time when they were expected – namely within the emotionally and financially secure context of marriage and after their education was completed – the common practice of delaying childbirth and controlling reproduction turned against these women, who experienced hostility from many people in their close social environment. Planning reproduction and controlling the body is a good and historically well-established practice of professional women, on top of being encouraged by Christian sexual moralities, but when they fail to have children *at all* these good signs of elite behaviour turn into being a flaw and let them appear arrogant in the eyes of other women.

The issues of stigma, feeling excluded, and receiving hostility from their social environment that have been reported for childless women in Botswana (Upton 2001, 2003; Mogobe 2005) are a recurrent topic in the literature on infertility across the continent (Inhorn 1996; Feldman-Savelsberg 1999; Larsen 2000, 2003; Hollos 2008). Incorporating the biomedical preventive paradigm into their reproductive practices and relying on Christian-biomedical paradigms of controlling the procreative body have gained legitimacy in the Christian realm, as husbands' extra-marital affairs are reinterpreted as 'cheating',[7] and educated professionals are supported in their decision to postpone childbirth. However, it does not shield women from the burden of stigma in cases of childlessness. This may reflect the paradoxes of reproductive Christian-biomedical morals that confront educated professionals. While such morals put a lot of emphasis on manipulating and monitoring fertility, the emphasis on childbirth remains intact. 'Having a child' is seen as a personal fulfilment as well as a social necessity, as childless women experience stigma and discrimination. Their belief in their right to remain healthy seems, in a few instances, to become stronger than their personal and social fears of remaining without children. With the emphasis on monitoring fertility and their moral stance against 'cheating', Christian-biomedical discourses and reproductive moralities introduce elite women to a new dilemma: that of remaining childless.

[7] Urban educated professional women often do have extra-marital affairs and indicate that having pleasure is important in these relationships. This is only to indicate that 'cheating' is not limited to males' sexual behaviour.

Conclusion

Botswana's Christianity, and Pentecostal Christianity in particular, has been absorbing globally circulating biomedical ideas on reproduction, the body, and health. This chapter provides an analysis of how urban educated professionals' striving for fertility has been influenced by these Christian ethics. Taken together, this group of educated professionals are consumers of travelling Christian moralities and ethics of well-being and the controllable body; they are beneficiaries of travelling contraceptive technologies and are themselves transnational patients during their 'medical travels' (Inhorn and Shrivastav 2010; Kangas 2010). Thus, educated professionals are beneficiaries in a landscape of 'stratified reproduction' in which fertility care is privately provided in an otherwise well-functioning health-care system. Supported by the Christian medicalised, enchanted paradigm of the 'make-ability' of reproduction, the controllability of the body through biomedical technologies and faith, as well as the feminist-Christian reinterpretation of male patriarchal rights to extra-marital affairs as 'cheating', some elite women insist on *safe* conception. As the life courses of these women turned out, their second marriages offered them the financially and emotionally secure space for *safe* conception. Do rural women or those who work as shop assistants, bar staff, servants, or maids in Gaborone pursue paradigms of safe conception? And if so, how do they go about it? I do not know whether they would relate their childlessness to their husband's cheating or safe sex practices. Neither would I know whether they seek divorce soon after marriage and find a second husband, this time one who is supportive. However, they are certainly not able to pay the cost of intensive IVF technologies. I suggest that women of lower socio-economic status would have little agency to insist on condom use and may face difficulties in seeking divorce due to the husband's cheating.[8] Safe conception presents itself therefore as an emotional and financial privilege of these educated Christian groups of professionals supported by Christian teaching on reproduction and sexuality. Safe conception turns into a luxury good that not everybody appears to be able to afford in Botswana.

The 'choice of health' versus the 'choice of fertility' that some educated professionals appear to pursue seems to confirm Christianity's production of a liberal subject as the right-bearing, responsible, free individual as proclaimed by Comaroff and Comaroff (1997: 365–6; see also Beckmann *et al.*, Chapter 1, this volume). The previous discussion paints a much more complex picture of how choosing health versus choosing fertility is produced in educated professionals' lives. The medicalised, enchanted paradigm of the body's controllability that evolved from Christian-biomedical discourses put forward a notion of self-

[8] During a visit to Ramotswa, a rural town, I witnessed a discussion of a group of women aged around 50 during which one of the women complained about her husband's cheating but that her pastor would not allow her to seek a divorce.

governance in educated professionals' accounts. Educated professionals who have remained childless never present their choice as a positive choice against having children. Rather, educated professionals seem to apply moralities and doctrines of Christian sexual pureness and biomedical sexual safety. Therefore, their condition of not having children does not present itself as having been a conscious *decision*. The biographies of the women mentioned above rather seem to be a response to changing reproductive ethics, and women therefore paradoxically do not appear as the 'right-bearing, responsible, "free" individuals' that Christian doctrine proclaims them to be. Their 'choice of health' appears to be determined by several reproductive ethical principles – that of sexual pureness, that of postponing reproduction, that of prevention in the context of HIV/AIDS, and that of the controllability of the body – that are blending in the Christian sphere. The 'choice of health' is therefore multi-faceted and inclusive of several ethical principles that favour postponement. By introducing a new morality that prioritises reproductive control and sexual pureness over fertility, Christian ethics support individuals to make choices against *immediate* reproduction. This re-evaluation of the reproductive and sexual body ties into globally circulating biomedical ideas of reproduction as put forward by family planning programmes and HIV prevention programmes. By proposing strong ethics of body control Christianity bears the potential to translate these health ethics into moral practices. Furthermore, elites are especially prone to take on these ethics of body control and health, so that some of these choices can be regarded to be specific to individuals of a certain social position. As a transnational religion, charismatic Christianity thus launches a health ethic that is characteristic of the positionality of new middle-class subjectivities. Following these new doctrines and making these choices, however, does not free those who remain without children from social exclusion.

Acknowledgements

This research was only possible with the support of the Fritz-Thyssen-Foundation and the Max Planck Institute for Social Anthropology, Halle, and was conducted with the permission of the Ministry of Labour and Home Affairs as well as the Ministry of Health, the Gaborone Private Hospital (Dr Music and Dr Eaton), and Bokamoso Private Hospital (Dr Abebe). I thank all the institutions and people involved who have supported my research, and especially Günther Schlee for his intellectual support. My special thanks go to Abigail Morgan (Women's Health Nurse at Bokamoso) and Pastor Seithamo, who actively helped me make contact with patients and church members. Pearl Sechele and Abigile and John Hamathi assisted me during my research. I thank especially John Hamathi for inspiring conversations and his help in connecting me with the right people, as well as Sethunya Mosime, Godisan Mokoodi, and Treasa Galvin from the Department of

Social Science and Musa Dube and Francis Nkomasana from the Department of Theology and Religious Studies at the University of Botswana. Last but not least, I want to thank Rijk van Dijk from the ASC, Leiden, who introduced me to these colleagues.

References

Adam, V. and S.L. Pigg. 2005. *Sex in Development: Science, Sexuality, and Morality in Global Perspective*. Durham, NC: Duke University Press.

Adogame, A. 2005. 'African instituted churches in Europe: Continuity and transformation', in *African Identities and World Christianity in the Twentieth Century: Proceedings of the Third International Munich-Freising Conference on the History of Christianity in the Non-Western World* (15–17 September 2004). Munich-Freising.

Asamoah-Gyadu, K.J. 2007. '"Broken calabashes and covenants of fruitfulness": cursing barrenness in contemporary African Christianity', *Journal of Religion in Africa* 37: 437–60.

Becker, F. and W. Geissler (eds) 2009. *AIDS and Religious Practice in Africa*. Leiden: Brill.

Blystad, A. and K.M. Moland. 2009. 'Technologies of hope? Motherhood, HIV and infant feeding in eastern Africa', *Anthropology and Medicine* 16(2): 105–18.

Bochow, A. and R. van Dijk. 2012. 'Christian creations of new spaces of sexuality, reproduction and relationships in Africa: exploring faith and religious heterotopia', *Journal of Religion in Africa* 42(4): 325–44.

Caldwell, J.C. 1982. *Theory of Decline*. London: Academic Press.

Caldwell, J.C. and P. Caldwell. 1987. 'The cultural context of high fertility in sub-Saharan Africa', *Population and Development Review* 13(3): 409–37.

Chapman, R.R. 2010. *Family Secrets: Risking Reproduction in Central Mozambique*. Nashville, TN: Vanderbilt University Press.

Comaroff, J. and J. Comaroff. 1991. *Of Revelation and Revolution. Vol. 1 Christianity, Colonialism and Consciousness in South Africa*. Chicago: University of Chicago Press.

Comaroff, J. and J. Comaroff. 1997. *Of Revelation and Revolution. Vol. 2 The Dialectics of Modernity on a South African Frontier*. Chicago: University of Chicago Press.

Comaroff, J. and S. Roberts. 1977. 'Marriage and extra-marital sexuality: the dialectics of legal change among the Kgatla', *Journal of African Law* 21: 97–123.

Cornwall, A. 2007. 'Taking chances, making choices: the tactical dimensions of "reproductive strategies" in southwestern Nigeria', *Medical Anthropology* 26: 229–54.

Csordas, T.J. 1997. *The Sacred Self: A Cultural Phenomenology of Charismatic Healing*. Berkeley: University of California Press.

Delius, P. and C. Glaser. 2005. 'Sex, disease and stigma in South Africa: historical perspectives', *African Journal of AIDS Research* 4(1): 29–36.

Dube, M.W. 2002. *HIV/AIDS and the Curriculum: Methods of Integrating HIV/AIDS in Theological Programmes*. Geneva: WCC Publications.

Feldman-Savelsberg, P. 1999. *Plundered Kitchens, Empty Wombs: Threatened Reproduction and Identity in the Cameroon Grassfields*. Ann Arbor: University of Michigan Press.

Fernandez, J.W. 1978. 'African religious movements', *Annual Review of Anthropology* 7: 195–234.

Graeber, D. 2005. 'Fetishism as social creativity', *Anthropological Theory* 5(4): 407–38.

Guyer, J. 1994. 'Lineal identities and lateral networks: the logic of polyandrous motherhood', in C. Bledsoe and G. Pison (eds), *Nuptiality in Sub-Saharan Africa: Contemporary Anthropological and Demographic Perspectives*. Oxford: Clarendon Press, 231–55.

Haram, L. 2004. '"Prostitutes" or modern women? Negotiating respectability in Northern Tanzania', in S. Arnfred (ed.), *Re-Thinking Sexualities in Africa*. Uppsala: Almquist & Wiksell Tryckerei, 211–32.

Heald, S. 2006. 'Abstain or die: the development of AIDS policy in Botswana', *Journal of Biosocial Science* 38: 29–41.

Hollos, M. 2008. '(In)fertility and the modern female life course in two southern Nigerian communities', *Ethnology* 47(1): 23–43.

Hörbst, V. and S. Schuster. 2006. 'Reproductive disruptions: perspectives on African contexts', *Curare* 29(1): 1–5.

Hunt, N.R. 2005. 'Fertility fires and empty wombs in recent Africanist writing', *Africa* 75(3): 421–35.

Inhorn, M. 1996. *Infertility and Patriarchy: The Cultural Politics of Gender and Family Life in Egypt*. Philadelphia: University of Pennsylvania Press.

Inhorn, M. 2002. 'The "local" confronts the "global": infertile bodies and new reproductive technologies in Egypt', in M. Inhorn and F. van Balen (eds), *Infertility around the Globe: New Thinking on Childlessness, Gender, and Reproductive Technologies*. Berkeley: University of California Press, 263–82.

Inhorn, M.C. and P. Shrivastav. 2010. 'Globalization and reproductive tourism in the United Arab Emirates', *Asia-Pacific Journal of Public Health* 22(3 suppl.): 68–74.

Kangas, B. 2010. 'Traveling for medical care in a global world', *Medical Anthropology* 29(4): 344–62.

Klaits, F. 2010. *Death in a Church of Life: Moral Passion during Botswana's Time of AIDS*. Berkeley: University of California Press.

Klassen, P.E. 2011. *Spirits of Protestantism: Medicine, Healing, and Liberal Christianity*. Berkeley: University of California Press.

Krause, K. and G. Hüwelmeier (eds) 2010. *Traveling Spirits: Migrants, Markets and Mobilities*. New York: Routledge.

Landau, P. 1996. 'Explaining surgical evangelism in colonial Southern Africa: teeth, pain and faith', *Journal of African History* 37: 261–81.

Langness, L.L. and G. Frank. 1981. *Lives: An Anthropological Approach to Biography*. Navato, CA: Chandler & Sharp.

Larsen, U. 2000. 'Primary and secondary infertility in sub-Saharan Africa', *International Journal of Epidemiology* 29(2): 285–91.

Larsen, U. 2003. 'Infertility in Central Africa', *Tropical Medicine and International Health* 8(4): 354–67.

Leonard, L. 2002. '"Looking for children": the search for fertility among the Sara of Southern Chad', *Medical Anthropology* 21: 79–112.

Lesthaeghe, R.J. (ed.) 1989. *Reproduction and Social Organisation in Sub-Saharan Africa*. Berkeley: University of California Press.

Lock, M. and P.A. Kaufert. 1998. 'Introduction', in M. Lock and P.A. Kaufert (eds), *Pragmatic Women and Body Politics*. Cambridge: Cambridge University Press, 1–27.

Mannathoko, C. 1999. 'What does it mean to be a middle-class woman in Botswana?', in C. Zmroczek and P. Mahony (eds), *Women and Social Class: International Feminist Perspectives*. London: UCL Press, 9–23.

Mogobe, D.K. 2005. 'Denying and preserving self: Botswana women's experiences of infertility', *African Journal of Reproductive Health* 9(2): 26–37.

Nguyen, V.-K. 2009. 'Therapeutic evangelism – confessional technologies, antiretroviral and biospiritual transformations in the fight against AIDS in West Africa', in W. Geissler and F. Becker (eds), *Aids and Religious Practice in Africa*. Leiden: Brill, 359–78.

Nieswand, B. 2005. 'Charismatic churches in the context of migration: social status, the experience of migration and the construction of selves among Ghanaian migrants in Berlin', in A. Adogame and C. Weissköppel (eds), *Religion in the Context of African Migration*. Scheßlitz: Rosch Buch, 243–67.

Ojo, M.A. 1997. 'Sexuality, marriage and piety among Charismatics in Nigeria', *Religion* 27: 65–79.

Ojo, M.A. 2007. 'Religion and sexuality: individuality, choice and sexual rights in Nigerian Christianity', in E. Maticka-Tyndale, R. Tiemoko and P. Makinwa-Adebusoye (eds), *Human Sexuality in Africa beyond Reproduction*. Auckland Park, South Africa: Action Health Incorporated, 131–49.

Oyedepo, D.O. 1998. *You Shall Not Be Barren*. Ota, Nigeria: Dominion Publishing House.

Paxson, H. 2005. 'Family planning, human nature, and the ethical subject of sex in urban Greece', in V. Adam and S.L. Pigg (eds), *Sex in Development: Science, Sexuality, and Morality in Global Perspective*. Durham, NC: Duke University Press, 95–124.

Pearce, T.O. 1995. 'Women's reproductive practices and biomedicine: cultural conflicts and transformation in Nigeria', in F.D. Grinsburg and R. Rapp (eds), *Conceiving the New World Order: The Global Politics of Reproduction*. Berkeley: University of California Press, 195–208.

Pearce, T.O. 1999. 'She will not be listened to in public: perceptions among the Yoruba of infertility and childlessness', *Reproductive Health Matters* 7(13): 69–79.

Sadgrove, J. 2007. '"Keeping up appearances": sex and religion amongst university students in Uganda', *Journal of Religion in Africa* 37: 116–44.

Schapera, I. 1933. 'Premarital pregnancy and native opinion. A note on social change', *Africa: Journal of the International African Institute* 6(1): 59–89.

Schapera, I. 1966. *Married Life in an African Tribe*. Evanston, IL: Northwestern University Press.

Steen, T.W., K. Seipone, *et al*. 2007. 'Two and a half years of routine HIV testing in Botswana', *JAIDS: Journal of Acquired Immune Deficiency Syndromes* 44(4): 484–8.

Sundby, J. and U. Larsen. 2006. 'Health care service for infertility in sub-Saharan Africa: the case of Moshi in Northern Tanzania', *Curare* (Special Issue: *Reproductive Disruptions? Perspectives on African Contexts*) 29(1): 47–57.

United Nations. 2013. 'UN data. Age of first marriage'. http://data.un.org/Data.aspx?d=GenderStat&f=inID%3A20 (accessed January 2013).

Upton, R.L. 2001. '"Infertility makes you invisible": gender, health and the negotiation of fertility in northern Botswana', *Journal of Southern African Studies* 27(2): 349–62.

Upton, R.L. 2003. '"Women have no tribe": Connecting carework, gender, and migration in an era of HIV/AIDS in Botswana', *Gender and Society* 17(2): 314–22.

van Dijk, R. 1997. 'From camp to encompassment: discourses of transsubjectivity in the Ghanaian Pentecostal diaspora', *Journal of Religion in Africa* 27(2): 135–59.

van Dijk, R. 2010. 'Social catapulting and the spirit of entrepreneurialism: migrants, private initiative, and the Pentecostal Ethic in Botswana', in K. Krause and G. Hüwelmeier (eds), *Traveling Spirits: Migrants, Markets and Mobilities*. New York: Routledge, 101–17.

Vaughan, M. 1991. *Curing Their Ills: Colonial Power and African Illness*. Cambridge: Polity Press.

Way, A.A., A.R. Cross, *et al.* 1987. 'Family planning in Botswana, Kenya and Zimbabwe', *International Family Planning Perspectives* 13(1): 7–11.

Werbner, R. 2004. *Reasonable Radicals and Citizenship in Botswana: The Public Anthropology of Kalanga Elites*. Bloomington: Indiana University Press.

Wilcher, R., W. Cates, *et al.* 2009. 'Family planning and HIV: strange bedfellows no longer' (editorial), *AIDS* 23(1): S1–6.

Woliver, L.R. (ed.) 2002. *The Political Geographies of Pregnancy*. Urbana: University of Illinois Press.

Part 4

TRANSNATIONAL IDENTITIES AND HOMOSEXUALITY

13

'Decadent Imports', 'Vile Abominations'

Transnational Discourses on Male–Male Sex and the Missionary Position in Buganda, 1875–1910

LINDSAY EHRISMAN

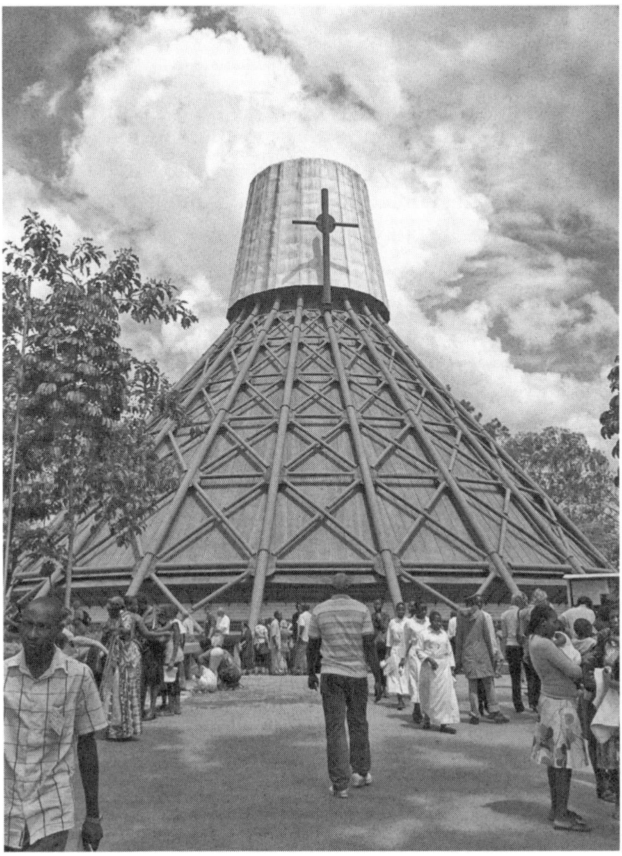

'Uganda Martyrs' Shrine': church built at the site of the 1886 Uganda Martyrs in Namugongo

Proceedings of the British Academy **194**, *271–288.* © The British Academy 2014.

Introduction

On 3 June 2010 Ugandan president Yoweri Museveni addressed a vast crowd gathered to commemorate Martyrs' Day at the Uganda Martyrs' Shrine at Namugongo. According to British missionary accounts and Ugandan collective memory, it had been 124 years since *kabaka* Mwanga, king of Buganda, stood at the same site, and sentenced thirty of his royal pages to death after they allegedly refused to submit to his sexual desires and denounce their new Christian faith (see Faupel 1962: 160–9). 'The church in Africa is very strong', boasted Museveni, 'and has been at the fore in fighting homosexuality and moral decadence' (Kasozi and Ahinbisibwe 2010). Using the historical narrative as a catalyst for contemporary political discussion, Museveni's speech reinforced the hegemonic notion that male-male sex was unnatural in Ugandan social tradition – a meme that undergirded the proposed 2009 anti-homosexuality bill, discussed by Alexandra Müller in greater detail in the next chapter (see Chapter 14, this volume). Instead, male–male sex has been, and continues to be, understood as a 'decadent import' that contaminates Ugandan morality and social progress, just as male–male sex 'contaminated' Buganda's royal court in the years leading up to 1886. Museveni concluded by warning that if Ugandans follow the sexual practices of foreign cultures, '[they] shall be headed for Sodom and Gomorrah' (Kasozi and Ahinbisibwe 2010).

The link between homophobia and Christian morality explicit in Museveni's speech is not new, nor is it solely Ugandan. As we shall see, such rhetoric – a ubiquitous feature of British social discourse during the nineteenth century – was introduced by British missionaries entering the Buganda kingdom situated along the northwestern shore of Lake Victoria in 1877, and used by them to legitimise Protestant hegemony and Baganda subjugation to metropolitan audiences. However, British assumptions, fears, and intolerance of male–male sex were not simply imported and superimposed onto Africans, as scholars such as Murray and Roscoe asserted in their anthology *Boy-Wives and Female Husbands: Studies in African Homosexualities* (1998).[1] Nineteenth-century European racialisation of male–male sex, moreover, cannot be reduced solely to 'Orientalist fabrications', as Marc Epprecht (2006: 191) has argued, although it was part of it. While considerable scholarly attention has been paid to the issue of contemporary homophobia and MSM (men who have sex with men) in Africa within anthropological and biomedical fields, historical scholarship remains relatively limited. Problematically, this limited corpus of historical scholarship has been broadly focused on the African continent at large, and has overwhelmingly cast Africans as detached, non-

[1] The editors state in the opening sentence, 'Among many myths Europeans have created about Africa, the myth that homosexuality is absent or incidental in African societies is one of the oldest and most enduring.' Later, the authors claim, 'The colonialists did not introduce homosexuality to Africa, but rather intolerance of it . . .' (Murray and Roscoe 1998: x, xvi).

participants in the development of homophobic discourse until after independence. In taking this approach, historians risk replacing one set of assumptions with another, and ultimately reproduce rather than challenge colonial images of Africans as monolithic sexual beings or helpless victims lacking historical agency. The transnational scope of this chapter, narrow in both time and space, underscores the active participation of Baganda Protestant converts in discursive productions of male–male sex between 1875 and 1910, and recasts this group of literate, Ganda elites as equal stakeholders alongside their British counterparts in such productions.

At first glance, this chapter marks a point of departure from the contemporary, anthropological focus of this anthology. As a historian, my contribution to this volume offers a historical perspective and proposes one possible origin of contemporary homophobia in Uganda, which developed long before the emergence of the AIDS pandemic, present human rights discourse, or modern sexual categories like 'homosexual' entered Ganda as well as Western vocabularies. This chapter is a necessary cohesive, which binds contemporary debates about transnational influences, homophobia, and notions of 'traditional' African sexuality presented in this volume, particularly in this section, to complex histories. Other contributors have expertly revealed the myriad ways in which ideas move across geographical, political, religious, and social terrains, and how transnational connections in Africa have informed responses to AIDS, sexual politics, and conservative moral epistemologies. The purpose of this chapter is to provide a historical analysis that traces the development of hegemonic transnational constructions of male–male sex through time.

This chapter will revisit the years surrounding the 1886 executions of Baganda Christian converts and analyse the missionary rhetoric that pertained to perceived male same-sex sexual acts. I will advance three main arguments. In the first section, I contend that British constructions of race, sexuality, and geography in the nineteenth century (mis)informed missionary interpretations of Baganda as exclusively and inherently heterosexual. While male–male sexual acts were believed to be racially and geographically determined in the British popular imagination, the notion that 'immoral' sexual acts could be 'imported' by 'decadent' outsiders featured prominently in the discourse and served as a major source of colonial anxiety. The latter becomes of particular importance in the second section, in which I argue that British missionaries proselytising in Buganda between 1875 and 1910 reconciled their metropolitan preconceptions about African sexuality as well as their own utopian visions for the region and its people with the same-sex relations they witnessed or heard about, by implicating 'decadent' Arabs as the importers of 'unnatural vice'. British missionaries somewhat opportunistically utilised and exacerbated anxieties about male–male sex to garner support from the colonial government during a time when a violent clash between religious sects (Catholics, Protestants and Muslims) compromised the Protestant missionary project. Claiming Protestant moral superiority over Baganda, and more importantly, over Arabs, in the missionary record proved vital to the survival and success of the missionary project and to British colonialism in Uganda. In the final section, I claim that homophobia was not simply a European import, and argue that Baganda Christian converts, like Apolo Kaggwa,[2] asserted themselves at the forefront of the development and proliferation of homophobic discourse in Buganda at the turn of the twentieth century.

Homophobia is understood here as a process that developed over time. There are many layers of this process that still need to be explored, both before and after the time period of this chapter. My work represents the first step in a wider project aimed at unearthing the discursive links between nineteenth-century and present-day same-sex sex denial and discrimination in B(U)ganda. It is important to note that the present work will only address British influences on sexual discourse in Buganda. Certainly, myriad influences shaped sexual attitudes, including the writings and teachings of the French Catholic White Fathers. More importantly, it goes without saying that Baganda had their own understandings of sexual normativity that require further exploration, and it is possible that intolerance toward male-male sex pre-existed the colonial encounter. Notwithstanding, I will make the argument that while intolerance of male–male sex may not have been new, the specific way in which male–male sex came to be understood, stigmatised and articulated at the end of the nineteenth century in Buganda was a new phenomenon. The unique circumstances caused, in part, by missionary interventions in Buganda fostered renegotiations of cultural meaning ascribed to male–male sex, which were intimately connected to structures of power. It is not my goal to come to definitive conclusions about contemporary Ugandan homophobia, but rather to open paths of exploration into this sensitive issue by examining the possible origins and pathways of contemporary homophobic discourse.

British constructions, missionary dreams: imagining African sexuality in the metropole

British scholars during the eighteenth century began 'mapping' same-sex sexuality, speculating that male–male sex did not exist in African cultures or geographic space. This was long before any contemporary African leader made the claim that homosexuality was 'un-African', or any missionary had come into contact with Baganda. In 1781, Edward Gibbon wrote, 'I believe . . . that Negroes, in their own country, were exempt from this moral pestilence', when referring to 'pederasty' in his *History of the Decline and Fall of the Roman Empire* (1844: 187). British

[2] I use the now widely accepted spelling of his name. However, his name appears as 'Apolo Kagwa' in early writings, which I will use in citations and reference information.

adventurer William Browne reaffirmed Gibbon's fabrication in 1799 when he recorded that men of the Sudan, 'exceed[ed] in indulgences with women . . . but however unbridled their appetites in other respects may be, pederasty, so common in Asia and North Africa, is in Sudan little known' (Browne 1799: 293). British discourse on inherent African heterosexuality continued to gain currency in the latter half of the nineteenth century when Sir Richard Burton described in his terminal essay to *A Thousand and One Nights* what he called the 'sotadic zone', or 'region where [male–male sex] was presumably indigenous'. Burton believed that 'the negro race [was] mostly untainted by sodomy' and therefore the sotadic zone 'did not extend south of the Sahara in Africa' (Murray and Roscoe 1998: xii). It was clear by the nineteenth century that imagined connections between race, geography and sexuality constructed sub-Saharan Africans as homogeneously heterosexual and North African Arabs as indulgent sodomites in the British imagination.[3]

While the idea that male–male sex was specific to certain peoples and cultures had become a well-established British trope by the end of the nineteenth century, it was a 'vice' that could move, contaminate, and ultimately destroy modern civilisation. It was believed to be 'anomalous to nature', but also 'contagious under certain conditions' from the British scientific gaze (Epprecht 2006: 190). The perceived infectious nature of male–male sex caused imperial concerns about the health and fitness of Empire. British colonisers looked back to former empires, and believed that their demise was in direct relation to decadent sexual indulgences. Marc Epprecht has asserted that Ancient Roman, Arab and Turkish empires were understood as 'proof' that 'decadence [led] to widespread homosexuality, effeminacy and pacification among men, [and ultimately] military defeat and humiliation by more virile societies' (2008: 40). Isaac Land's (2006) illuminating study of the treatment of what he calls the 'homosocial community of shipmates' within the colonial British navy engenders such anxieties. According to Land, British naval commanders strictly policed and commonly 'flogged' seamen who engaged in sexual acts with other shipmates in an attempt to 'protect the integrity of metropolitan culture from seaborne vectors of infection from the periphery', and to maintain an image of 'manliness' among the so-called 'defenders of civilization' (2006: 92). In the context of an expanding British Empire, sexual morality became not only a domestic priority but also an instrument of foreign policy. Sodomy needed to be contained to its 'indigenous' locations to protect the geographic spaces and peoples uncontaminated by perceived sexual indecencies.

The fear of perversions contaminating British subjects, or worse, British citizens, prompted imperial efforts to curtail native sexual immoralities in the periphery. Missionaries, more than any other group, believed it was their (religious) duty to

[3] These examples can be found in numerous publications. For an example see Epprecht (2006: 189–90).

police such sins by inculcating 'proper' gender and sexual behaviours through Christianity and bourgeois mores in the 'heathen' peoples of the world (Wilson 2004: 42). Africa became the region that was in the greatest need of missionary attention. The 'dark' continent, after all, was predominantly unharmed by same-sex sex, but also most susceptible to its endemic nature. Consequently, the missionary project in Africa during the nineteenth century became one of protection from dangerous, morally 'decadent' outsiders as well as guidance into proper evolutionary 'adulthood'. As Catherine Hall has argued, 'Black people were "sons of Africa," "babes in Christ," [and] . . . missionaries were the parents who would act as their teachers and guides' (2002: 98).

The missionary project was not completely selfless, however. Missionaries, deeply affected by the changing social conditions and moral decline in industrial Great Britain, had their own utopian visions of creating new Christian communities in lands untainted by the social ills of the metropole (Ahlberg 1994: 228). Early explorers in the inter-lake region of central east Africa, like Speke and Grant in 1862, portrayed such a place to eager missionaries at home. During an expedition to Lake Victoria Nyanza, Speke claimed that the lake was the source of the Nile and one of several lakes that surrounded and 'disclosed villages and hamlets, their brown thatched roofs contrasting with the emerald of the beautiful milk-bush, the coral branches of which clustered around cottages, and formed alleys and hedgerows equal to the choicest of English shrubberies'. He concluded simply that, 'This was a happy-looking secluded nook' (Swayne *et al.* 1868: 98). Another traveller later wrote of the region that it:

> is practically an island lying at the very heart of Africa. Its boundaries are the mighty lakes . . . which are almost linked up by broad fast-flowing rivers. Probably on account of its unique geographical position, its peoples have retained an exclusivism against the barbarous races all around. Approach it from whatever direction you will, tribes of abject savages, including pigmies and cannibals, will be found.
>
> (Fisher 1911: 2)

There was something special and enchanting, quaint and heavenly about Ganda's secluded, and temporally, displaced landscape. Though there may have been 'evils' in close proximity, somehow in this small pocket of the African interior, the people embodied a Rousseau-like quality of innocence and potential that seemed to provide the ideal setting for their missionary dream.

No one was more influential in animating British missionaries or stoking British popular imagination than Henry Morton Stanley. Stanley wrote extensively about his experiences in the Great Lakes region as well as his relationship with *kabaka* Mutesa (Mwanga's father). Though he was not a missionary, in 1874, Stanley took it upon himself to enlighten the Buganda hegemon on 'the wonders of civilization and the benefits of Christianity', largely because of what he called the 'Muslim threat' from the north (Faupel 1962: 10). Notwithstanding dangerous Arab influence, Stanley made explicit romantic notions of noble savages and his expressed admiration for the *kabaka* in his accounts and British print culture. Noting Mutesa's impressive power, sophisticated bureaucracy, and welcoming nature, Stanley wrote, 'I see that Mtesa [*sic*] is a powerful Emperor with great influence over his neighbours . . . and [I] witnessed with astonishment such order and law as is obtainable in semi-civilized countries' (Stanley 1878: 194). The *kabaka*'s positive first impressions led the traveller to believe that Mutesa could be 'the light that shall lighten the darkness . . . a prince well worthy of the most hearty sympathies that Europe can give him' (ibid.: 193). The coupling of Mutesa's 'interest' in Christianity and a perceived Muslim threat gave impetus to Stanley's call to missionaries in the *Daily Telegraph* on 15 November 1875, urging them that their work was needed, and would be welcomed by Baganda who were eager to embrace Christianity and 'undermine Islamism' (Stanley 1878: 194; Faupel 1962: 11). The Church Missionary Society (CMS) responded immediately, and in 1877, a group of eight missionaries penetrated the African interior to protect the Baganda from 'evil' Arab influence, to guide them into modern civilisation, and create an ideal Christian community for themselves and their adopted African children.

The missionaries' initial observations of indigenous social behaviours were influenced by British metropolitan constructions of race, geography and sexuality. In 1877 CMS missionary Alexander Mackay wrote in an initial letter home:

> God has blessed, and is still blessing, our work here . . . The king and I are great friends, and the chiefs also have great confidence in me; and I hope to be able to guide them in the way of a more humane policy than has existed hitherto. Cruelty, slavery, polygamy, [and] witchcraft . . . are the evils to be combated.
>
> (Harrison [1890] 1970: 103–4)

Mackay's assessment vividly illustrated African stereotypes as well as the initial tensions within the missionary project. British missionaries had to become 'friends' with possible converts, as it was imperative for missionaries to have open dialogue with non-believers in order to create opportunities to teach the gospel. However, because missionaries lived closely among indigenous peoples, it was vital that they utilised cultural differences to delineate racial boundaries and establish moral hierarchies. In these 'intimate transfer points', as Ann Stoler (1995: 10) has called them, missionaries tended to establish racial distinctions by pointing out the 'heathen' customs that were closely linked to improper sex and gender roles. They saw such customs as socially and morally inferior to their own civilised conduct, and by highlighting certain practices as 'heathen', missionaries justified their imposition on a foreign culture and legitimated their religious project.

Polygamy was the most noted Baganda sexual custom in the early missionary record that needed to be 'combated'. One observer recorded that the king had so many wives that he must have 'possessed over 1,000 children', and that 'princes and princesses [were] almost as plentiful as mosquitoes' (Fisher 1911: 43). On several occasions Mackay noted Mutesa's inability to resist polygamy and to make moral decisions 'for Him and not for the flesh' (Harrison [1890] 1970: 134). Rev.

Robert Pickering Ashe similarly reported in disbelief that during his illness Mutesa refused to follow the advice of (European) doctors after they suggested a 'new regimen [that] prevented him from enjoying the society of his wives' (Ashe 1889: 71). Depictions of Mutesa's seemingly untameable sex drive stood in stark contrast to the emerging social and moral ethos that undergirded British bourgeois culture and Victorian sexual suppression, yet also reinforced preconceived notions of licentious, heterosexual Africans.

Similar to racialised and gendered constructions of polygamy, British missionaries utilised gendered associations with 'witchcraft' to reaffirm Baganda cultural and sexual differences from British Christians. Witchcraft particularly concerned missionaries in the last year of *kabaka* Mutesa's fatal illness in 1883.[4] One report suggested that he had been 'persuaded by his female relatives to seek advice of a wizard or medicine man, professing to have intercourse with the *lubare*, or spirit, of the great Nyanza' (Mockler-Ferryman 1903: 278). The perceived gender-ambiguous territorial spiritual entity was 'Mukasa, the powerful spirit associated with Lake Victoria' (Kodesh 2010: 38). According to Mackay, Baganda strongly believed that 'the remains of ancestors [were] being preserved by certain persons who were either regarded as holding converse with the departed spirits of the kings, or were themselves possessed of certain spirits' (Harrison [1890] 1970: 149). Spirit possession was not exclusive to males, however. The commonality of female mediums or 'spirit wives' represented the power 'related to the general connection between women, fertility, and the continuity in life' in Ganda culture (Kodesh 2010: 58). The perceived gendered fluidity of spiritual entities and the prominence of females in Ganda spiritual space threatened a patriarchal hierarchy that British missionaries associated with 'rational' and 'civilised society'.

The repugnance expressed in missionary accounts toward cultural customs like polygamy and witchcraft reaffirmed African sexual and gendered stereotypes in the British imagination. In the case of polygamy, missionaries expected to encounter sexually lax, hyper-masculine African men, as they had been conditioned through various British mediums to believe that Africans were 'primitive', 'close to nature', and 'animal-like'. Natural scientists in Europe had even made connections between African sexuality and physical traits. For instance, male Africans' 'larger genitals were equated with smaller brain size [and] sexual excess became the mark of inferiority' (Levine 2004: 136). Furthermore, the practice of witchcraft underpinned popular British tropes of African irrationality, which reinforced theories about Africans' 'child-like' nature, their vulnerability, and sexual moral unawareness. Though polygamy and witchcraft were considered to be horrifying symptoms of backward societies, they were presupposed and treatable. Through conversion, rigorous moral instruction, and inculcation of Western values, Africans could be

[4] Evidence suggests that Mutesa died of gonorrhoea in 1884.

cleansed of such immoralities. In the British missionary imagination, Africans, like children, did not know any better, and it was the responsibility of Christian fathers (i.e. missionaries) to be their moral guides. Thus, missionaries wanted to write explicitly about these fixable 'immoralities' to reaffirm their preconceptions and justify their role in the 'civilising mission' to both themselves and their supporters at home.

Anticipated cultural 'symptoms' such as polygamy and witchcraft were not the only 'immoralities' that missionaries encountered in Buganda. Sexual relations between male, high-ranking members of Buganda's royal court and boy pages were repeatedly implied, though not explicitly described, in missionary accounts throughout the reign of both *kabaka* Mutesa and his successor Mwanga. Unlike other 'inferior' and 'immoral' practices, however, same-sex sexual allegations were written in coded language such as 'unnatural' or 'vile' 'crimes' and 'vice'. Additionally, and without exception, instances of male–male 'evil doings' were deemed circumstantial, not indigenous, and attributed to Arab presence and influence in the royal court.

In this section I have demonstrated that metropolitan discourses of African sexuality (mis)informed the missionary record. However, male–male sex denial similarly permeated British social and imperial discourses. In the following section I will link the discursive transformations of male–male sexual anxieties in imperial Great Britain to the rhetorical ambiguities in missionary accounts in regard to Baganda male–male sex as well as the explicit criminalisation of 'Arabs'.

'A crime unfit to be named'

'Sodomy' or 'buggery' had been punished in British law since the sixteenth century. The Buggery Act of 1533 made sodomy punishable by death under King Henry VIII, and it remained in effect to be re-emphasised in the Offences Against the Person Act of 1828, which stated, 'Every person convicted of the abominable crime of Buggery, committed either with Mankind or any Animal, shall suffer death as a felon' (*Statutes of the United Kingdom of Great Britain and Ireland* 1828: 105). However, in 1885 sodomy was hazily redefined as 'gross indecency' under the Labouchere Amendment of the Criminal Law Amendment Act, and was reduced to a misdemeanour and a two-year jail sentence (White 1999: 25). Though 'gross indecency' was generally interpreted as any same-sex sexual act, the law did not make a direct reference to same-sex sexual activity. By the late nineteenth century, it appeared that there was an increase in same-sex sexual denial in British legal language.

While legal definitions of same-sex relations were less pronounced, the rhetoric of British political commentators on the issue of sodomy evidenced the rising influence of bourgeois morality and evangelical fervour. In Edward Deacon's 1831 book, *A Digest of the Criminal Law of England*, he wrote, 'sodomy is that horrible sin against nature, and the ordinance of the Almighty'. Similarly, in 1857, William Blackstone lamented that sodomy was 'a crime unfit to be named' as it went against the laws of 'nature and of reason, and the express law of God'. The deeply disturbed tone in both statements suggests that the very mention of sodomy was too traumatic for Britons to endure. Disapproval of same-sex sex had become intrinsically connected with Christian values and common sense, hence there was little need to discuss such obscenities. The Protestant emphasis on 'self-improvement' and 'self-discipline' created a shift in how sodomy should be punished. Beginning in the mid-nineteenth century, same-sex relations were to be morally, not legally, policed, and punished not by death, but eternal damnation.

In the British popular imagination, however, Africans lacked reason and rationality and did not have the ability to understand such anomalies, and thus missionaries dismissed what they understood as Baganda sexual aberrance as childish moral unawareness. One missionary wrote that inside the royal court, a chief of Budu in a room with other men 'was amusing himself and the company with obscene jests. I told him it was a shame for a great man so to lower himself and he accordingly refrained' (Ashe 1889: 104). Like children who unknowingly act inappropriately, British missionaries assumed Baganda were sexually naïve. Thus, missionaries disregarded male sexual acts among Baganda as primitive ignorance rather than intentional sexual exchanges between men, and remedied the situation through moral inculcation rather than punishment.

In particular circumstances, however, even the most 'civilised' Briton risked succumbing to 'irrational' sexual behaviours. Rudi Bleys (1995) theorises that male–male sexual 'silences' in the historical record resulted from masculine 'imperial anxieties'. According to Bleys, European men colonising in West Africa had reported that there was an 'apparent increase of homosexual contacts within the army or between soldiers and indigenous men' (1995: 148). Rumours of men having sex with men in South African mine camps also permeated reports, stoking masculine anxieties among missionaries whose similar tropical, male milieu made them especially 'susceptible' to sexual perversions. Bleys's theoretical assertions can be historically grounded in Buganda. Before 1898, female European missionaries were strictly prohibited from proselytising in Buganda, and it was not until after 1900 that British women could settle in Uganda (Tripp 2004: 129). Protestant missionary Frank Rowling, for example, wrote a series of letters requesting that the CMS permit him to marry Miss Browne, a British woman and fellow missionary living in Great Britain. His requests were repeatedly postponed due to marriage regulations. In 1897 he lamented, 'I have already served five years loneliness in Busoga, which has tried me.'[5] The ways in which loneliness 'tried'

[5] Letter from Frank Rowling to Rev. Fox, 12 November 1897, CMS G3 A7/0 1898/26.

Rowling must have resonated with CMS officials because his request was subsequently approved, and he married Miss Browne the following year. From 1877 to 1898 missionaries could not travel with their families to Africa, and scholars like Bleys have highlighted nineteenth-century European fears that the lack of (European) women in hot and exotic African colonial settings 'caused' otherwise respectable and moral European men to act in inappropriate ways.

'Tropicalisation' seemingly affected Rev. Ashe as his accounts of boy pages verge on homoerotic. In arousing language he described two of Mutesa's pages as 'handsome boys, their bodies shining in a superabundance of oil' (Ashe 1889: 59). In another instance, he described falling into a trance-like state after 'a skilled male dancer went through the surprising evolutions and contortions of the strange body dance, which [he] had seen women of Unyamwesi performing'. 'The mazy motion of the dance, [coupled with] the heat of the reception hall', Ashe wrote, had hypnotising affects, nearly lulling him to sleep (ibid.: 61). Ashe also wrote repetitively about his unusually close and 'special' relationship with a young convert and former slave, Mugaju Lugalama, whom he referred to as his 'favourite' and physically described as a 'handsome Muhuma boy' (ibid.: 126). His affection for the young convert was evident when Lugalama later became one of the 'Uganda Martyrs'. An entire chapter in his book is dedicated to Lugalama's death. Among several comments about his execution, Ashe wrote, 'The butchers do their work and mar what was so wonderfully made' (ibid.: 146). Whether Ashe had a romantic relationship with Lugalama is unclear, but he could have been conflicted with his own 'unnatural' sexual desires, which possibly skewed how he recorded (or did not record) same-sex acts.

Above all, same-sex sexual denial in the missionary record was linked to the British belief that decadent foreigners must have imported male–male sex into African geographic and social space. The British notion that Arabs and Arab geographies were predisposed to sodomy was deeply couched in Orientalist discourse, and Britons widely subscribed to such salient racist and sexual stereotypes. Protestant missionaries in Buganda consistently rationalised male same-sex acts with the presence and influence of Muslims within the royal court. The influence of racial and sexual British ideologies was evident in Ashe's reflection on *kabaka* Mutesa after his death in 1884. Ashe wrote that Mutesa's 'vilest abominations, I believe, he committed by the advice of the Arabs' (ibid.: 82). The criminalisation of Arabs allowed missionaries to doubly employ the method of 'othering' on both Arabs and Baganda, as highlighting Arab alterity and accusing Arabs of having negative influence over Baganda concomitantly implied that Baganda were easily influenced and highly impressionable.

Concern over 'impressionability' was a common justification for paternalistic, colonial interventions in Africa. Such paternal tropes cast Africans as easily swayed children who needed protection from harmful outside influences. Missionaries suggested that members of the Buganda royal court were somehow tricked into following Arab advice and culture. 'The Arabs had tried to prevail upon Mutesa', wrote Ashe, 'to copy their own customs with reference to the custody of his harem' (ibid.: 65). British missionaries commonly portrayed Muslims in Buganda as deceitful and conniving. In another description, Ashe characterised Muslims as 'men who can smile and smile and be villains with it all' (ibid.: 57). According to missionaries, both *kabaka* Mutesa and *kabaka* Mwanga were too naïve to see through the Arabs' deceptive and decadent nature, and, as a result, were influenced to behave in immoral and improper ways. *Kabaka* Mutesa, Ashe lamented, had 'followed [the Arabs'] evil counsel in the case of a few of his pages', and this 'training in cruelty, brutality, and lust' led the king to 'such vile obscenities as make daylight ashamed' (ibid.: 82). In another observation Ashe alleged that Mwanga 'had allowed himself to fall completely under the influence of Arab traders' (Ashe 1894: 68). The young king even began to mimic 'all the [subtlety] of Arabs, he adopted their dress [and] learned their language' (Ashe 1889: 105). Through rhetorical methodologies, missionaries implicated Muslims as immoral and unfit 'fathers' to African 'children'.

According to both Ashe and Mackay, Mwanga's rage and the dangers of Arab influence had reached a climax in late May 1886. In Ashe's accounts, Mwanga allegedly ordered one of his royal pages, Matia, to 'participate in some of those evil doings' with a 'Muhammedan chief, named Kauta'. Matia, a recent convert, refused to follow orders, and an enraged Mwanga charged all Christian converts within his court with 'disobedience' and 'gave the order that that all Christians in [Buganda] should be seized and put to death'. 'The fact was', Ashe speculated, that '[the pages] had begun to set themselves against the evil practices of Mwanga's shameful court', which ultimately led the converts to martyrdom. Missionaries depicted a bloody and barbaric scene of the pages' arrests in which Christians 'were clubbed to death and speared, and many were seized and put in the stocks; many were mutilated in a manner which in some cases proved fatal' (Ashe 1889: 80). The event culminated on 3 June 'at the Namugongo execution ground where thirty two victims were burned to death on a single pyre' (Rowe 1964: 55). Missionaries rhetorically linked sexual deviance to Muslim influence and Mwanga's subsequent 'irrational' behaviour.

News of the mass killings made its way back to England, giving further credence to the dangers of decadent societies, and the need for the British 'civilising mission' in sub-Saharan Africa. In the aftermath of martyrdom, Ashe wrote:

> This is Africa left to herself. Livingstone, Stanley, and Cameron have told us what Africa is when left to the Arabs. If such recitals as these have any meaning, it is that the most powerful appeal is made to civilised nations to take African tribes under their fostering care. It is an appeal to England to do for Africa what she has so triumphantly affected for the peoples of India.
>
> (Ashe 1889: 124)

The British East Africa Company took command over the region in 1894, the British Uganda Agreement was signed in 1898, and in 1900 Uganda officially became a British Protectorate. Upon signing, one British representative said of Mwanga, 'Perhaps he might have still been king had not his vicious propensities taken a turn which disgusted even his Negro people' (Hoad 2007: 5). When unpacked, this statement implies that Mwanga's behaviour was a rare exception among an over-generalised and singular African people. Despite their knowledge of male same-sex relations, missionaries maintained that Mwanga's behaviour was directly related to Muslim influence, and was not representative of normative Baganda sexual practices.

The indigenisation of homophobia

Ideas about sexual norms were not exclusive to missionary accounts or British minds. Instead ideas moved in multidirectional patterns, flowing back and forth, not only from metropole to periphery, but also between missionaries and Baganda, and among Baganda. While British constructions of Baganda heterosexuality skewed data in the historical record, early homophobic discourse could not have developed and intensified without Baganda participation. I assume, as Carolyn Hamilton (1998) asserted in a different context, that 'the colonial worldview was not simply imported from the metropole and imposed on the colonized, nor was a new worldview suddenly "invented". Rather it emerged out of the colonial experience, through a process of transformation and rearrangement' (Hamilton 1998: 27). British colonisation and missionary intervention refashioned the social, moral and political terrain in Buganda, creating new frameworks for Baganda Christian converts to work within in order to access previously unattainable power.

After 1886, *kabaka* Mwanga fled to Tanganyika, and Prince Chua, the legitimate successor, was deemed too young to rule by the British colonial government.[6] In the same year, British missionaries started making note of 'helpful' converts they believed would sufficiently lead the native population. Based on these lists, missionaries acting as colonial agents wrote in a report to Her Majesty's Government in 1898:

> As Prince Chua is only a child, it is necessary that, until he is old enough to rule the country, a Council be formed to act for him, and for this purpose the following Chiefs have been elected:
>
> Apollo Kagwa, Katikiro.
> Mugwanya, Katikiro.
> Zachariah, Kangao.[7]

[6] 'Uganda Papers: Recent Events in the Uganda Protectorate', CMS G3 A7/0 1898/56, January 1899, 13.
[7] Ibid.

Apolo Kaggwa and his cohorts represented an emerging class of literate Christian converts. Seeking to legitimise their rapid political ascendance, the former royal pages wrote down testimonies and refashioned Ganda histories, 'in a way that would both reinforce [their] positions of power in the [new] volatile Ganda political order and satisfy Western tastes and sensibilities', as Neil Kodesh (2010: 3) has convincingly argued. In his testimonies, for example, Andrew Kiwanuka claimed that, '[a]t that time the Kabaka practiced the works of Sodom. Muslims and pagans were prepared to do those things with him, but the [Christians] absolutely refused' (Faupel 1962: 83). Apolo Kaggwa, arguably the most outspoken convert, echoed both missionary rhetoric and British medicalisation of male–male sex when he claimed that, 'these Arabs introduced to us, along with numerous disorders, an abomination which we had never practiced and which had never heard spoken of' (ibid.: 9). Another convert, and former royal page, Ham Mukasa, wrote:

> I think I must have been about twelve years old when I entered [Mutesa's] household. I found the king's court full of the vilest customs, introduced by the Arabs and Turks (the people who came from Egypt). I was much afraid, for my parents had told me not to agree to such things; for they told me if I did such things I should die at once. But in spite of this I was compelled to join with the rest.
>
> (Mullins and Mukasa 1904: 176)

After his 'sinful' experiences in Mutesa's Arab-influenced court, Mukasa confessed, he 'lusted after evil things, and the only thing that saved [him] from doing them was that earnest Christian men always lived with [him] at [his] house' (ibid.: 202). The Church Missionary Society published his narrative in *The Wonderful Story of Uganda* in 1904. The testimonies of converts gave credence to missionary constructions of Baganda sexuality, and the absence of same-sex relations in traditional Buganda, and further promoted British discourse of same-sex sex.

Subsequently, these converts formed the basis for Ganda historiography. In 1901, Apolo Kaggwa published *Bakabaka Bebuganda* (*The Kings of Buganda*), the first dynastic history of Buganda written in Luganda, which was 'printed privately with financial assistance from an Anglican missionary friend' (Twaddle 1974: 86). Interestingly, Kaggwa's dynastic genealogy ends with Mutesa; no information regarding Mwanga's reign is provided in the text whatsoever. Though Kaggwa does mention the 1886 executions, his version places Mukasa, Mwanga's chief adviser and a man who 'practised Islam', as the person responsible for the fatal persecution of Baganda converts. According to Kaggwa, Mukasa announced to missionaries, 'You are our guests, but those boys are our sons. As many as you teach, we shall kill' (Kagwa 1971: 184). In his portrayal, sodomy was left out of the narrative entirely, and the executions were solely the result of religious strife between a Muslim man and his Christian adversaries who challenged Baganda patriarchal social and dynastic structures.

In 1918, Kaggwa published *Mpisa za Baganda* (*The Customs of the Baganda*), a book that described pre-colonial Baganda customs and oral traditions. Throughout the book, Kaggwa linked a number of imported 'vices' to Arab influence (Twaddle 1974: 87). 'The Arabs', he wrote, 'caused the breakdown of [Baganda] customs. They also introduced sodomy' (Kagwa 1934: 98). Though his second book did not completely silence male–male sex in Buganda history, it did reinforce and perpetuate British conceptions of African heterosexuality and influential Arab sexual immorality. His published 'histories', funded by British missionaries, provided 'empirical' support to British constructions of Baganda sexuality.

Testimonies and written histories produced by converts proved problematic, as British officials and missionaries rewarded converts for being 'devout Christians'. Kaggwa along with fellow convert Honorat Nyonyintono, for example, were made 'commanders of two powerful regiments . . . and given royal license to pillage and raid anywhere in the kingdom without restraint. It was a greater privilege than that enjoyed . . . under Mwanga or Mutesa' (Rowe 1964: 58). Converts were also given large pieces of land and political power (Twaddle 1974: 86). Sir Apolo Kaggwa, as he was later titled, was appointed to the position of prime minister (Katikkiro) in 1890, which he retained until 1926, and as early as 1888, all 'the chief offices were taken over by Christian converts' (Mockler-Ferryman 1903: 281).

Conclusion

In this chapter, I have analysed written documents produced by British explorers, adventurers, intellectuals and missionaries, and these documents suggest that British missionaries entered Uganda with certain preconceptions about race, geography, and male–male sex, which skewed their understanding of Baganda sexuality. Missionaries could not break from their imagined perceptions of African-ness, resulting in male–male sexual constructions that were closely linked to what they saw as Arab decadence. Caused in part by missionary inculcation and incentive, Baganda converts became active participants and equal stakeholders in the development and proliferation of homophobic discourse in the context of a rapidly transforming colonial reality.

In this chapter I intended to deconstruct a particular set of historical assumptions about 'traditional' Ganda sexuality, and contextualise those assumptions within a specific transnational, historical process, which gave the assumptions hegemonic power. Ideas about so-called 'traditional' Ganda sexuality presented in the writings of British missionaries or Ganda elites should not be accepted as historical 'truth' or as representative of commonly held Baganda beliefs about normative sexual behaviour during the time period discussed here. In fact, it is unlikely that the vast majority of Baganda (non-elites) subscribed to or had knowledge of this new moral code, which stigmatised male–male sex, until much later. Even Ganda elites who rhetorically adopted Christian moral discourse 'did not stop being Baganda', as historian Holly Hanson put it (2003: 105). In other words, Baganda Christian elites did not completely abandon traditional practices or ways of knowing, spiritually or otherwise, even after they converted.

However, recovering pre-colonial or pre-Christian Ganda moral epistemologies and sexual practices is a challenging and complicated task. While there was much recorded about 'traditional' customs, these sources were produced either by European missionaries or by the first generation of literate Ganda elites under the tutelage of British missionaries within the context of an emerging colonial order. In their early published works 'Baganda intellectuals', Neil Kodesh tells us, 'struggled to present their past in a manner that was palatable to those in power in order to win legitimacy in the colonial world' (2010: 31). These histories thus distort and limit our knowledge about the Ganda distant past, including our perceptions of Ganda pre-colonial sexual practices and attitudes. In order to get closer to an 'authentic' past, Kodesh as well as other scholars of pre-colonial Buganda insist that we must first deconstruct written texts and clear the 'colonial clutter' obscuring our historical view. It is only then that historians can begin to reconstruct a version of the Ganda past without strings attached to its colonial legacy.

References

Ahlberg, Beth Maina. 1994. 'Is there a distinct African sexuality? A critical response to Caldwell', *Africa: Journal of the International African Institute* 64(2): 220–42.

Ashe, Robert Pickering. 1889. *Two Kings of Uganda.* London: Frank Cass & Co. Ltd.

Ashe, Robert Pickering. 1894. *Chronicles of Uganda.* London: Hodder & Stoughton.

Blackstone, William. 1857. *Commentaries on the Laws of England*, vol. 4. Oxford: John Murray.

Bleys, Rudi. 1995. *The Geography of Perversion: Male-to-Male Sexual Behavior Outside the West and the Ethnographic Imagination, 1750–1918.* New York: New York University Press.

Browne, William. 1799. *Travels in Africa, Egypt, and Syria, From the Year 1792 to 1798.* London: T. Caldwell & W. Davie.

Deacon, Edward E. 1831. *A Digest of the Criminal Law of England*, vol. 2. London: Saunders & Benning.

Epprecht, Marc. 2006. 'Bisexuality and the politics of normal in African ethnography', *Anthropologica* 48(2): 187–201.

Epprecht, Marc. 2008. *Heterosexual Africa? The History of an Idea from the Age of Exploration to the Age of AIDS.* Athens, OH: Ohio University Press.

Faupel, Fr. J.F. 1962. *African Holocaust: The Story of the Uganda Martyrs.* London: Geoffrey Chapman.

Fisher, Ruth. 1911. *Twilight Tales of the Black Baganda.* London: Frank Cass & Co. Ltd.

Gibbon, Edward. 1844. *History of the Decline and Fall of the Roman Empire*, vol. III. New York: Harper & Brothers.

Hall, Catherine. 2002. *Civilizing Subjects: Metropole and Colony in the English Imagination 1830–1867.* Chicago: University of Chicago Press.

Hamilton, Carolyn. 1998. *Terrific Majesty: The Powers of Shaka Zulu and the Limits of Historical Invention*. Cambridge, MA: Harvard University Press.

Hanson, Holly Elizabeth. 2003. *Landed Obligation: The Practice of Power in Buganda*. Portsmouth, NH: Heinemann.

Harrison, Alexina Mackay. [1890] 1970. *A. M. Mackay: Pioneer Missionary of the Church Missionary Society to Uganda*. London: Frank Cass & Co. Ltd.

Hoad, Neville. 2007. *African Intimacies: Race, Homosexuality, and Globalization*. Minneapolis: University of Minnesota Press.

Kagwa, Apolo. 1934. *The Customs of the Baganda*. Trans. Ernest B. Kalibala, ed. May Mandelbaum Edel. New York: Columbia University Press.

Kagwa, Apolo. 1971. *The Kings of Buganda*. Trans. M.S.M. Kiwanuka. Nairobi: East African Publishing House.

Kasozi, Ephraim and Patience Ahinbisibwe. 2010. 'Uganda: opposed to homosexuality – Museveni', *The Monitor*, 4 June. http://allafrica.com/stories/201006040263.html.

Kodesh, Neil. 2010. *Beyond the Royal Gaze: Clanship and Public Healing in Buganda*. Charlottesville: University of Virginia Press.

Land, Isaac. 2006. 'Sinful propensities: piracy, sodomy, and empire in the rhetoric of naval reform, 1770–1870', in Steven Pierce and Anupama Rao (eds), *Discipline and the Other Body: Correction, Corporeality, Colonialism*. Durham, NC: Duke University Press.

Levine, Philippa. 2004. 'Sexuality, gender, and empire', in Philippa Levine (ed.), *Gender and Empire*. Oxford: Oxford University Press.

Mockler-Ferryman, A.F. 1903. 'Christianity in Uganda', *Journal of the Royal African Society* 2(7): 276–91.

Mullins, Rev. Joseph Denis and Ham Mukasa. 1904. *The Wonderful Story of Uganda*. London: Church Missionary Society.

Murray, Stephen O. and Will Roscoe (eds) 1998. *Boy-Wives and Female Husbands: Studies in African Homosexualities*. New York: Palgrave.

Rowe, J.A. 1964. 'The purge of Christians at Mwanga's court: a reassessment of this episode in Buganda history', *Journal of African History* 5(1): 55–72.

Stanley, Henry Morton. 1878. *Through the Dark Continent*. New York: Harper & Brothers.

The Statutes of the United Kingdom of Great Britain and Ireland 1828. London: His Majesty's Statute and Law Printers.

Stoler, Ann Laura. 1995. *Race and the Education of Desire: Foucault's History of Sexuality and the Colonial Order of Things*. Durham, NC: Duke University Press.

Swayne, George, John Speke and James Grant. 1868. *Lake Victoria*. London: William Blackwood & Sons.

Tripp, Aili Mari. 2004. 'A new look at colonial women: British teachers and activists in Uganda, 1898–1962', *Canadian Journal of African Studies* 38(1): 123–56.

Twaddle, Michael. 1974. 'On Ganda historiography', *History in Africa* 1: 85–100.

Uganda Anti-Homosexuality Bill. 2009. http://www.ukgaynews.org.uk/Archive/09/Nov/Bill-No18-Anti-Homosexuality-Bill-2009_Uganda.pdf.

White, Chris (ed.) 1999. *Nineteenth Century Writings on Homosexuality: A Sourcebook*. New York: Routledge.

Wilson, Kathleen. 2004 'Empire, gender, and modernity', in Philippa Levine (ed.), *Gender and Empire*. Oxford: Oxford University Press.

Archival material

Church Missionary Society Archives.
Special Collections, University of Birmingham.

14

Transnational Moralities and Invisible Sexual Minorities

Human Rights Discourse and Religion in Uganda

ALEXANDRA MÜLLER

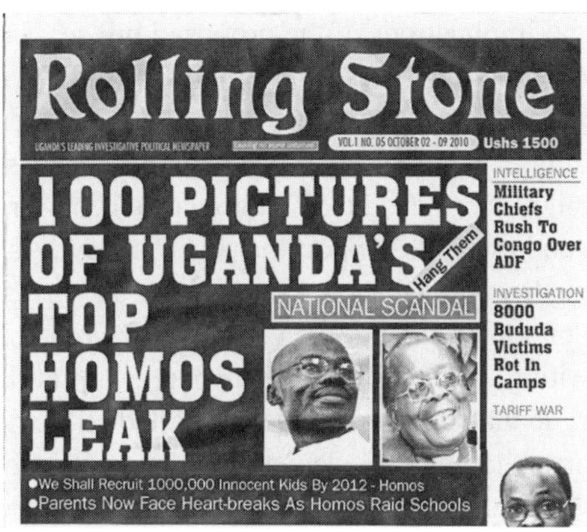

Ugandan newspaper, *Rolling Stone*, calls for the 'hanging' of 'homosexuals'. David Kato, whose name was published among many others on this list, was murdered shortly afterwards.

Introduction: transnational governmentality and the international HIV discourse

THIS CHAPTER SEEKS TO ANALYSE the transnational connections, conservative moral agendas and expressions of contestation that are at play in the current discourse around sexual and reproductive rights of sexual minorities in Uganda.[1]

[1] I would like to thank Talia Meer and Fiona Ross for their comments, criticisms, suggestions and support in shaping the argument of this chapter. I would also like to thank the participants of the UCT Anthropology departmental seminar for illustrative comments and constructive suggestions.

Proceedings of the British Academy **194**, *289–310*. © The British Academy 2014.

After Uganda had been hailed for its political commitment to reducing the prevalence of HIV, the country again drew international attention in 2009 on issues related to sexual and reproductive health and rights. However, this time it provoked an outcry of criticism due to the parliamentary debate of a bill which proposed the death penalty for 'repeated homosexual offences'. A member of parliament, David Bahati, proposed to tighten the existing Ugandan legislation on homosexuality, which would make Uganda the third country on the continent to punish same-sex sexual acts by death.[2]

Currently, under a penal code that dates back to colonialism, same-sex sexual acts are punishable by prison sentences up to life imprisonment.[3] The draft of the revised bill proposed the death penalty for 'aggravated homosexuality', which it defined as repeated offences and consenting same-sex sexual acts when one partner is HIV-positive. The revised bill also proposed to outlaw public education on homosexuality, and it would legally oblige ordinary Ugandans to report people whom they know to be gay to the authorities within twenty-four hours (for a discussion of the legal implications of the proposed bill see Sander 2010).[4]

The introduction of the bill sparked international outcry and condemnation, including threats by European donors to withhold development aid, and this led the Ugandan parliament to temporarily suspend its discussion.[5] However, in February 2012 the bill was re-introduced without provision for the death penalty,[6] and most MPs in Uganda seem to support the proposed law. As a woman MP said: 'We abhor homosexuality and value our God, culture and there is no way we shall allow a man to step on top of another man or a woman to lie on top of another.'[7]

At the time of writing, it remains unclear whether or not the bill will pass. In this chapter I will argue that Uganda's widely extolled HIV/AIDS strategy and its internationally abhorred homophobic legislation are inextricably related, and that both can be traced back to transnational religious and conservative movements, most notably evangelical organisations in the United States and Uganda. I contend that these Christian movements use prevention messages to veil moral discourses that aim to restrain what they view as sexual deviance. As Adams and Pigg write

[2] Currently, homosexuality is punishable by death in Mauritania and Sudan, as well as in parts of Nigeria and Somalia.

[3] Section 145–148 of the Penal Code Act of 1950 (Chapter 120). The text of the law is available at http://www.ulii.org/ug/legis/consol_act/pca195087 (accessed 14 September 2011).

[4] The full text of the proposed bill can be accessed at http://wthrockmorton.com/wp-content/uploads/2009/10/Bill-No-18-Anti-Homosexuality-Bill-2009.pdf (accessed 29 August 2011).

[5] See 'Uganda shelves anti-gay bill', *Mail & Guardian*, South Africa, 14 May 2011. http://mg.co.za/article/2011-05-14-uganda-shelves-antigay-bill (accessed 14 September 2011).

[6] http://www.guardian.co.uk/world/2012/feb/08/uganda-gay-death-sentence-bill.

[7] Statement made by Ms Ogwal, leader of Uganda's delegation to the Pan African Parliament, at the celebration of the fiftieth anniversary of Uganda's independence, on 9 October 2012. http://www.nation.co.ke/News/africa/Uganda+s+anti+gay+laws+blots+jubilee/-/1066/1529392/-/7r8cs5/-/index.html.

in the introduction to *Sex in Development: Science, Sexuality and Morality in Global Perspective*:

> No longer imagined indirectly through the proxy of fertility, sexuality has become scripted through the imperative of disease prevention and in some cases, remains attached to concerns about family planning. Discussions of who is having what sorts of sex with whom are routed through an ultimate concern with disease vectors, echoing an earlier era when venereal diseases were central to moral debates that linked health and national strength . . . Yet compared with social hygiene campaigns of the late nineteenth and early twentieth centuries, today's focus on disease and sexuality is more explicit about sexual acts, pairings, and identities; more precise in its scientific elaboration of the physiological, even molecular, mechanisms of risk, more exacting and elaborate.
>
> (2005: 19)

The chapter provides a critical feminist analysis that builds upon the notion of 'power topographies', locating the various actors within a framework of transnational dynamics of financial and political influence, which transcend the power distributions between civil society and the state (Ferguson and Gupta 2002; Ferguson 2006). This framework extends 'the discussion of governmentality to modes of government that are being set up on a global stage', and includes 'transnational alliances forged by activists and grassroots organisations and the proliferation of voluntary organisations supported by complex networks of international and transnational funding and personnel' (Ferguson and Gupta 2002: 990). Through an analysis of both Ugandan and international media sources and policy frameworks, I seek to provide an example of the localised consequences of the shortcomings in transnational human rights approaches and expose the underlying heteronormative assumptions about sexuality, masculinity and femininity in these transnational alliances and networks.

Based on an analysis of media sources (*The Daily Monitor*, *Rolling Stone*, *New Vision* in Uganda, *Mail and Guardian*, *Sunday Times*, *The Sowetan* in South Africa, pan-African internet-based media portals, *The New York Times*, *Huffington Post*, *Guardian*), policies and academic literature, as well as participant observation in international policy processes, this chapter uses critical discourse analysis, notably the line of discourse-as-social-practice (Fairclough 1992). Discourse-as-social-practice examines the broader realm of discourse, including its ideological effects and the hegemonic processes in which it exists. Hegemony in this context refers to the 'power that is achieved through constructing alliances and integrating classes and groups through consent' (Blommaert and Bulcaen 2000: 449).

The chapter will question the 'strings attached' to international funding and the role of faith-based NGOs in shaping public discourse around homosexuality in an African context. It will also highlight the ways in which the current human rights discourse perpetuates the invisibility of non-heteronormative sexualities. It is notable that I use the term 'African sexualities', not to suggest a homogeneous essentialism of sexualities based on the continent, but 'politically to call attention to some of the commonalities and shared historical legacies inscribed in cultures and sexualities within the region by forces such as colonialism, capitalism, imperialism, globalisation and fundamentalism' (Tamale 2011: 1). By taking a political position I follow Adams and Pigg in arguing that these 'often mundane programs [also] frequently function as the instruments through which neo-colonial, nationalist and identity politics are articulated' (2005: 2).[8]

My analysis begins with a focus on the increase in the transnational religious funding for HIV programmes and then shifts to an analysis of the local impact in Uganda, a country that has received substantial international aid to fight its HIV/AIDS epidemic. I then move on to examine the rights-based international HIV response and the invisibilities and discourses that it produces.

US policies: PEPFAR and the increased funding of FBOs

The emergence of a multi-faceted international HIV response with numerous non-state players has led to new dynamics in transnational governmentality. With new provisions for the funding of, among others, faith-based organisations (FBOs), the spheres of influence of conservative moralities have expanded. FBOs have become an integral part of the civil society response in many African countries, yet their network of influence and power exceeds local contexts (Ferguson and Gupta 2002). In this section I will explore the impact of these transnational organisations on the flows of moralities.

There is a strong connection between far-right religious groups and the former US Republican administration of George W. Bush, who initiated the United States President's Emergency Plan for AIDS Relief (PEPFAR), at the time the largest funding programme for the HIV response in African countries. Girard (2004) lists more than eight extremely conservative religious organisations which she identifies

[8] Since my chapter speaks explicitly to transnational dynamics of ideology and power, I cannot ignore the historical and contemporary hegemony of knowledge production, which is acutely and painfully visible in the academic discipline. Given that my chapter, as well as the whole volume, speaks to sexualities and moralities in Africa, it is imperative to articulate the forces of colonialism, imperialism, capitalism and patriarchy that have historically shaped the knowledge on 'African' sexualities – Northern voices, or voices coming out of Northern institutions. With the discourse moving beyond the simplistic binary of coloniser and colonised, and recognising the intersecting ways that colonisation and neo-colonisation operate through ideologies, resources and social capital, it remains a fact that the hierarchy of knowledge production (and dissemination) is still rooted in the North. This is most noteworthy in light of the dominance of Western theories and perspectives on sexuality studies, of historical objectifications and derogations, as well as the fact that the main languages of academia are colonial. This book (and my chapter) is yet one more example. As a White, European, queer woman working at a South African university I am still of and writing to the centre, even though I write from a position of the periphery.

as key actors in policy decisions around sexual and reproductive health in the Bush administration.[9] Since 1960, US domestic politics have heavily defined the country's policies on global reproductive health (White and Pope 2007). The debates have been heavily influenced by a discourse of moralities and rights: 'Reproductive health and rights, and specifically women's bodies, have become the site of the battle between the powerful moralist agents and people who advocate a human rights approach to public health' (Ahlberg and Kulane 2011: 324). At the national level, the alliance of the Republican Party with the religious right as 'one of the main precipitants of this new [conservative] morality' (Susser 2009: 49) has provided financial support to policies that impose conservative moralities on matters related to sexuality. The linkages between domestic and foreign policy have been most widely researched with regard to reproductive health and abortion rights, and are illustrative of the influence and power of the conservative religious right on these policies (Chamberlain 2006; White and Pope 2007).

An early example can be found in the 1970s: three years after the US Supreme Court recognised women's rights to abortion in *Roe vs. Wade* in 1973, the Republican-dominated House of Representatives passed the Hyde Amendment, which cut federal funding for most abortions. By doing so, the allocation of funds clearly served a political agenda, and resulted in reducing the abortion services offered to low-income American women covered under state-sponsored Medicaid (Boonstra and Sonfield 2000). The consequence of this shift in domestic politics for foreign policy became clear when later, in 1973, Congress passed the Helms Amendment to the Foreign Assistance Act (FAA). This amendment prohibited the direct use of money received through FAA funding for the provision of abortion services, and effectively withheld funding from organisations in other countries if they provided abortion services to women. The Republican agenda further regulated foreign policy by what is known as the Global Gag Rule: in 1984, Republican President Ronald Reagan stopped USAID funding to organisations that carry out abortions (White and Pope 2007). USAID could also withdraw funding from organisations that included discussion of abortion as part of family planning options. It is thus for a long time that the religious right has had influence on foreign policy, with a particular focus on (but not limited to) exporting pro-family values on women's reproductive rights. Martin remarks that the

> same values that underlie the Christian Right's domestic policies also drive its international agenda. Religious activists have consistently opposed any foreign-policy [*sic*] initiative that might weaken parental control over children, facilitate abortion, expand the rights of homosexuals, or devalue the role of the conventional housemaker and mother.
>
> (1999: 74)

[9] These include, among others, Focus on the Family, the Family Research Council, the Traditional Values Coalition and the Wilberforce Forum/Prison Fellowship.

With the creation of PEPFAR in 2003, George W. Bush began to channel USAID funding to fifteen countries to support scaling up HIV prevention and treatment programmes. PEPFAR promotes what is known as the 'ABC' approach to prevention: **A**bstinence-only, **B**e faithful, use a **C**ondom. The programme placed much more emphasis on the 'A' than the 'C' – indeed, earlier versions of the funding conditions required organisations to spend at least 33 per cent of the received prevention money on the promotion of abstinence.[10] These conditions are eerily reminiscent of the ones on abortion funding promulgated by the Global Gag Rule during the Reagan administration, and PEPFAR became known as the 'Bush Global Gag Rule':[11]

> Neoconservative policies promoted by the US are being spread dramatically to poor countries by US funding for AIDS. The faith-based, fundamentalist platform of the United States Republican regime – with its particular restrictions on women and reproduction as well as neglect of comprehensive sex education and stigmatization of sexual orientation, sex workers, and drug users – may be leading to the deaths of many people.
>
> (Susser 2009: 63)

More bluntly, as Girard writes about the global impact of US policies on sexuality, 'the focus, then and now, was to *regulate and control nonorthodox expressions of sexuality* – that is, anything except the conjugal and heterosexual kind – in the context of traditional gender roles' (2004: 4). From the beginning of PEPFAR, Uganda was to become a model country in its implementation of the 'ABC' approach, and indeed, funds from the US to Uganda increased by 50 per cent from 2004 to 2005. In 2006, Uganda's total spending on HIV/AIDS equalled just short of $200 million – 73 per cent of which was provided by PEPFAR (Oommann *et al.* 2007: 9). The remaining $45 million came from the Global Fund, the World Bank, other donors, and the Ugandan government (ibid.). As the contributions from the Ugandan government to HIV prevention remained at around 5 per cent of the total funds available (ibid.), PEPFAR, through its financial power, could effectively control a large part of the HIV response in the country, including the selection of which organisations could receive PEPFAR funding.[12] Within the first few years of PEPFAR, funds were withheld from progressive family planning organisations like the United Nations Population Fund (UNFPA) and the International Planned Parenthood Federation (IPPF). Instead, money was increas-

[10] See Kaiser Family Foundation, 'Reauthorization of PEPFAR, The United States Global Leadership Against HIV/AIDS, Tuberculosis and Malaria Act: a side-by-side comparison to prior law'. http://www.kff.org/hivaids/7799.cfm (accessed 10 September 2011).

[11] 'The Bush Global Gag Rule: endangering women's health, free speech and democracy', Fact Sheet from the Center for Reproductive Rights, June 2003. http://www.crlp.org/pub_fac_ggrbush.html (accessed 14 July 2011).

[12] The amount of funding by other international and bilateral donors such as UNICEF, UNFPA and DFID was significantly lower – no agency provided more than 8 per cent of the total amount (Uganda AIDS Commission 2009).

ingly directed to faith-based organisations, with the effect that 'NGOs [mission organisations] have become valuable partners in implementing US objectives' (Hearn 2002: 56).[13]

Under the administration of President Obama, little has changed in the implementation of PEPFAR, despite the president's more progressive political stance on the rights of sexual minorities (see Schoepf, Chapter 3, this volume). With its integration into the president's Global Health Initiative, PEPFAR's targets for 2014 still fail to mention non-heterosexual transmission or prevention of HIV, and only identify women and children as vulnerable groups.[14] While the earmarked funding for abstinence programmes was removed from the legislation in 2008, Congress still needs to approve programmes that spend less than 50 per cent of funding on abstinence and fidelity programmes.[15] With the current Republican stronghold in the House of Representatives, it is likely that ideologically motivated political decisions will continue to characterise PEPFAR's spending on HIV prevention. This is shown in the most recent debate over suggestions that the funding may not be used to purchase family planning commodities.[16]

The increased funding of faith-based organisations is not a novelty. Since neoliberal policies and Structural Adjustment Programmes have conditioned the privatisation of health services, faith-based NGOs have rapidly taken up the delivery of these services, and thus come to play an ever more prominent role in development cooperation (De Waal 2006). Hofer notes that 'even the highly appraised new anti-HIV/Aids [*sic*] scheme appears to be a continuation of this line, channelling funds to unilateral programmes carried out increasingly by the private sector and especially by "faith-based organisations", i.e. NGOs run by religious organisations' (2003: 381). The novelty under PEPFAR, however, was that the US government allocated and increased special funds for faith-based organisations that often had no previous experience in delivering HIV prevention services (Stockmann *et al.* 2006). As a result, US-based churches with fundamentalist moral agendas could set out to provide HIV care and prevention services at grassroots level: there are over 2,000 accredited HIV/AIDS projects in Uganda, and the majority are affiliated

[13] While not all FBOs aggressively promote conservative and homophobic views, a review of the literature suggests that those that do are presented as the models for future involvement. For example, Green (2001) concludes that FBOs who promote abstinence and fidelity have had a significant impact on the rate of decline of HIV prevalence since 1992. Where FBOs do not actively promote conservatism and homophobia, Parry (2002) notes that their voices are 'muted' in relation to key issues such as access to treatment and care, human rights, and other factors that underpin HIV transmission, such as gender discrimination and domestic violence.

[14] *U.S. President's Emergency Plan for AIDS Relief: Five-Year Strategy of the U.S. President's Emergency Plan for AIDS Relief*, p. 2. http://www.PEPFAR.gov/documents/organization/149857.pdf (accessed 31 October 2012).

[15] See www.PEPFARwatch.org (accessed 30 October 2012).

[16] As reported by Serra Sippel, 22 October 2012. http://www.huffingtonpost.com/serra-sippel/short changing-womens-rights_b_1989638.html (accessed 31 October 2012).

with an evangelical church (Hofer 2003; Lacey 2003). These FBOs have established HIV prevention education projects, home-based care centres, orphanages and support groups, and increased the influence of fundamentalist evangelism in a country that was already characterised by strong Pentecostal churches in HIV/AIDS programmes (Gusman 2009).

Many of these churches' responses to HIV/AIDS reflected broader concerns of Ugandans about the immorality of modern life, and are based on a move in Ugandan society towards embracing born-again Christianity and its values of strict sexual morality and conservative family values (Gusman 2009). As Dilger (2007) has shown in Tanzania, the values of neo-Pentecostalism may provide meaning and orientation in a time of economic, political and physical incertitude due to HIV/AIDS. Within a year of the start of the PEPFAR programme, religious revivalism emerged in Uganda and quickly gained ground.[17] The ideology of many faith-based organisations fitted within the religious discourse of restricting sexuality and cautioning against moral decay in the region (Gusman 2009; Beckmann 2009), and they quickly became major pillars in the provision of HIV prevention and care. The values promoted by the new revivalists were strictly 'pro-family' – that is, opposing women's reproductive rights, comprehensive sex education and any expression of unorthodox sexualities or sexual orientation.

Intertwining religion and homophobic politics

In this section, I will illustrate how the religious values of the transnational revivalist networks were intimately linked with Ugandan government policies and increasingly expressed in public discourse. Thomas Muyunga, a physician working in HIV care in Kampala, reflects that:

> [r]eligious organisations had never received any form of funds until it was Bush's time. [. . .] 8 years is big for an organisation to get on its feet and to be able to say something. All of a sudden you are here and they have mobilised in getting over 300 people in the street. Within 3 days you see a street covered with anti-homosexuality posters and pamphlets.
>
> (Alsop 2009: 2044)

The rhetoric of these anti-homosexuality protests that Muyunga describes relies heavily on US-based conservative, at times fundamentalist, religious networks. In a recent radio interview, Frank Mugisha, the chairperson of the Ugandan gay rights

[17] Helen Epstein (2005) remembers her visits to Uganda in 2004, one year after the introduction of PEPFAR, and the involvement of evangelical revivalism: 'A large number of new faith-based abstinence organizations like Ssempa's Campus Alliance to Wipe Out AIDS (CAWA) and Mrs. Museveni's UYF have sprung up in Uganda in recent years, including the Glory of Virginity Movement (GLOVIMA), the Family Life Network (FLN), and American groups such as True Love Waits. [. . .] US law forbids organizations receiving federal funds from evangelizing, but every abstinence event I attended involved much praying and discussion of Jesus.'

NGO 'Sexual Minorities Uganda' (SMUG), related a conversation he had with the editor of *Rolling Stone*, the newspaper that exposed 'Uganda's top homos' and called to 'Hang Them!'[18] According to Mugisha, the editor was adamant that homosexuals needed to be outed, because 'homosexuality is against the culture of Uganda, because it is a sin and because homosexuals will recruit Ugandan children into their lifestyle'.[19]

The debate about whether or not homosexuality is 'un-African' is familiar to many African countries, and it continues to go on in spite of scholarly works which highlight the pre-colonial existence of transgressive sexualities and expose how these debates are based on colonial myths and Western representations of African sexualities (Epprecht 2008; Lewis 2011). Recent legal scholarship has documented that 'anti-sodomy' laws were introduced during British colonialism and became the first legislation against homosexuality on the African continent (Hollander 2009/10). It is not homosexuality that is a product of Western, colonial, or neo-colonial influences, but rather homophobic legislation. The introduction of British law in the British colonies is one example of how hegemonic discourses have shaped contemporary conceptions and constructions of sexuality. It is therefore not surprising that the editor of *Rolling Stone* uses the argument of 'Ugandan culture' to express his disapproval of homosexuality. However, the deeply religious moralised argument that homosexuality is a sin, together with the accusation that homosexuals 'recruit children', has fuelled the recent increase in aggression, and appears more and more often in the public discourse. Pastor Martin Ssempa from Makerere Community Church, a leading clerical voice in support of the anti-homosexuality bill, has repeatedly warned against homosexuals 'converting and recruiting' innocent children.[20] The provenance of this rhetoric of 'gay recruitment' points to the United States, where there are clear parallels with the main propagators and funders.[21]

[18] For a picture of the front page, see http://www.boxturtlebulletin.com/btb/wp-content/uploads/2010/10/Rolling-Stone-Cover-e1286223527879.jpg; also http://www.timeslive.co.za/africa/article718887.ece/Hang-them—Ugandan-paper-publishes-photos-of-Top-100-gays.

[19] The complete interview with Frank Mugisha can be found at http://whyy.org/cms/radiotimes/2011/01/21/being-gay-persecuted-in-uganda-with-frank-mugisha/ (accessed 25 August 2011).

[20] Mariana van Zyl, 'Missionaries of Hate'. Vanguard documentary, first aired 26 May 2010. http://current.com/shows/vanguard/episodes/season-four/missionaries-of-hate/ (accessed 10 October 2010). See also Pastor Ssempa's letter to *Christianity Today*, in which he defends the proposed anti-homosexuality bill: http://www.christianitytoday.com/ct/special/pdf/1217ssempaletter.pdf (accessed 1 September 2011).

[21] Local homophobia in East African and southern African countries is rife and can be attributed to many things, including colonial legislation, perceptions of 'imported' gay identities, nationalist discourses around 'African identities', etc. (Epprecht 2008). I am not contesting this local homophobia and its causes. Rather, I am pointing out that its aggressive, public display is reminiscent of US evangelical homophobia, and that links between the two are increasingly pointing towards a systematic transnational network. The rhetoric of 'gay recruitment' was, to my knowledge, not present in local homophobic discourses before the turn of the millennium.

Between 1995 and 2000, USAID channelled 35 per cent of its funding through NGOs.[22] Hofer (2003) outlines that in 2001, the majority of Uganda's accredited HIV/AIDS projects were affiliated with an evangelical church. This involvement of evangelical-linked NGOs in Uganda's political and civil society landscape has been bolstered by the increased funding made available through PEPFAR from 2003 onwards. An important example is the involvement of the evangelical 'Family Life Network' (FLN), a 'family-centred' broadcasting ministry with its base in New York City.[23] In the early 2000s it opened a branch office in Kampala, and it has since emerged on numerous occasions in the Ugandan capital to promote 'pro-family' values that encompass anti-abortion advocacy, and, as I will show in the following paragraph, massive mobilisation against homosexuality and the rights of sexual minorities. In 2003, 'the Family' organised a large rally in Kampala in protest against pornography in the media. The regional newspaper *The East African* reported that the crowd demanded, 'parliament, save us from pornography', and claimed, 'Joseph Koney and Richard Tusiime [Ugandan porn-magazine editor] are the Axis of Evil!'[24]

Scott Lively, one of the rally's main speakers, is a representative of the FLN in the United States, where he has written several books against homosexuality, including one that instructs parents on how to shield their children against 'recruitment by homosexuals' (Lively 1998). His rhetoric links concerns for children and adolescents, rather blatantly, with onslaughts on the rights of sexual minorities. For example, he declared that Uganda's high rate of teenage pregnancies was to be blamed on 'increased consumption of pornography' and claimed that the FLN was 'just beginning to lay the foundations for a national campaign to teach Christian living as the answer to this nation's many problems'.[25] Similarly, he accuses same-sex sexuality of inducing sexual violence against children (Lively 1998). This rhetoric has been picked up by Ugandan religious leaders. For instance, Pastor Martin Ssempa, once a volunteer Africa coordinator for the organisation Family Watch International, another evangelical think-tank that lobbies to undermine the rights of sexual minorities in Africa, has been a leading figure in Ugandan anti-homosexual campaigns.[26]

The FLN held a conference in one of Kampala's leading hotels in 2009, where its executive director Stephen Langa and members of parliament met with key

[22] US Agency for International Development, *President Bush Approves Faith-Based Office for USAID*, USAID Press Release 138 (2002), 12 December 2002.

[23] See www.fln.org.

[24] *The East African*, 19 May 2003. See also *AllAfrica*, 13 May 2003.

[25] See online journal of the American Family Association, July 2002. http://www.afajournal.org/2002/july/noi.asp (accessed 10 September 2011).

[26] W. Throckmorton, 'American anti-gay campaign in Africa opposes "fictitious sexual rights"'. http://www.religiondispatches.org/archive/sexandgender/4996/american_anti-gay_campaign_in_africa_opposes_%22fictitious_sexual_rights%22/ (accessed 9 September 2011).

members of the American evangelical fundamentalist movement.[27] Amongst them was Scott Lively, accompanied by Don Schmierer, a board member of Exodus International (an organisation whose mission is 'mobilizing the body of Christ to minister grace and truth to a world impacted by homosexuality') and Caleb Lee Brundidge, who describes himself as a former gay man and leads 'healing seminars'. At this meeting of American and Ugandan evangelists with members of the Ugandan legislative, the attendees discussed measures to marginalise, ostracise, and prosecute homosexuals. As SMUG learned through their network, this included 'lobbying the police, the government, Members of Parliament and other law enforcement agencies to get rid of homosexuals in Uganda in disregard to human rights' and 'encouraging the public to use violence against homosexuality in case the law fails to work in their favour'.[28]

These connections between US fundamentalist movements and the instigators of state-sponsored homophobia in Uganda illustrate how an aggressive religious discourse was imported into a country that already had outlawed non-heteronormative sexualities. They further increased the longstanding linkages between fundamentalist religious institutions and the state, often facilitated through concerns about HIV:

> At present in Uganda it is difficult to tell the 'secular' and religious campaigns apart. There are intimate links between the government of Uganda and born-again Christians in Uganda. Many of the most influential Ugandans at government level are born-again Christians; not least the woman who is doing much to rally the abstinence-only campaigns amongst the youth, Janet Museveni, wife of the president.
>
> (Sadgrove 2007: 121)

Uganda, like many African societies, '[was] and remain[s] powerfully heteronormative, with little public space or unambiguous vocabularies for people who openly did not conform to the virile and fecund marital ideal' (Epprecht 2008: 162). Far from being oversimplified expressions of 'innately African homophobia' (Sadgrove 2007: 105), the contestations around the proposed bill place sexuality and sexual activity 'at the core of Uganda's current nationalising project' (ibid.), where 'elite actors (including government officials, the media and religious leaders) are able to further particular ends by manipulating social anxieties' (ibid.: 106). Where sexual minorities were not invisible, they were often referred to using

[27] J. Gettleman, 'American's role seen in Uganda anti-gay push', *New York Times*, 4 January 2010. http://www.nytimes.com/2010/01/04/world/africa/04uganda.html (accessed 1 September 2011); see also the press release by the International Gay and Lesbian Human Rights Commission: 'Uganda: the U.S. religious right exports homophobia to Africa'. http://www.iglhrc.org/cgi-bin/iowa/article/press room/pressrelease/868.html (accessed 15 August 2011).

[28] These and other outcomes of the meeting were reported by Frank Mugisha, chairperson of SMUG, in a letter to the Minister of Ethics and Integrity, in which Mugisha expressed his concern about a hate campaign launched by the FLN.

derogatory terms, and denied societal belonging by being considered 'un-African' (Epprecht 2008). The new radical US discourse was inculcated into this public opinion, and has contributed to the radicalisation of all layers of Ugandan society. It targeted two specific societal levels: members of the legislature and other powerful positions in public office, and grassroots community members. David Bahati serves as a prime example of this process: besides his involvement in the FLN conference to brief Ugandan members of parliament about the 'dangers of homosexuality', he has been one of the driving forces to establish the FLN in Uganda.[29] Through his double affiliation, he illustrates how US-driven, locally established evangelical movements reach deep into state power and influence legislative decisions on all levels, and thus significantly further weaken the divide between church and state.

In addition to the interrelationship between church and state, this approach is based on individual moral-religious obligations. Whilst it was partly enabled by the mushrooming of faith-based organisations across the country and the new societal landscape of conservative Christian involvement through HIV prevention and care, it nevertheless needed the infusion of the missionary zeal of organisations such as the FLN to bring its full power to bear. The broad consensus for the anti-homosexuality bill rests on the values and morals of an inherently conservative social contract, but it has been brought to culmination by populist incitement of hatred. Pastor Martin Ssempa, as one of the key conduits between Uganda's clerics and the US evangelical movement, has mobilised support for the bill in church services, prayer meetings and at public worship. In addition to using the same rhetoric so often used by the FLN and other US evangelicals, he screened hard-core pornographic material depicting male same-sex sexual acts at a Sunday service whilst asking the congregation of 300 people: 'The major argument homosexuals have is that what people do in the privacy of their bedrooms is nobody's business but do you know what they do in their bedrooms?'[30]

With this rhetoric the Ugandan evangelical movement – supported by powerful networks from the United States and operating in a social environment shaped by the heteronormative moralities from Ugandan society and international institutions – incited a wave of aggressive homophobia. In early 2011, David Kato, an openly gay man and one of Uganda's most outspoken gay rights activists, was murdered in his home. There is large consensus in the gay community that he was killed because of his sexual orientation.[31] In as much as the complex transnational dynamics of sexuality and moralities have shaped Ugandan society, they have

[29] See J. Sharlet in 'The secret political reach of the family'. NPR interview transcript at http://www.npr.org/templates/transcript/transcript.php?storyId=120746516 (accessed 10 September 2011).

[30] See 'Martin Ssempa, anti-gay Ugandan pastor, shows church gay porn videos', at http://www.huffingtonpost.com/2010/02/18/martin-ssempa-anti-gay-ug_n_467157.html (accessed 15 September 2011).

[31] See J. Gettleman, 'Ugandan who spoke up for gays is beaten to death', *New York Times*, 27 January 2011. http://www.nytimes.com/2011/01/28/world/africa/28uganda.html?_r=1 (accessed 13 April 2011).

also contributed to the climate within which his murder, and doubtless several others, have taken place.[32]

Global governance of health rights: invisibility of sexual minorities

This section focuses on the dynamics that have contributed to the invisibility and persecution of sexual minorities in Uganda. In an award presentation speech in 2002, President Museveni brought this invisibility to the point by claiming that 'there are no homosexuals in Uganda'.[33] Although he subsequently acknowledged that sexual minorities always existed in Uganda, albeit 'not encouraged',[34] his first statement nonetheless reflects common national and regional discourses that promote the idea that homosexuality is an imported practice and a sign of moral deterioration, and as such foreign to 'traditional' Ugandan culture. The debate about whether or not homosexuality is 'un-African' has long raged in Uganda and other countries in the region, from Kenya to Zimbabwe, and is historically rooted in colonialism (Epprecht 2008; see also Ehrisman, Chapter 13, this volume). As Epprecht (2008) has argued, anthropologists, colonial officials and African elites have constructed a singular, heterosexual identity for the entire continent. He details that this essentialising heterosexual identity flourished under the conditions of the early responses to HIV, and that sexual minorities have been made invisible in the African HIV pandemic. Early research into the epidemiology of HIV systematically disregarded evidence for same-sex activities, either due to bias in the methodology of data collection or because of conscious decisions by researchers. Regardless of the reasoning, the consequence was a lack of knowledge about HIV among sexual minorities.

An analysis of how the current policy framework has contributed to these invisibilities must attend to the rights discourse, which forms a basis for the international HIV response. The rights commonly invoked in the discourse are part of what is termed 'positive rights' – rights on which citizens of a country can hold claims from their government and that fall under the category of socio-

[32] While there is no collected evidence of homophobic killings in Uganda, it can be argued that widespread homophobia leads to hate crimes, the consequences of which are currently painfully visible in South Africa's homophobic murders. With the existing homophobia in all of Uganda's state systems including the police, it is unlikely that murders would be reported as homophobia-related. It is also of note that a lot of the international outcry about David Kato's death can be attributed to his active involvement in international advocacy work and his work with international organisations.

[33] This was first reported by the Ugandan newspaper *Daily Monitor*, see http://allafrica.com/stories/200203060386.html.

[34] Museveni pointed this out at the inaugural Young Achievers Awards Ceremony by saying: 'They [homosexuals] were not persecuted but were not encouraged either' (*Daily Monitor*, Uganda, 16 November 2009, p. 2).

economic rights (Mann *et al.* 1994). The right to health asserts a citizen's right to receive health care from the state in order to guarantee the highest possible standard of health. Propounded by such emerged global governing bodies as the United Nations and the World Health Organization (WHO), these rights are enshrined in numerous international treaties and documents and can be envisaged as new instruments of global governance (Ferguson and Gupta 2002). As such, the documents appear to be new forms of regulation and control, which, through their origin and propagation by influential transnational institutions, bypass and transcend the sovereignty of the nation-state. The rights discourse in the international HIV response centres around the right to the highest attainable standard of health. This right was first reflected in the constitution of WHO (1946), reiterated in the Declaration of Alma Ata (WHO 1978) and adopted by the World Health Assembly in 1998.[35] It is also included in article 16 of the African Union's Charter on Human and People's Rights (African Union 1986).

As African countries battled with the pervasive HIV pandemic, their struggle highlighted the massive global inequalities in health and access to health care. Through the immediacy of the life-threatening, incurable disease, it became evident that most people living with HIV in the global South could neither access nor afford life-saving antiretroviral HIV drugs, while HIV-positive people in the global North benefited from the newest HIV medicines, provided to them through the safety net of health insurance and comprehensive medical schemes. In response to these blatant inequalities, human rights language became an integral part of the response of the international community, which focuses on issues of access to antiretroviral treatment and the reduction of vulnerabilities to infection by strengthening the rights of the groups most affected by HIV (Mann 1997). However, in Uganda as in most African countries, the response operates mostly within the paradigm of heterosexual HIV transmission and ignores the existence of non-heteronormative sexualities.

WHO and the UN share a broad approach to the definition of sexuality, which includes sexual orientation, sexuality education, reproduction, and marriage. The rights of sexual minorities (people who do not fall under the heterosexual, monogamous paradigm) that are most often mentioned in the discourse led by the actors in international development and funding are called sexual rights, which WHO defined comprehensively in 2002.[36] However, the violations experienced

[35] The 51st World Health Assembly in 1998 recognised the importance of obtaining 'Health for All' and re-committed to the right to health (resolution 51.7).

[36] Sexual rights embrace human rights that are already recognised in national laws, international human rights documents and other consensus documents. These include the right of all persons, free of coercion, discrimination and violence, to: (i) the highest attainable standard of health in relation to sexuality, including access to sexual health including reproductive health care services; (ii) seek, receive and impart information in relation to sexuality; (iii) sexuality education; (iv) respect for bodily integrity; (v) choice of partner; (vi) decide to be sexually active or not; (vii) consensual sexual relations; (viii) consensual marriage; (ix) decide whether or not, and when to have children; and (x) pursue a satisfying,

by sexual minorities in Uganda go well beyond a violation of sexual rights – they are, indeed, violations of the right to health and, more gravely, the right to life.[37] It is an ironic twist that the very same programmes that are mandated to decrease HIV transmission have contributed to an increase in transmission among criminalised and stigmatised groups (Senior 2010; Tocco, Chapter 15, this volume). In Uganda, as in thirty-five other African countries, homosexuality is illegal (Bruce-Jones and Itabohary 2011). A recent survey estimates that HIV prevalence among men who have sex with men is at 14 per cent, much higher than the 6 per cent prevalence in the general population (Crane Survey Report 2010). However, no HIV prevention programme has yet addressed the structural and legal causes of higher prevalence among criminalised groups. This has significant implications for the right to health of Ugandan sexual minorities, as gay men, lesbian women, bisexual and transgender people do not access health care as much as heterosexual patients due to fear of criminalisation, stigmatisation and discrimination (Alsop 2009).

Since the first reported cases of HIV in the 1980s, Uganda has been praised as a success story in Africa. Uganda was the first country to reduce its HIV prevalence and incidence (the overall number of people infected with HIV and the number of new infections per year), and it did so through a concerted public campaign that put HIV and AIDS in the spotlight. Celebrities and government representatives openly talked about HIV and safer sex – a novelty in East Africa. For instance, in the early years of the response, the Ugandan government, under President Yoweri Museveni, partnered with international organisations such as UNAIDS in a campaign to create open societal dialogue and increase the willingness to speak about HIV at all levels of society, which included the widespread disbursement of male, and even female, condoms. At the African Development Forum, held at the United Nations Economic Commission for Africa in Addis Ababa in 2000, Museveni declared the Ugandan model a success: '[M]ost of all, the stigma attached to people living with HIV/AIDS has virtually evaporated' (De Waal 2006: 96). The claim that stigma has been erased for most Ugandans living with HIV is dubious at best, but for sexual minorities, the HIV response has been decidedly abysmal.

A Ugandan general practitioner working in HIV care since the early 1990s remembers how international health bodies and donors had insisted that the African HIV/AIDS epidemic was a heterosexual one: only after a gay friend of his tested positive for HIV did he realise that the epidemic also had a non-heterosexual face

safe and pleasurable sexual life. The responsible exercise of human rights requires that all persons respect the rights of others. See WHO, *Defining Sexual Health. Report of a Technical Consultation on Sexual Health*. www.who.int/reproductivehealth/.../sexual_health/defining_sexual_health.pdf (accessed 7 September 2011).

[37] The Yogyakarta Principles (International Commission of Jurists 2007), a legal framework applying international human rights law to sexual orientation and gender identity, outline among others the fundamental right to life of people who engage in same-sex activities.

(Alsop 2009). This experience illustrates that the perception of HIV transmission in African countries is strongly focused on a heteronormative and opposite-sex centred approach to sex. It is striking that non-heterosexual sexualities are absent in the discussions of HIV prevalence and modes of transmission in medical journals. The following excerpt from the widely cited *British Medical Journal* illustrates the issue:

> Heterosexual intercourse is the most common mode of transmission of HIV in poor countries. In Africa slightly more than 80 percent of infections are acquired heterosexually, while mother-to-child transmission (5–15 percent) and transfusion of contaminated blood account for the remaining infections.
>
> (Lamptey 2002: 207)

This discourse has been adopted by Ugandan institutions such as the Uganda AIDS Commission, and led to an invisibility of non-heterosexual HIV transmissions:

> In Uganda, some of the factors driving the epidemic include behavioural factors, social-cultural, socio-behavioural, economic and geographic factors. These include higher risk sex (which include non-marital sex, extra-marital sex, non-consensual sex, commercial sex, transactional sex, intergenerational sex and sex for survival), mother to child transmission, HIV discordance and non-disclosure, poverty, early marriage, glorification of non-marital sex, multiple sexual partners, stigma, discrimination and Sexually Transmitted Infection (STI) prevalence.
>
> (Uganda AIDS Commission 2008: 3)

It is curious that a disease that originated as 'gay-related immune deficiency syndrome'[38] is still seen as an almost exclusively heterosexual pandemic on the African continent (Susser 2009). Uganda is not an exception: for example, the current National Strategic Plan on HIV/AIDS does not acknowledge lesbian, gay, bisexual and transgender (LGBT) people as one of the most at-risk groups (Uganda AIDS Commission 2007). In fact, homosexuality is only mentioned once in the entire document.[39]

This invisibility of non-heterosexual sexualities is also notable in reports and guidelines from international organisations and donors. For example, the 2010 report on the Millennium Development Goals (MDGs), with MDG 6a being 'Have halted by 2015 and begun to reverse the spread of HIV/AIDS', only presents the prevalence and the prevention efforts made for heterosexual HIV transmission (UN 2010). There is no mention of non-heterosexual sex in the report. A brief paragraph addresses gender inequalities as an important area of policy intervention (UN 2010: 44), again implying that most HIV transmission takes place between people of the opposite sex.

[38] 'GRIDS' became AIDS in 1982, after researchers became concerned with the accuracy of the name. Until then, it was colloquially also known as the 'gay plague'.

[39] For the 'uniformed services', mentioned as one of the 'most-at-risk' populations, the document states that 'rarely, transmission may happen due to homosexual acts and intravenous drug use'.

This approach to HIV prevention has translated into a selective approach of rights-based interventions. The current discourse thus focuses on women's rights, and though it is crucial to address gender inequalities that fuel the spread of HIV, it neglects the rights of sexual and gender minorities who are equally at risk. The failure of the international community to address the rights of these groups creates a space for national governments to continue violating the rights of sexual minorities.

In more recent years, international bodies have recognised that the HIV epidemic in Africa extends beyond the heterosexual population – but this was often limited to 'key affected groups' such as 'men who have sex with men'. Furthermore, the response generated by the realisation was not one that consequently comprehensively embraced (and thus protected) sexual diversity. At its Youth Summit in Bamako, Mali, in 2011, UNAIDS brought together young HIV activists from all over the world with the ambitious goal of 'revolutioniz[ing] the AIDS response'.[40] The summit was meant to serve as a mobilising event in the lead up to the United Nations General Assembly High Level Meeting on AIDS (UNGASS), with a strong focus on new social media to spread the message and 'mobilize young people'.[41] The outcome document of the summit was highly contested, mostly for its failure to include progressive definitions of high-risk groups (including definitions of sexualities that went beyond the jargon of 'men who have sex with men'). A drafting committee made up of progressive summit delegates[42] reworked the document to ensure that it comprised a comprehensive approach to sexual and reproductive rights. This included, among other things, the acknowledgement of gay, lesbian, bisexual, transgender and queer people as most-at-risk populations, and a call to repeal all punitive laws that target these key affected populations. The summit delegates approved the revised document; however, the version that UNAIDS published on its website did not include all the changes made with respect to progressive and comprehensive definitions of sexuality, but relegated these to a footnote.[43]

[40] The UNAIDS 'Mali Youth Summit' took place in Bamako, Mali from 15 to 18 April 2011. See: 'Young people convene in Mali to revolutionize the AIDS response'. http://www.unaids.org/en/resources/presscentre/featurestories/2011/april/20110415amali/ (accessed 12 September 2011).

[41] The 'Call for Action' that was developed at the Mali Youth Summit was published online after the summit in April 2011, with the aim of collecting 100,000 signatories before the UNGASS meeting in June 2011. http://www.whatabouthiv.org/?p=145 (accessed 12 September 2011).

[42] These were elected by the summit delegates and included representatives from the Global Youth Coalition on AIDS (GYCA), HIV Young Leaders Fund (HYLF), World AIDS Campaign (WAC) and the Youth Coalition on Sexual and Reproductive Rights (YC), all of which advocate for progressive rights with regard to sexual and reproductive health as well as sexual orientation and gender identity.

[43] In the main document, 'key affected populations' are still defined as 'young people who use drugs, young men who have sex with men, young people living with HIV, young transgender people and young sex workers', while it is only in a footnote to the introductory paragraph that other sexualities are acknowledged: '[1] 'Young key affected populations' is defined as: young people living with HIV; young men who have sex with men; young women; lesbian, gay, bisexual, transsexual and queer youth; young sex workers; young people who use drugs; young migrants, refugees and internally displaced people; young people in detention; indigenous young people; and young people with disabilities.' http://www.whatabouthiv.org/?p=145 (accessed 12 September 2011).

The Mali Youth Summit was progressive in the sense that its delegates clearly pointed to the risk of HIV transmission in Africa among sexual minority groups. However, the process that I described above also illustrates the shortcomings of the current 'human rights-based' approaches. By placing heterosexual orientation at the pinnacle, above gay male sexuality, and by largely ignoring other sexualities, international bodies recreate a discourse of hierarchies of sexualities. As Rubin (1993) has argued, this hierarchy of sexual value both stems from and serves ideological systems, and is imbued with religious and political interests. The international HIV response is located in such a situational hierarchy, and, by not challenging its foundations, implicitly leads to its perpetuation and reproduction. Its discourse is rooted in Western concepts of hegemony, including hegemony of sexuality and sexual identities, which are universally applied through its transnational policy framework. As such, the conception of sexual minorities in HIV prevention programmes reinforces both a hierarchy of sexualities as well as Western concepts of 'gay identity' that focus on public identities determined by sexual orientation and sexual practice (as the term 'men having sex with men' illustrates).[44]

By excluding non-heteronormative sexualities from the discourse of the human rights response, sexual minorities have been marginalised and thus remain invisible: 'International donors too often greet this unacceptable situation [the criminalisation and discrimination of same-sex practising people] with equivalent muteness; even some human rights defenders still exclude sexual rights from human rights' (Cameron 2007: viii). This void in the international HIV response has allowed the Ugandan government to continue to violate the rights of sexual minorities, and is a failed opportunity to address human rights comprehensively.

Conclusion

The discourses that I have delineated here, influenced by transnational dynamics of moralities and sexualities, align with the characteristics of the moral panics that Rubin (1993) describes. She argues that moral panics are the most important and consequential kind of sexual conflict. They are the 'political moment' in which diffuse attitudes are channelled into political action and from there into social change. Thus it is vital that the consequences of political action and social change are examined through a framework of transnational governmentality and with a particular focus on the impact of a hegemonic normativity. The exclusion and ostracism of sexual minorities in Ugandan society has implications beyond the health of this group of sexual minorities.

[44] For a discussion of non-Western same-sex sexualities and the hegemonic imposition of gay identity, see Joseph Massad's *Desiring Arabs* (2007) for example.

A recent landmark study[45] determined that the HIV prevalence among Ugandan men who report sexual encounters with men was 14 per cent, which is more than double the estimated prevalence of 6 per cent in the general population (Crane Survey Report 2010). As many of these men also have sex with women, any HIV prevention programme that fails to address the needs of sexual minorities will ultimately fail.[46] A report of the International Gay and Lesbian Human Rights Commission takes this point further:

> The vulnerability of same-sex practicing men and women is not due to any biological predisposition, but is the result of an interlocking set of human rights violations and social inequalities that heighten HIV risk. Anti-gay discrimination is fueling the African HIV/AIDS epidemic.
>
> (Johnson 2007: 2)

The vulnerability of gay, lesbian, bisexual and transgender people in African countries can only be addressed if the international HIV response makes them visible in the discourses informing strategies and programmes, and challenges the legal and structural marginalisation of sexual minorities. If the right to health is a right that can only be accessed by a certain 'appropriate' group, it remains merely shallow discourse, selective, and ultimately more harmful than beneficent. Furthermore, if rights-based health intervention programmes allow themselves to be hijacked by religious moralities and foster human rights violations, this challenges their legitimacy in the most fundamental way.

In this chapter, I have analysed two main influences at play in the current conflict around the rights of sexual minorities in Uganda: institutions of transnational governmentality and the hegemony of their discourse. The articulation of hegemonic, conservative moralities in HIV prevention programmes in Uganda has contributed to a moral panic against sexual minorities. Cheney reaches a similar conclusion; however, she proposes that a key strategy to address this moral panic is 'cultivating renewed respect for human rights' (2012: 77). I contest her assertion that the anti-homosexuality bill 'signifies regression from adherence to universal human rights standards' (2012: 89). Instead, I have pointed out that the invisibility perpetuated by the human rights-based HIV response has led to the failure to protect

[45] The Crane Survey from 2010, conducted by the School of Public Health at Makerere University, in collaboration with the AIDS Control Programme of the Ministry of Health.

[46] The 'Ugandan Health and Science Press Association' (UHSPA) analysed the implications of the anti-homosexuality bill for the health of LGBT people and the success of HIV prevention programmes. At a meeting with the Legal and Parliamentary Committee of the Ugandan Parliament, Kivumbi Kikonyogo, the executive secretary of UHSPA, noted that 'Uganda risked creating a briding [sic] population of new infections if LGBTI people were intentionally kept off the health access radar on the basis of their sexual orientation' and that the threat of being reported by their health-care workers had already led to 'a sharp decline in many gay people seeking treatment'. See http://www.uhspa.org/2011/06/uhspa-pleads-with-parliamentary-legal-and-parliamentary-affairs-committe-bahati-bill-will-fuel-new-hiv-infections/.

the rights of sexual minorities. Current configurations of power, be it the state, NGOs or other civil society actors, have increasingly been influenced by the power of transnational movements and dynamics, whose hegemony is often based on ideology and thus operates in complex and covert spheres. The violent backlash against sexual minorities in Uganda can thus be seen as both a product of and an act of resistance against 'imported' knowledge, the hegemony of transnational knowledge production and the invisibility of African theories of homosexuality.

References

Adams, V. and S.L. Pigg. 2005. 'Introduction: the moral object of sex', in V. Adams and S.L. Pigg (eds), *Sex in Development: Science, Sexuality and Morality in Global Perspective*. Durham, NC: Duke University Press.

African Union. 1986. African (Banjul) Charter on Human and People's Rights.

Ahlberg, B.M. and A. Kulane. 2011. 'Sexual and reproductive health and rights', in S. Tamale (ed.), *African Sexualities: A Reader*. Cape Town: Pambazuka Press.

Alsop, Z. 2009. 'Ugandan bill could hinder progress on HIV/AIDS', *The Lancet* 374: 2043–4.

Beckmann, N. 2009. 'AIDS and the power of God: narratives of decline and coping strategies in Zanzibar', in F. Becker and P.W. Geissler (eds), *Aids and Religious Practice in Africa*. Leiden: Brill.

Blommaert, J. and C. Bulcaen. 2000. 'Critical discourse analysis', *Annual Review of Anthropology* 29: 447–66.

Boonstra, H. and A. Sonfield. 2000. 'Rights without access: revisiting public funding of abortion for poor women', *The Guttmacher Report on Public Policy* 3(2): 8–11.

Bruce-Jones, E. and L.P. Itaborahy. 2011. 'State-sponsored homophobia: a world survey of laws criminalising same-sex sexual acts between consenting adults', ILGA Report. http://ilga.org/ilga/en/article/1161 (accessed 14 September 2011).

Cameron, E. 2007. 'Preface' to *Off the Map: How HIV/AIDS Programming is Failing Same-Sex Practising People in Africa*. New York: International Gay and Lesbian Human Rights Commission.

Chamberlain, P. 2006. *UNdoing Reproductive Freedoms: Christian Right NGOs Target the United Nations*. Somerville, MA: Political Research Associates.

Cheney, K. 2012. 'Locating neocolonialism, "tradition", and human rights in Uganda's "gay death penalty"', *African Studies Review* 55(2): 77–95.

Crane Survey Report. 2010. 'The Crane Survey Report: high-risk group surveys conducted in 2008/9, Kampala, Uganda'. http://www.uhspa.org/wp-content/uploads/downloads/2011/06/Crane-Survey-Report-Round-1-Dec10.pdf (accessed 14 September 2011).

De Waal, A. 2006. *AIDS and Power: Why There Is No Political Crisis – Yet*. London: Zed Books.

Dilger, H. 2007. 'Healing the wounds of modernity: salvation, community and care in a neo-Pentecostal church in Dar Es Salaam, Tanzania', *Journal of Religion in Africa* 37(1): 59–83.

Epprecht, M. 2008. *Heterosexual Africa? The History of an Idea from the Age of Exploration to the Age of AIDS*. Pietermaritzburg: University of KwaZulu-Natal Press.

Epstein, H. 2005. 'God and the fight against AIDS', *New York Review of Books*, 28 April. http://www.nybooks.com/articles/archives/2005/apr/28/god-and-the-fight-against-aids/?pagination=false (accessed 11 January 2013).

Fairclough, N. 1992. *Discourse and Social Change*. Cambridge: Polity.

Ferguson, J. 2006. *Global Shadows: Africa in the Neoliberal World Order*. Durham, NC: Duke University Press.

Ferguson, J. and A. Gupta. 2002. 'Spatializing states: toward an ethnography of neoliberal governmentality', *American Ethnologist* 29(4): 981–1002.

Girard, F. 2004. 'Global implications of U.S. domestic and international policies on sexuality', SPW Working Papers, No. 1, June.

Green, E.C. 2001. 'The impact of religious organizations in promoting HIV/AIDS prevention'. Paper presented at 'Challenges for the Church: AIDS, Malaria & TB', Arlington, VA, 25–26 May 2001.

Gusman, A. 2009. 'HIV/AIDS, Pentecostal churches, and the "Joseph Generation" in Uganda', *Africa Today* 56(1): 67–86.

Hearn, J. 2002. 'The "invisible" NGO: US evangelical mission in Kenya', *Journal of Religion in Africa* 32(1): 32–60.

Hofer, K. 2003. 'The role of evangelical NGOs in international development: a comparative case study of Kenya and Uganda', *Africa Spectrum* 38(3): 375–98.

Hollander, M. 2009/10. 'Gay rights in Uganda: seeking to overturn Uganda's anti-sodomy laws', *Virginia Journal of International Law* 50(1): 219–66.

International Commission of Jurists. 2007. 'Yogyakarta Principles – Principles on the application of international human rights law in relation to sexual orientation and gender identity'. http://www.unhcr.org/refworld/docid/48244e602.html (accessed 12 August 2011).

Johnson, C.A. 2007. *Off the Map: How HIV/AIDS Programming is Failing Same-Sex Practising People in Africa*. New York: International Gay and Lesbian Human Rights Commission.

Lacey, M. 2003. 'AIDS war in Africa: invitation to fraud', *New York Times*, 10 July.

Lamptey, P. 2002. 'Reducing heterosexual transmission of HIV in poor countries', *British Medical Journal* 324: 207–11.

Lewis, D. 2011. 'Representing African sexualities', in S. Tamale (ed.), *African Sexualities: A Reader*. Cape Town: Pambazuka Press.

Lively, S. 1998. *Seven Steps to Recruit-Proof Your Child: A Parent's Guide to Protecting Children from Homosexuality and the 'Gay' Movement*. Keizer: Founders Pub. Corp.

Mann, J. 1997. 'Medicine and public health, ethics and human rights', *The Hastings Center Report* 27(3): 6–13.

Mann, J. *et al.* 1994. 'Health and human rights', *Health and Human Rights* 1(1): 6–23.

Martin, W. 1999. 'The Christian Right and American foreign policy', *Foreign Policy* 114: 66–80.

Massad, J. 2007. *Desiring Arabs*. Chicago: University of Chicago Press.

Oommann, N., M. Bernstein and S. Rosenzweig. 2007. 'Following the funding for HIV/AIDS: a comparative analysis of the funding practices of PEPFAR, the Global Fund and the World Bank MAP in Mozambique, Uganda and Zambia', HIV/AIDS Monitor and the Center for Global Development.

Parry, S. 2002. *Responses of the Churches to HIV/AIDS: Three Southern African Countries*. Harare: World Council of Churches, Ecumenical HIV/AIDS Initiative in Africa, Southern Africa Regional Office.

Rubin, G. 1993. 'Thinking sex: notes for a radical theory of the politics of sexuality', in H. Abelove, M. Borale and D. Halperin (eds), *The Lesbian and Gay Studies Reader*. New York: Routledge.

Sadgrove, J. 2007. 'Keeping up appearances: sex and religion amongst university students in Uganda', *Journal of Religion in Africa* 37: 116–44.

Sander, B. 2010. 'A nation at war with itself: the potential impact of Uganda's anti-homosexuality bill', University of Westminster, Centre for Capital Punishment Studies Reports.

Senior, K. 2010. 'HIV, human rights and men who have sex with men', *The Lancet Infectious Diseases* 10(7): 448–9.

Stockmann, F., M. Kranish and P. Canellos. 2006. 'Changing the rules: exporting faith – Bush brings faith to foreign aid', *Boston Globe*, 8 October.

Susser, I. 2009. *AIDS, Sex and Culture: Global Politics and Survival in Southern Africa*. Chichester: Wiley-Blackwell.

Tamale, S. 2011. 'Introduction', in S. Tamale (ed.), *African Sexualities: A Reader*. Cape Town: Pambazuka Press.

Uganda AIDS Commission. 2007. 'Moving toward universal access: national HIV & AIDS strategic plan 2007/8 – 2011/12', Uganda AIDS Commission, Republic of Uganda. http://siteresources.worldbank.org/INTHIVAIDS/Resources/375798-1151090631807/2693180-1151090665111/2693181-1155742859198/UgandaNSP25Oct07.pdf (accessed 30 October 2012).

Uganda AIDS Commission. 2008. 'UNGASS Country Progress Report Uganda'. http://data.unaids.org/pub/Report/2008/uganda_2008_country_progress_report_en.pdf (accessed 20 August 2011).

Uganda AIDS Commission. 2009. 'Uganda HIV modes of transmission and prevention response analysis', Final Report, March. http://siteresources.worldbank.org/INTHIVAIDS/Resources/375798-1103037153392/UgandaMoTCountrySynthesisReport7April09.pdf (accessed 3 August 2011).

United Nations. 2010. *The Millennium Development Goals Report 2010*. New York: United Nations.

White, R. and C. Pope. 2007. 'Global impact: US sexual health and reproductive policy', in G. Herdt and C. Howe (eds), *21st Century Sexualities: Contemporary Issues in Health, Education, and Rights*. New York: Routledge.

World Health Organization. 1946. *Constitution of the World Health Organization*. Geneva: WHO.

World Health Organization. 1978. *Declaration of Alma Ata*. Geneva: WHO.

World Health Organization. 2002. 'Questions and answers around health and human rights', Health & Human Rights Publication Series, No. 1, July. Geneva: WHO.

15

The Mode of Transmission That Dare Not Speak Its Name: Islam, AIDS and the Public Secret of Homosexuality in Northern Nigeria

JACK UME TOCCO

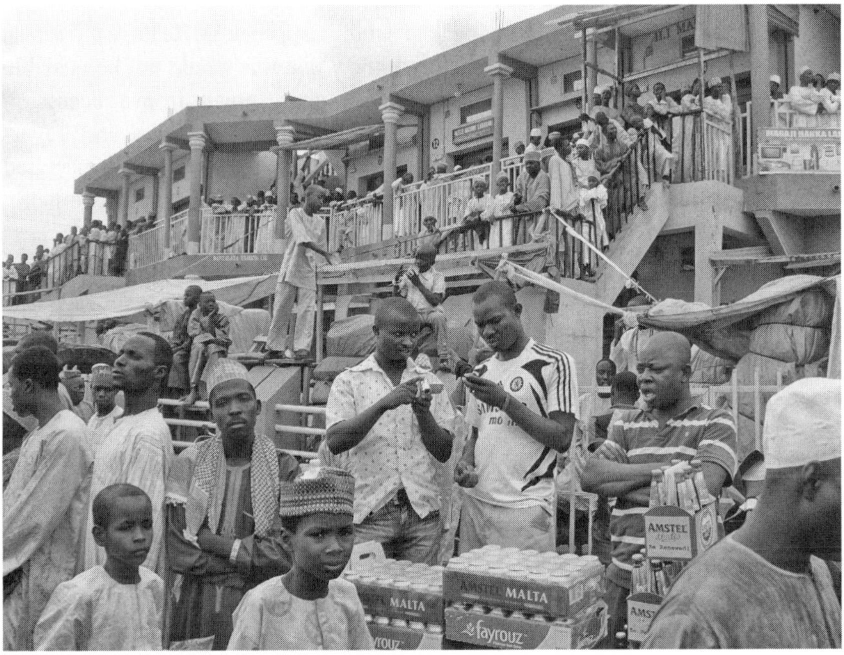

Men and boys at a market in Kano during Eid-al-Adha, an Islamic festival. Social life is largely gender-segregated among Muslims in Northern Nigeria (photograph by author).

Proceedings of the British Academy **194**, *311–335*.

Introduction

I NEVER SUSPECTED THAT El Haji Salisu has sex with men.[1] We meet in 2008 in Kano, Northern Nigeria's largest city, at the office of a support group for HIV-positive people where I am conducting research. The first thing I notice about him is his easy, bright-eyed laugh that reveals a flash of teeth; a *haƙorin Maka*, or gold-plated 'Mecca tooth', covers one of his top incisors. More than merely fashionable, this signifies social status: these gleaming gold teeth are one of the most obvious markers of having performed the *hajj* in Saudi Arabia, which all observant Muslims aspire to do.

Salisu tells me he is 33 years old and has known he is HIV-positive for seven months. He had been living and working in Saudi Arabia for several years, but when he took an HIV test to renew his Saudi residence permit and found out he was positive, he knew that his visa would not be extended. As a foreign national, he would also be denied HIV treatment in Saudi Arabia.

He returned to Nigeria not knowing what would happen next. He hoped to return to his well-paying job in Saudi Arabia, but knew that this would not be possible so long as he was HIV-positive. He began seeking out treatments from a succession of individuals who claimed that they could cure HIV with various herbal and prayer-based preparations, but his health steadily worsened. When he became emaciated and weak, his mother took him to a government hospital, where he was quickly started on antiretroviral drugs. His recovery was dramatic.

We continued to see each other at support group meetings over the next few years whenever I was back in Kano, and occasionally called and text-messaged to greet each other from overseas. As we became better acquainted, I came to think of Salisu as something of a ladies' man. At the end of the monthly support group meetings when members briefly socialise in mixed-sex groups – a rarity among Muslims in Kano, for whom opposite-sex socialisation with non-family is generally proscribed – he often flirted with one or more women, teasing and laughing and flashing his golden smile.

Salisu has two wives and is also looking to marry a third. He is divorced from another woman who still lives in Saudi Arabia, and was widowed by his first wife, who died of AIDS. Sharing a box of wine one evening at his favourite outdoor drinking spot in Kano's predominantly Christian Sabon Gari neighbourhood, Salisu admits that he also has ongoing sexual relationships with several other women, including a long-term girlfriend he has no intention of marrying.

Two years pass before Salisu and I reveal to each other, almost by accident, that we are both involved in *harka*. The standard meaning of the Hausa word *harka* (plural: *harkoki*) is 'matters', 'affairs', or 'business dealings'. Secondarily, *harka*

[1] Names and identifying characteristics of some individuals have been changed to preserve anonymity.

connotes the sex trade and other activities considered immoral. Among Hausa-speaking men who have sex with other men (MSM), the word has a related in-group meaning of which many Hausa speakers are unaware: for such men, *harka* means homosexual sex. More expansively for *masu harka* ('men who have sex with men' in the in-group lexicon; singular: *mai harka*), *harka* is the carefully concealed culture that surrounds sex among men.

Sexual acts that occur outside of marriage are considered *haram* (forbidden) in Islam and are addressed publicly by Northern Nigerian Muslims only in the context of condemnation. Public discussion of homosexuality is avoided, and initiatives addressing the male-to-male sexual transmission of HIV have been virtually non-existent. This chapter is about the social and epidemiological implications of these avoidances and inactions. I argue that dominant rights-based approaches to sexual health which are predicated on admission of risk-specific identity – on 'coming out' – have failed to meet the needs of *masu harka*, for whom public avowal of homosexual behaviour is inconceivable. Most *masu harka* are unaware that HIV prevalence among MSM in Nigeria far exceeds general population prevalence, and underestimate the transmission risk from unprotected anal intercourse.

Living in a society where marriage is a fundamental marker of respectable adulthood, *masu harka* nearly always marry women and have children while keeping their homosexual relationships hidden. This *de facto* bisexuality has under-appreciated consequences: well integrated into larger sexual networks, such men contribute disproportionately, if unwittingly, to Northern Nigeria's AIDS epidemic. This underscores the need for HIV initiatives that address *masu harka*, while recognising the challenges and risks of backlash that such efforts face.

This chapter is based on ethnographic participant observation and interviews conducted in 2009–10 in the course of a larger research project about Islamic responses to AIDS in Northern Nigeria. Secondarily, I draw on previously published documents such as newspaper articles and epidemiological studies. As the vignette about my friend Salisu that begins this chapter suggests, many of the insights I develop were predicated on *masu harka* acquaintances' recognition of me as a similarly inclined man.[2] Given the secrecy with which *masu harka* guard their homosexual behaviours from outside purview, my ethnographic research among *masu harka* was in many instances dependent upon my perceived insider status among this stigmatised community.

[2] While ethnographers' sexual subjectivities were long elided from published accounts, there has been increasing recognition that ethnographers negotiate their sexual positions within the communities they study – particularly when sexuality and gender are explicit research themes (Kulick and Wilson 1995; Lewin and Leap 1996; Markowitz and Ashkenazi 1999).

The limits of gay transnationalisation

In writing about *masu harka* I privilege (and also expose to outside purview) an in-group term and translate it roughly as 'men who have sex with men'. Aside from a general ethnographic preference for emic terms, why do this? Why not refer to such men in terms that are more widely known, such as 'homosexuals', 'bisexuals', or 'gay'? Why not simply refer to them as 'MSM', the *de rigueur* category in global public health discourse? Why not use a more mainstream Hausa term such as *'yan ludu* ('sodomites'), or *'yan daudu*, a term central to Rudolf Gaudio's 2009 monograph on feminine men in Kano? More broadly, what is at stake politically, epidemiologically, even morally, in the terms a researcher uses to represent non-normative sexualities?

Foucault's (1978) thesis that 'homosexuality' first came to be understood as a distinct and pathological sexual sensibility in Western societies beginning in the late nineteenth century has been foundational to much subsequent social scientific enquiry into sexuality.[3] Although Foucault did not go very far towards theorising the transnational exchange of culture and identity, sexual or otherwise, subsequent scholars have built on his work by situating the history of European sexual discourse within the political economic history of European imperialism. Drawing both on Foucault and on Edward Said's (1978) contention that Europeans measured Western masculinity and rationality against an irrational, feminised, Oriental 'other', Ann Stoler (1995) asserts that the history of nineteenth-century European sexuality is inextricable from the histories of colonial expansion and racial classification. Relatedly, historians have analysed the many possibilities that the colonies provided European men to escape the strictures and opprobrium of European societies with regard to homosexuality and to use their relative wealth and power for sexual exchanges with colonised subjects (Bleys 1995; Aldrich 2003).

Whereas 'homosexual' originated in late nineteenth-century Europe to delimit a certain sexual personhood deemed pathological, the designation 'gay' did not become prominent until the early 1960s. 'Gay' has increasingly come to denote what Gilbert Herdt and Andrew Boxer have called 'a full spectrum of social life: not only same-sex desires but gay selves, gay neighbourhoods, and gay social practices that are distinctive of our affluent, postindustrial society' (1992: 4). The seeming fixity and stability which characterises Western gay personhood is in large part the result of gay civil rights strategies in the West, which have emphasised sexual identity as a pseudo-ethnic identity over and above sexual desire or conduct (Halperin 2012). Egalitarianism among sexual partners has been noted as another

[3] Not all scholars have corroborated this position. Stephen Murray (1995), for instance, critiques the postulation that 'homosexual' was invented by late nineteenth-century Western medical discourse as 'special creationism', arguing that this orthodoxy evinces a northern European and American will not to know that recurrent homosexual desire was indeed recognised in other times and places.

distinctive feature of many 'gay' sexual relationships, in contrast to the age-structured, gender-differential, and profession-defined homosexualities that have predominated in many non-Western societies (Adam 1986).

There is little doubt that 'gayness' as an identity and set of social practices emerged from particular socio-economic conditions. Yet as more recent ethnographic research evinces, self-consciously 'gay' identities and movements have flourished around the world and even in places afflicted by pervasive poverty (Drucker 2000). The past decade has seen considerable scholarly attention to the so-called 'globalisation of gayness' – how Western-styled gay identities and cultural formations have moved across national and cultural settings.[4]

The global circulation of entertainment and news media has propelled the notion of gayness and gay rights politics around the world with increasing speed. Asked to date the start of the gay movement in Soweto, for instance, some young black men there named the appearance of a gay character on the American programme *Dynasty* on South African television (McLean and Ngcobo 1995: 180). Nor is it only sexual minorities who encounter sexual identity concepts through transnational media. I can recall an evening in 2002 when, as a US Peace Corps volunteer, I was eating dinner with local friends at an open-air restaurant in Maradi, the second most populous city in Niger. An episode of the gay-themed American sitcom *Will and Grace*, dubbed into French, was playing on a small TV as we ate. For me it was a moment of great cultural dissonance. I had heard little public mention of homosexuality in Niger, yet here was a programme depicting the lives and relationships of gay American men garnering nonchalant chuckles from a viewing audience of urban Nigeriens. My first sense was that what was being depicted was culturally untranslatable; that a publicly declared sexuality based on exclusive homosexuality was inconceivable in the local context. In Hausa I asked my friends, married men in their thirties, 'Do you know what this TV show is about? These men don't have sex with women, only with other men.' 'Well of course,' my friends replied unfazed, 'that's what gay means!'

Diaspora communities in Western countries also facilitate ideas about gay personhood and culture back to their countries of origin, sometimes influencing the adoption of Western-styled gay identities – such as the role of Latin American migrants in the United States in the Westernisation of queer sexual identities in Latin America (Drucker 2000), and that of Asians living in North America, Australia and Britain in spreading consciousness of gay life back to Asia (Altman 2000). Holidaymaking and international business trips also afford (non-Western) travellers an emotional distance from home that has the potential to affect sexual behaviours and identities (Cox 2002).

[4] This attention has followed on from more general theorising about impacts of global processes on local cultural formations, e.g. Appadurai 1996; Hannerz 1992; Urban 2001.

Yet mere exposure to notions of gay personhood does not necessarily result in the adoption of gay self-identity for same-sex desiring people. Encountering gay sensibilities may create a sense of 'complex loyalties', whereby gay identities are balanced with ethnic, racial, and national identities that may seem incompatible (Cant 1997: 14). The extent to which 'gay' has been conceptually adopted by sexual minorities and by society-at-large, or constructed as culturally 'other', has varied considerably across societies. Recent ethnographies in countries as diverse as Bolivia (Wright 2005), South Africa (Donham 1998), Japan (Suganuma 2007), and the Philippines (Johnson 1998) demonstrate that differently structured queer sexual typologies often co-exist in the same society.

'MSM', a category coined by public health practitioners in the context of AIDS to disaggregate sexual behaviour from sexual identity and thus correct the Western presumption that all men who have sex with men necessarily identify as gay or with some other non-heteronormative identity, has yielded certain complications. On the one hand, the term obscures the social dimensions of sexuality, undermines self-labelling, and ignores epidemiologically relevant variations in sexual behaviours beyond one's partner's gender (Young and Meyer 2005). On the other hand, 'MSM' has morphed into a subject position, the very thing the term was coined to avoid (Boellstorff 2011: 298). In Nigeria, where (implicitly immoral) 'MSM' are constructed in official discourse as outside the (implicitly moral) 'general population', the consequences of this can hardly be overstated. The problem, as I will explain further, is that almost all 'MSM' in Nigeria are sexually integrated into the (implicitly heterosexual) 'general population' as the husbands or other sexual partners of women (Merrigan *et al.* 2011).[5]

Queer sexual personhoods in Nigeria are increasingly, if geographically unevenly, influenced by the transnationalisation of lesbian, gay, bisexual and transgender (LGBT) identity politics. The country's LGBT movement has grown slowly since Alliance Rights, the first indigenous gay advocacy organisation, formed in 1999. Today several small LGBT groups exist, mostly in the southern commercial megalopolis, Lagos, and the central federal capital, Abuja. These groups largely adopt the language and rights-based strategies of the transnational LGBT movement, even though many people in culturally and linguistically diverse Nigeria who have same-sex sex do not self-identify as lesbian, gay, bisexual, or transgender. Nigeria's LGBT groups receive limited monetary and strategic support

[5] Just over half of the 1,545 MSM surveyed during Nigeria's 2010 Integrated Bio-Behavioural Surveillance Survey said they had had at least one female sex partner in the past year, meaning that a majority of those surveyed were behaviourally bisexual. However, only 12.4 per cent of those surveyed had ever been married. In a country where marriage rates are very high, this cohort is thus unrepresentative of Nigerian MSM in regard to marriage. Older and married men are particularly unwilling to risk exposure by coming forward to participate in a survey of MSM, and over half of MSM respondents were under the age of 25. We should infer, then, that a much greater proportion of MSM in Nigeria are behaviourally bisexual than this sample indicates.

from organisations such as the International Gay and Lesbian Human Rights Commission and various AIDS NGOs.

As in other countries where homosexuality is criminalised and pursuing broad human rights protections has been dangerous, Nigerian LGBT organisations and their allies have concentrated efforts on AIDS. This 'AIDSification of homosexuality' (Odets 1995) reflects a growing realisation of the gravity of the epidemic among (especially male) sexual minorities in Nigeria. Focusing on AIDS is also a pragmatic decision: Nigerians overwhelmingly disapprove of homosexuality, and prospects for non-AIDS-related advocacy are poor.[6] Although few Nigerians would favour directing AIDS resources to a group considered as immoral as homosexuals are, working on AIDS prevention and service delivery for sexual minorities has been the *least intolerable* strategy for local and international LGBT and LGBT-supportive organisations.

Nigerian LGBT groups – indeed, anyone who in any way works for the rights of sexual minorities in Nigeria – operate in the context of serious opprobrium and legal restriction. Despite already having among the world's most stridently anti-homosexual laws,[7] Nigeria has seen forceful national and state-level efforts to legislate against gay relationships and organisations since the mid-2000s. This new batch of anti-gay legislation has reflected transnational debates and anxieties over same-sex marriage. As of November 2013, the Nigerian legislature has nearly finalised a bill that will criminalise two people of the same sex living together 'as husband and wife or for other purposes of same sexual relationship'. The bill further calls for punishing anyone who 'witnesses, abet[s] and aids' such a union with up to ten years' imprisonment, and outlaws advocacy for LGBT rights. This last provision could be used to target organisations that support sexual minorities in any way, including HIV/AIDS prevention.[8]

The blind and the sighted

My friend Salisu and I reveal to each other that we both do *harka* several years into our acquaintance, after he sees me socialising one day with another man who

[6] In a 2007 survey by the Pew Global Attitudes Project, 97 per cent of Nigerians said that homosexuality should be rejected by society (Pew Research Center 2007).

[7] Chapter 21, Articles 214 and 217 of the Nigerian penal code – vestiges of colonial-era British sodomy laws – make male homosexuality punishable by imprisonment for up to fourteen years throughout the country. Similar laws exist in many countries that were colonised by Britain.

[8] Similar legislation has been introduced in several African countries, most notably in Uganda where anti-gay evangelical Christians from the United States were instrumental in the introduction of anti-gay legislation that would, among other things, make homosexuality punishable by death in certain instances (cf. Müller, Chapter 14, this volume).

he knows does *harka*. When we meet for lunch later that week, Salisu makes subtle allusions to homosexuality using words from the '*harka* dialect' that have double meanings generally known only to *masu harka* (Gaudio 2009). When I pick up on these hints and return in kind, Salisu becomes even more obvious and asks if I can connect him with anyone sexually – a common expectation among *harka* friends and sexual partners. I play coy, telling him I don't know if we're interested in the same type of people. 'So what type do you like?' he asks me in Hausa, winking and using the masculine form for the phrase 'what type'. With the secret seemingly out of the bag, we admit to each other that we both like men.

Salisu tells me he has many boyfriends and tends to go for men in their mid-twenties, about ten years younger than his own age. As in the broader (heterosexual) society, *masu harka* have few qualms about inter-generational sexual relationships, and substantial age differences among partners are common. I ask how he normally meets other men involved in *harka*. 'Ah, there are plenty!' he exclaims, as if my question is rather naïve. 'There are at least one million in Nigeria. And anybody who sees me, you know, I'm handsome. If I say I like it, they won't reject me. And if they don't agree, I will use my money to interest them', he tells me with a sly laugh. Sex-for-benefit exchanges are common and even valorised among *masu harka*, particularly when age and status differences exist between sexual partners. 'But normally', he continues more seriously, '*harka* here is considered a sort of abomination. If somebody finds out you are in the act, people will hate you. It's not like America, where a person can show that "I am gay". Here, if you show it, it's going to be a big problem.'

As Salisu alludes, the idea of liberating oneself by 'coming out' to family and acquaintances has become a cornerstone of gay experience in the United States and other Western countries. Whereas homosexuals in the era preceding the gay liberation movement generally strove to keep their same-sex proclivities hidden from the broader society, the promise of gay liberation involved asserting one's same-sex sexuality as a fixed and recognisable public identity. For many this entails the exemption from heterosexual marriage and, increasingly, the right to legally sanctioned union with a same-sex partner.

In contrast, attitudes and legal sanctions against homosexuality in Northern Nigeria are such that intentionally and publicly revealing oneself is considered unfathomable. Even in the southern Nigerian metropolises where LGBT identity politics have had the greatest relative influence in the country, very few people claim gay identities publicly. In the predominantly Islamic north, homosexuality is rarely discussed in public and has not formed the basis of any rights-based political movement.

In addition to the nationwide sodomy statutes and more recently introduced anti-gay legislation, since 2000 anal intercourse has been technically punishable by death for married and divorced Muslim men and by 100 lashes and imprisonment for never-married Muslim men in the twelve predominantly Muslim northern states that have adopted *sharia* (Islamic law).[9] Aware of these potential legal repercussions and of disapproving social attitudes towards homosexuality, *masu harka* maintain a sharp distinction between *masu ido* (literally, 'those with eyes/those who see', metaphorically, 'those who do *harka*') and *makafi* (literally, 'the blind', metaphorically, 'those who do not do *harka*'). *Masu harka* use richly developed coded language and non-verbal cues to subtly suss out the *harka* status of unknown men, guard against inadvertently revealing themselves to the uninvolved, and discuss sexual matters without being detected. So subtle are these codes that words are not necessary. For instance, where a man known to one *mai harka* but unknown to the others present enters the social space, the man's status could be ascertained by pointing to one's own eye and then glancing at the person in question as a way of asking, 'Does he do *harka* too?' The person who knows the man would then respond to the query with a quick nod 'yes' or 'no'.

I have argued that calls for sexual minorities' rights in Nigeria – and opposition to recognising such rights – overwhelmingly follow the identity-based strategies of the transnational LGBT movement. But are *masu harka* gay men? Rudolf Gaudio addresses this question in his monograph on *'yan daudu*[10] ('feminine men') in Northern Nigeria:

> The answer is not so straightforward. In the earliest days of my research, when all I knew about *'yan daudu* was what other people had written or said about them, I imagined I might, as a gay man, be able to become involved in their largely hidden social world. I was intrigued the first few times I saw *'yan daudu* strolling and dancing at nightclubs and outdoor parties, and could not help but compare these images to gay life at home. Although subsequent events forced me to reconsider, but not reject outright, the naive idea that *'yan daudu* were men with whom I could communicate on the basis of a shared sexuality, my interactions with them introduced me to a thriving social world of men who acknowledged and acted upon their sexual attraction to other men. These men comprise what could arguably be called a Hausa homosexual community, though their social life differs in important ways from gay life in the West. (2009: 9)

[9] To my knowledge, no sentences of capital punishment for homosexuality have been meted out since *sharia* went into effect. The stringent burden of proof demanded by *sharia* requires either a confession by the accused or that four adult male witnesses independently testify to having witnessed the act in question. In addition, Northern Nigerian governments have demonstrated little will in carrying out judicial killings since the international outcry over the (eventually overturned) 2002 stoning conviction of Muslim woman Amina Lawal for adultery.

[10] During the time of my research in the late 2000s, *meƙa* (an in-group term without independent meaning but which roughly equates to the gay usage of 'queens'; plural, *meƙoki*) was more commonly used among *masu harka* when referring to feminine men. My sense is that *'yan daudu* increasingly carries a pejorative connotation with which few wish to be identified. *'Yan daudu/meƙoki* are thus the subset of feminine men within the larger category of *masu harka*, 'a "secret" code term' (Gaudio 2009: 9) that encompasses both *'yan daudu/meƙoki* and more conventionally masculine men who have sex with other men (known variously in the *harka* lexicon as 'civilians' (*fararen-hula*), *'yan aras*, or simply as 'men' (*maza*)).

Similarities in sexual behaviour and sociality aside, there are considerable differences in what it means to be gay in the Western sense and what it means to be a *mai harka*. The most formidable difference is that,

> unlike most Western men who describe themselves as gay, *masu harka* do not see homosexuality as incompatible with heterosexual marriage or parenthood, or vice versa. At some point in their lives most *masu harka*, including a majority of *'yan daudu*, marry women and have biological children.
>
> (Gaudio 2009: 10)

In societies where kinship ties and social pressure to marry are strong, the public insistence on a gay identity exclusive of heterosexual marriage is figured as a serious threat to the family (Aarmo 1999). Thus, 'the African lesbian or gay man is figured outside the clan, the tribe, the race, the nation-state' (Pincheon 2000: 47).

Even more importantly for Nigerian Muslims, a public gay identity that excludes marrying someone of the opposite sex puts someone outside the faith community. Sexual-minority Christian Nigerians risk similar ostracisation from their religious communities. However, at least some Christian Nigerians have formed gay-affirming church congregations, and the members of Nigeria's LGBT organisations have overwhelmingly been Christians. Hausa people see marriage foremost as a religious and social obligation, a critical stage in the attainment of social adulthood (Cooper 1997; Gaudio 2009). A man's lack of innate sexual desire for women does not exempt him from the obligation of marriage, and *masu harka* do not see a necessary connection between marriage and heterosexual desire (Gaudio 2009: 10). It is no overstatement to say that given the centrality of marriage in Islamic teachings, Northern Nigerian Muslims consider the refusal to marry as deeply threatening to Islamic society.

Some married men who do *harka* feel little emotional or sexual connection to their wives; others profess a strong affinity. (This, of course, is also true of men not involved in *harka*.) It is difficult, moreover, to disambiguate the various desires that structure *masu harka* attitudes towards marriage. Contemporary Western discourses on marriage privilege romantic love, sexual fulfilment, and emotional connection between spouses. These discourses and their associations with modernity increasingly influence marital ideals around the world (Padilla *et al.* 2007), including in Africa (Cole and Thomas 2009). Northern Nigerians are certainly concerned with love and sexual fulfilment in marriage. Yet they are equally likely to emphasise the desire to fulfil religious obligations, please their family of orientation, and become a respectable adult as motivating the decision to marry.

One day a *harka* friend in his late twenties and I were looking at photos on my laptop computer in my apartment in Kano. We came upon a photograph I had taken of two of my friends, a gay American couple in their fifties. In the photo, one friend was kissing the other on the cheek with a loving look on his face. 'Do they do *harka*?' my friend asked. 'Yes, they're married to each other', I responded. A look of unpleasant surprise registered on his face. 'There should be a retirement age!' he exclaimed. In actuality, many men continue to have male sexual partners after they marry. But the notion that same-sex romance should be publicly exhibited and supplant heterosexual family life is remote to *masu harka*.

Having children is an especially strong reason for *masu harka* to marry, as it is for Nigerians in general. *Harka* friends frequently asked me when I planned to end my bachelorhood. When I replied candidly that I was unlikely to ever marry a woman, I invariably received the mystified response, 'But don't you want to have children?' That one would allow one's homosexual orientation to force one to forgo family life makes little sense. As one married *mai harka* reasoned, 'Everyone wants to have children for the sake of leaving a legacy. When you have children, they will pray for you even after your death. And if you die without leaving any children, I think you won't be remembered at all.'

The exposure of one's homosexual behaviour is a source of generalised anxiety for *masu harka*, who fear the dissolution of relational ties with family, neighbours, friends, and colleagues. An unmarried man in his mid-twenties explained what he thought would happen if the word got out that he was having sex with men:

> My family would feel depressed if they knew. They would stop treating me the way they do now. They might even disown me. They would say I would spoil the family's image, or spoil other people's children. People in the area would warn their children to stop talking to you or going on errands for you, and things like that. All this would happen because of what you are accused of. I really don't want to be exposed. It would honestly be devastating.[11]

A married man in his early thirties said in an interview that he initially aspired to stop doing *harka* upon getting married, and expressed exasperation at the persistence of his sexual desires for other men. Because exposure of his same-sex extra-marital relationships would constitute a serious threat to his marriage, he was at great pains to keep his extra-marital homosexual encounters hidden from his wife:

> If my wife knew, she would not like it at all. I would say it's not a good thing when it comes to Muslims. I'm not sure about Christians, whether it's okay or not in their religion. But if it were a Muslim, I would say it was a bad thing. And if a person's wife found out, she would probably leave and ask for a divorce. So a person should be very careful. If you have a family, he should never let them find out what he does, because that would be really bad.

[11] Homosexuality is commonly associated with pederasty in Nigeria; it is widely assumed that older men coerce boys and adolescents into homosexuality.

‘We could not come across any Nigerian with such sexuality’: secrecy, sexual transgression, and human rights

Despite these steep social and legal consequences, homosexuality is ironically reputed in popular Nigerian sentiment to be most prevalent among northerners, particularly among men of the Muslim ruling class. Extensive social-sexual networks of men who have sex with men indeed exist and, ironically, have flourished under *sharia*. I became acquainted with *masu harka* of all different ages and socio-economic statuses. Once, when I expressed surprise at how extensive *harka* networks seemed to be, a middle-aged friend quipped, ‘If you know one guy who does *harka*, you know a thousand.’

Scholarship on homosexuality and globalisation has focused overwhelmingly on how Western identities, discourses, and cultural productions affect non-Western people. Yet to the extent that homosexuality is ‘othered’ by Northern Nigerians, it is *Larabawa* (Arabs) who are more commonly professed to be its progenitors than *Turawa* (Europeans/Whites). That this is the case is unsurprising: Islam and other longstanding trade and cultural connections have meant that Middle Eastern influences are much more pronounced in Northern Nigeria than Western influences.

Harka acquaintances who had spent time in the Middle East disabused me of my half-surprise that same-sex pick-ups in that region were so brazen. A man in his mid-twenties, responding during a focus group discussion I held with *masu harka* involved in sex work, professed, ‘Men do *harka* in Mecca more than any other place. I have videotape from Jidda where such things happened. Sometimes, you will be approached by them [Saudi men] while just walking or on your way home.’ Another participant added wryly, ‘Whenever *meƙoki* [feminine men] travel to Mecca, everybody knows what they are going there to do.’ A married friend who travelled occasionally on business to Cairo enjoyed recounting tales of Egyptian men who brazenly picked him up on train platforms, in markets, and on the street.

Male homosexuality in Northern Nigeria in the *sharia* era must be understood in the context of Islamic norms of gender segregation and women’s exclusion from the public sphere. These norms constrain opposite-sex socialisation among unrelated adults and promote homosociality. While illicit heterosexual relationships certainly occur, the social separation of unrelated men and women exerts considerable limitations on sexual opportunity structures with unmarried opposite-sex partners. Whereas women are largely restricted to the domestic sphere, men have substantial freedom of movement and pursue close social relationships with other men. Since little suspicion is cast on close male friendships and sociality, there is considerable leeway for discreet homosexual relationships. Unmarried men – both those who would prefer sex with women and those who would prefer it with men – find sexual experiences more readily with other men.

Such patterns have been observed across Islamic-majority societies. In Vern Bullough's formulation, homosexuality is 'a natural outgrowth of a sex-positive, sex-segregating religion in which women had little status or value' (1976: 238). Writing about Pakistan, Badruddin Kahn claims that from the perspective of family life it is less of a risk for a man to have sexual affairs with other men than with women, since infidelity with women may result in penalties that are far worse (1992: 95). Stephen Murray and Will Roscoe contend that in Islamic societies, 'Boys are much more available and their sexual use less serious than the expropriation of women's bodies to which some other man might have the rights or responsibility for conserving' (1997: 309). In each of these accounts, homosexuality is seen as widespread and 'tolerated' in Islamic societies to the extent that it is easier and less damning than extra-marital heterosexual sex.

Punishment, tolerance, and protection: shifting cultural responses to homosexuality

Much has been written about *liwat* (generally translated as 'sodomy') in Islamic scripture and jurisprudence, and in contemporary scholarship. The precise meaning of *liwat* has been a matter of considerable disagreement. Several scholars argue that translating *liwat* as 'homosexuality' is inaccurate insofar as it is anachronistic, imposing a broader contemporary concept onto a more narrowly understood and older term (see especially Schmitt 1992). Although no specific penalty is prescribed in the Qur'an, several *hadith* (sayings and acts attributed to the Prophet Muhammad) have been interpreted as calling for the severe punishment of those who engage in *liwat,* although some progressive Muslim scholars, such as Scott Kugle (2003: 219) and Aleardo Zanghellini (2010: 288), have challenged this position. Dissenting exegeses notwithstanding and definitional indeterminacies aside, the orthodox Islamic position is that *liwat* is a punishable offence.

Scriptural injunctions notwithstanding, the legal status of homosexuality in contemporary Muslim-majority countries ranges widely, from incurring the death penalty in some countries to no penalty whatsoever in others. There is, in short, no universal Islamic response to homosexuality. In general, however, and in contrast to how it is now dealt with in most Western countries, homosexuality in African and Muslim-majority societies is what Michael Taussig (1999) has termed a 'public secret': that which is generally known but cannot be easily articulated. Homosexuality (similar to AIDS-related death and domestic violence) is generally considered a secret best confined to the private sphere (Reid and Walker 2005: 185). As Marc Epprecht argues, the key proviso for the *de facto* tolerance of 'non-normative sexuality [is that it] not be named as such, but take place under the umbrella of heteropatriarchal constructions of faith, family, and African identity – don't ask, don't tell, in other words' (2012: 226).

The condemnatory treatment of homosexuality in Nigeria, as elsewhere, has come under mounting challenge by Western-led efforts to grant 'LGBT' people human rights protections. In a December 2011 speech before the United Nations Human Rights Council in Geneva, and following a memorandum in which President Barack Obama wrote that he was 'deeply concerned by the violence and discrimination targeting L.G.B.T. persons around the world', US Secretary of State Hillary Clinton declared the intention to use the tools of American diplomacy to promote gay rights internationally: 'Some have suggested that gay rights and human rights are separate and distinct, but in fact they are one and the same' (Myers and Cooper 2011). In a policy statement derided by several African governments as an affront to African autonomy and cultural mores, British Prime Minister David Cameron announced in 2011 that future development aid to African countries would be contingent on recognition of gay rights.

However modest their aims, campaigns for sexual rights are typically perceived in many African societies as Western cultural imperialism and have provoked patriotic, patriarchal and religious antipathy (Epprecht 2012; Müller, Chapter 14, this volume). Advocates for 'LGBT rights' have seemed to assume that 'gay, 'lesbian', 'bisexual', and 'transgender' identity categories obtain, or are at least culturally translatable, around the world. Like their counterparts in several other African and Middle Eastern countries, Nigerian political leaders have denied the existence of 'gays', arguing that such people do not exist in their country and are instead emblematic of a morally depraved West. In 2009 – the same year that the National Assembly began debating new anti-gay legislation – Nigerian Minister of Foreign Affairs Ojo Madueke told the United Nations Universal Periodic Review on Human Rights that there was no LGBT community in Nigeria: 'We went out of our way to look for the gay, lesbian and transgender group, but we could not come across any Nigerian with such sexuality.'[12] In 2011, Nigeria joined a large minority of African and predominantly Islamic countries that voted against the United Nations' first successfully adopted declaration to condemn discrimination against LGBT people.

The limits of 'heterosexual African AIDS'

The assumption that AIDS in Africa is spread through heterosexual sex has driven approaches to addressing the pandemic on the continent. Epidemiologists and government officials – both African and foreign – have generally rejected the notion

[12] The minister's claim is implausible, as self-proclaimed gay activists delivered a petition and speech to the National Assembly during debates over the bill. This action was reported in a front-page article in Nigeria's most widely read English language newspaper, dramatically titled 'Homosexuals storm National Assembly' (*Daily Trust*, 12 March 2009).

that male homosexual transmission plays any serious role in Africa's epidemics. Noting nearly equivalent ratios of HIV infection among males and females across Africa, epidemiologists posited that transmission in sub-Saharan Africa was overwhelmingly heterosexual, in contrast to the homosexually driven epidemics in much of the rest of the world (e.g. Chin and Mann 1988). This epidemiological hypothesis was buttressed by the cultural assumption that homosexuality is rare or non-existent in African societies.

An estimated 3.1 million Nigerians are living with HIV or AIDS, making it the country with the world's second largest population of HIV-positive people. However, research on the epidemic among MSM has been quite minimal. Government justifications for neglecting MSM in AIDS research and programmes vacillated, contradictorily, between denying that male–male sexual transmission happens and vilifying MSM for intentionally spreading the virus. Pressed in a 2004 interview about homosexual transmission, the then Chairman of Nigeria's National Action Committee on HIV/AIDS (NACA), Professor Babatunde Osotimehin, responded:

> The point I want to make very clearly is that the major cause of infection in Nigeria is by heterosexual transmission. I don't think we should detract from that because if we detract from that, we may have problems with the prevention of HIV/AIDS.
> (Abdullahi 2004)

The following year, NACA's project manager asserted that, 'Homosexuals are only interested in spreading HIV/AIDS. They are a serious threat to human existence anywhere in the world' (Akanji 2005).

The academic literature on AIDS in Nigeria largely followed suit in its reticence on MSM. For instance, the extensive section on HIV/AIDS in Nigeria in *The International Encyclopedia of Sexuality* (2001) makes no mention whatever of homosexuality, instead claiming that '95 percent of all infections are by heterosexual intercourse, 4 percent are through blood transfusions, and one percent are through mother-to-child transmission' (Esiet 2001; cf. Müller on Uganda, Chapter 14, this volume). In *AIDS in Nigeria*, a 2006 edited volume that is otherwise the most comprehensive publication to date on AIDS in Nigeria, scant attention is paid to homosexual transmission. In the epidemiology chapter, Nasidi and Harry state only that, 'Homosexual intercourse does not appear to contribute significantly to the HIV epidemic in Nigeria' (2006: 21), without offering any further explanation or evidence to support this assertion.

It is clear, more than thirty years into the pandemic, that heterosexual sex *is* the primary mode of HIV transmission in Africa. It is also increasingly clear that homosexual transmission was excluded from the African AIDS narrative until recently not because African MSM do not exist, but because few were willing and able to conduct epidemiological research among them. More recent studies demonstrate that across the continent HIV prevalence rates for MSM are substantially higher than general population prevalence. A systematic review of data from thirty-eight low- and middle-income countries, including several African countries, found that MSM were nineteen times more likely on average to have HIV than the general population (Baral *et al.* 2007). While very few HIV prevalence studies among African MSM were conducted before 2005, recent research from sites spanning more than a dozen African countries has found prevalence among MSM to greatly exceed general population prevalence, frequently by factors of ten or more (Smith *et al.* 2009).

NACA with a team of research partners conducted an Integrated Bio-Behavioural Surveillance Survey (IBBSS) on HIV/AIDS in 2007, and again in a more expanded version in 2010 (Federal Ministry of Health 2010). The purpose of the survey was to estimate HIV prevalence and bio-behavioural correlates of 'most at-risk populations' (MARPs), including female sex workers, injection drug users, armed forces and police, and transport workers and, for the first time, MSM. Whereas national adult HIV prevalence in Nigeria is estimated at 4.1 per cent, the 2010 survey found that prevalence among 1,545 MSM in the six study cities was 17.2 per cent – the second highest prevalence of any group after female sex workers. Furthermore, MSM were the only group out of the seven studied that showed an increase in HIV prevalence from the 2007 study. Among the seven groups under study, MSM were also the population least likely to know that they were positive – only 36.9 per cent did.

The public secret as policy directive

I have asserted that the price for the tacit toleration of homosexuality in Northern Nigeria is that it stays out of sight, unannounced, and that *masu harka* fulfil the expectations of heterosexual marriage. What has this meant for the efforts to intercede in the male homosexual transmission of HIV?

Dr Ashiru Rajab is Deputy Director of the Kano State Ministry of Health's AIDS Control Programme. He is a medical doctor, a Muslim, and a lifelong resident of Kano city. When he is not travelling for conferences in Nigeria or internationally, Dr Rajab's small and mercifully air-conditioned office on the third floor of Kano's Ministry of Health is constantly busy with a stream of visitors and phone calls; CNN seems always to be playing on his wall-mounted TV.

During our second recorded interview, Dr Rajab talked at length about the significance of MSM in Kano's epidemic and expressed strong interest in addressing this population in the state's AIDS research and programming. He is also aware that the religious and political climate in which he works constrains his ability to carry out programmes based on what he believes is best epidemiological practice. He explained the controversy that arose during the IBBSS in 2007, the first time anyone attempted to estimate HIV prevalence among MSM in Kano:

> We had to kind of downplay the information going into the community that this [2010] survey is happening or is going to happen. Uh, we usually keep quiet; remain low, conduct our survey, and then that is it – unlike other surveys that we are free to broadcast. And if I can remember, after the dissemination meeting of the last IBBSS survey in 2007 there was quite a controversy in Kano. Unfortunately one of the media houses that attended the dissemination meeting went ahead and wrote something that was not really what happened, uh, that 'An NGO came into Kano and they claimed that they have seen homosexuals, they have tested them [for HIV], that Kano has so-so much number of homosexuals, which is a lie, and the survey was not sanctioned, blah blah blah blah.' You know? So that information is of course on the national daily.[13]
>
> It got to the CDC,[14] the GHAIN project,[15] and the Federal Ministry of Health. What I learned later is that it went as high as to the presidency, and the governor of Kano was, uh, asked to clear the information, whether the state had actually rejected the results [of the survey]. Because if the state says that they have disowned the result it means they cannot go public; it's null and void. There was concern, serious concern. [. . .] So my own thinking was that this [newspaper reporter] was somebody [that's] so patriotic, maybe an indigene of Kano that doesn't want the name of the state to be spoiled, who on his own decided to change the news. [. . .] I suppose the person that wrote that article wanted to . . . maybe to him he was doing a service to Kano, so to say.

The IBBSS included several other groups that might be seen as tarnishing the state's reputation, including female sex workers and injection drug users. I asked Dr Rajab to clarify whether it was the issue of homosexuality that had provoked the denial:

> It's basically the homosexual component of it. Because they were saying, 'How can you say you come to Kano and you find them [homosexuals]? Where did you find them?' Because they know you can go and find prostitutes all over the place. But where did you find them [homosexuals]? Yeah, they don't believe, they don't want to believe. So I actually had to clear the story, that it wasn't true that we rejected [the survey results]. [. . .] [JT: *So the concern then was that someone from outside of Kano* . . .] Exactly. [. . . *was somehow tarnishing the reputation of the state by saying, 'There are homosexuals in Kano, they have this problem with HIV* . . . '] Exactly, exactly. So that's the way I read the situation. That's just to show you that this kind of high-risk survey, we are not free. Yeah, we are constrained because people are still not accepting the situation.

Dr Rajab continued by explaining how he perceives mainstream attitudes on homosexuality hindering his work:

[13] *Daily Trust*, Nigeria's national newspaper with the greatest circulation.

[14] The US Center for Disease Control and Prevention, which has worked in Nigeria since 2001.

[15] Global HIV/AIDS Initiative Nigeria, a large project begun in 2004 and funded by the US President's Emergency Plan for AIDS Relief through USAID.

> That is my challenge now: stigma generally against these certain populations, and still for now we don't have the means of tackling it. That is the most challenging aspect of it. How can you tell an imam to preach that an MSM is a normal person, just that he has deviated – just like somebody that goes and takes alcohol? It's deviation. It's really difficult. It's a crucial question, yeah. A real challenge, a real challenge.

The sense of challenge is not limited to government entities. The Nigerian Supreme Council for Islamic Affairs' AIDS Programme for the Muslim Umma has been similarly constrained in addressing homosexual transmission of HIV among Muslim men. In the following interview excerpt, the Programme Manager of the AIDS Programme for the Muslim Umma narrates what happened during the development of the Council's *National Islamic Policy on HIV/AIDS* in 2009 when a Western staff researcher with the United Nations Development Programme providing technical assistance for the new policy raised the question of male–male sexual transmission:

> She [the UNDP staff researcher] brought up the issue; they [the Nigerian Muslim scholars writing the policy] shouted her down. They said it's not an issue. So who am I [to contradict the scholars]? So you see, big problem. And the researcher, she showed me her research that it's more prevalent in the north, men having sex with men. And we know it, but we are just like the ostrich.[16] So it's a big challenge. It's not something I can address at my level. A whole lot of big people have to come to say, 'You can address it'. Because when she [the UNDP staff researcher] talked to me about it as the programme manager, I was like, 'Good, it's something I can do'. But when I spoke to my director, my director said, 'Don't talk about it'. So it's a big challenge – and you know it, having stayed in the north. But it's something I hope some day, *some* day, yeah – because if you want to address it, not here. I would have to go somewhere else.

Like state and federal governments and religious organisations, AIDS NGOs operating in Northern Nigeria have been similarly unable (or unwilling, depending on one's perspective) to address MSM. A programme manager in the Kano office of the Global HIV/AIDS Initiative Nigeria (a massive programme funded by the US President's Emergency Plan for AIDS Relief through USAID) said succinctly when I enquired about prevention initiatives for MSM, 'No known homosexual has ever come to identify himself in this office.' When I asked why he thought this was the case, he responded, 'Kano is a state practising *sharia*. If anyone admitted to any of those things, he would be a pariah. It hasn't been addressed. These are social taboos in the north. It would be difficult for anyone to come out and identify himself as a prostitute or a gay person.'

In sum, a code of silence has thus far prevented intervening in HIV transmission among MSM through institutional channels in Northern Nigeria. Some individuals

[16] I.e. burying heads in the sand and ignoring the problem.

working within the region's AIDS establishment *personally* recognise the need for a public health approach to the epidemic that includes addressing male–male sexual transmission. However, as the interviews excerpted indicate, these individuals find themselves and their organisations to be constrained by the religious conventions that govern public discourse and policy in Northern Nigeria.

What has this meant for perceptions of the epidemic on the part of *masu harka*? In places where it has long been recognised that MSM bear a disproportionate burden of HIV/AIDS and safer sex campaigns targeting such men exist, basic facts about same-sex transmission and risk reduction strategies are commonly known. By contrast in Northern Nigeria, *masu harka* remain largely unaware of their behaviour-specific risks and how these risks can be mitigated. In structured interviews and informal conversations, I found that *masu harka* as a group were overwhelmingly unaware that they carry a much heavier burden of HIV. Many further expressed the belief that anal sex posed little or no risk of HIV. This statement by a married 27-year-old father was representative of *masu harka* I interviewed:

> People who only sleep with women are more at risk of getting infected than those who sleep with men. That's the way I see it. People who sleep with women only are more infected. They come in contact with diseases like gonorrhoea more often, because it's easier to catch them from women.

Just over half of MSM surveyed in Nigeria's 2010 IBBSS reported using a condom at last anal sex.[17] However, MSM in Kano had by far the lowest self-reported condom use across the six sites: only 6.7 per cent reported consistent condom use with non-paying partners in the last six months. This is epidemiologically disquieting but culturally unsurprising: condoms are associated with adultery in the Northern Nigerian imaginary and are often avoided to deflect the perception of engaging in immoral behaviour. Moreover, condom-compatible lubricants are not easily found in Northern Nigeria, making effective condom use for anal sex particularly difficult. As a married *mai harka* in his thirties explained:

> Sometimes I feel too embarrassed to buy condoms or lubricants, because I am not the type of person who should be buying them – that's what they [the people selling condoms] will think. I look too respectable, and I'm a married man, so I shouldn't need condoms in the first place.

Conclusion: moral dilemmas of intervention

The ideology of human rights raises expectations that the rights apply to all people, irrespective of time and place. This aspirational universality imbues human rights

[17] As interviews were conducted face-to-face, responses to this and other sensitive questions may have been biased towards over-reporting socially desirable behaviours such as condom use.

with moral authority. Yet, 'human rights' emerged from and evolve in specific historical and cultural circumstances. Recognition of this fact is hardly new. During the 1947 drafting of the UN's Universal Declaration of Human Rights, the Executive Board of the American Anthropological Association asked, 'How can the proposed Declaration be applicable to all human beings, and not be a statement of rights conceived only in terms of the values prevalent in the countries of Western Europe and America?' (1947: 539).

Religions too are moral systems that emerge from specific historical and cultural conditions. Like human rights, religious authority is predicated on the assertion of universality. And like human rights, religious doctrines are contested in and adapted to diverse historical-cultural settings.

In this chapter I have explored the moral tensions between Islamic doctrines of virtuous sexuality, the health-as-a-human-right imperative, and assessments of epidemiological best practices as they are playing out in Northern Nigeria's AIDS epidemic for sexual minority men. This investigation has shown that the assertion that 'gay rights are human rights' has done little to address the male homosexual transmission of HIV – not least because the identity category 'gay' is minimally applicable to the organisation of sexuality in Northern Nigerian society. Furthermore, Muslim ethics of care have not been extended to *masu harka* because many perceive that doing so would constitute abetting socially deleterious moral transgression.

What can be done? Marc Epprecht (2012) argues that subtle, covert strategies that negotiate a path between rights activism and secretive bisexuality have the best chances for intervening in the AIDS epidemics of sexual minority men in Africa. The few international NGOs and local LGBT groups that have partnered to address male–male transmission of HIV in Nigeria have attempted to strike precisely this sort of delicate balance between engaging networks of sexual minority men with education and service delivery without inciting public backlash. However, even this covert approach to intervention has thus far seemed too risky to pursue in the northern region, where violence against activities perceived as threatening to the Islamic moral order has erupted with increasing frequency in recent years. Moreover, Nigeria's latest batch of far-reaching anti-gay legislation threatens to upend the already tenuous progress made in reaching sexual minority men with HIV interventions, decreasing the likelihood that such interventions will extend to *masu harka* in the north anytime soon. And as stated earlier, most members of Nigeria's LGBT organisations are Christians and live in southern cities.

I advocate a multi-faceted approach in beginning to address the HIV epidemic among *masu harka*. First, a process of advocacy and coalition building will be crucial. Programmes that do not have some institutional support within national and state government will surely fail. Programmes perceived to be imposed or initiated from outside the region will also likely fail. There are well-placed advocates for initiatives addressing MSM – generally those who have solid epidemiological and cultural understanding of *masu harka*'s role in the local epidemic. Garnering their support will be indispensable.

Second, peer education should be a main strategy for giving *masu harka*, and subsets of this population such as men who engage in transactional sex, the health information they need. The benefits of peer education are at least twofold: first, given the secrecy and stigma surrounding same-sex sexuality in Nigeria, *masu harka* are in the best position to reach out to other *masu harka* – especially to older men who are unlikely to be 'found' by government agencies and NGOs. Second, a peer education model recognises that with proper institutional support, *masu harka* can be empowered to effectively address the unmet needs that members of the group consider the most pressing. Just as cell phone technology is used by *masu harka* to discreetly arrange sexual and social connections, it should also be used as a tool to discreetly spread information about HIV and other STI prevention and services.

Masu harka should be involved in all aspects of planning, message development, and campaign roll-out in order for education campaigns to be effective – rather than used as 'implementing partners' when programmes have already been developed. A peer education model does not relieve the federal and state governments of their duty to protect the public health by shifting the programmatic onus to marginalised and under-resourced groups of MSM. Rather, it challenges the government and NGOs to forge meaningful alliances with MSM and recognises that programmes that do not incorporate MSM in all levels of decision-making are unlikely to succeed in the long term.

Third, *masu harka* need access to HIV testing, preventative technologies, psychosocial support, and treatment. No such programmes currently exist in Northern Nigeria, outside of Kaduna. *Masu harka* are unlikely to reveal their sexual behaviours to most medical practitioners due to stigma and likelihood of negative social consequences. It is also unlikely that, given prevailing attitudes towards homosexuality, most Nigerian medical practitioners would feel comfortable working with this population. Establishing a network of medical staff who have been trained in both the medical specificities and social sensitivities of working with *masu harka* will be crucial. At this time, the creation of *masu harka*-specific clinics is infeasible for reasons of social stigma. Rather, clinicians should be both easily accessible and in an environment where MSM feel safe from being exposed as MSM.

Ideally, clinical services should follow a 'one-stop shopping' model, with testing and treatment for STIs and HIV, condoms and condom-compatible lubricants, referrals to other clinical services, and MSM-specific health information all readily available. The cost of services is another major factor. Many *masu harka* are unable to afford appropriate health care when they need it. Such services should therefore be provided free of cost to maximise uptake. As identity management is a key concern for many MSM, service providers must also be trained in the importance of maintaining strict patient confidentiality.

There is no obvious or ready-made path towards addressing the AIDS epidemic among *masu harka*, but the best chances for intervention will entail drawing on pre-existing social-sexual networks and on the dexterity *masu harka* have with discretion and euphemism. While HIV interventions for MSM will be highly challenging in the current legal and socio-political climate, continued inattention to this high-prevalence population will have considerable epidemiological, economic, and social tolls in Northern Nigeria.

Acknowledgements

This chapter is based on research made possible by grants from the Institute of International Education Fulbright Program, and the Center for Afroamerican and African Studies, the International Institute, and the Global Health Research and Training Initiative at the University of Michigan. Some data is drawn from interviews conducted under the auspices of the Population Council. Thanks to Serena Owusua Dankwa, Nadine Beckmann, and two anonymous reviewers for their suggestions on this work.

References

Aarmo, Margarete. 1999. 'How homosexuality became "un-African": the case of Zimbabwe', in Evelyn Blackwood and Saskia Wieringa (eds), *Female Desires: Same-Sex Relations and Transgender Practices Across Cultures*. New York: Columbia University Press.

Abdullahi, F. 2004. 'To many, HIV/AIDS in not real', *This Day* (Nigeria), 16 November.

Adam, Barry. 1986. 'Age, structure, and sexuality: reflections on the anthropological evidence of homosexual relations', in Evelyn Blackwood (ed.), *Anthropology and Homosexual Behavior*. New York: Haworth Press, 19–33.

Akanji, M. 2005. 'Re: Abuja homosexuals are spreading HIV/AIDS'. http://www.mask.org.za/SECTIONS/AfricaPerCountry/ABC/nigeria/nigeria_14.htm.

Aldrich, Robert. 2003. *Colonialism and Homosexuality*. London: Routledge.

Altman, Dennis. 2000. 'The emergence of gay identities in Southeast Asia', in Peter Drucker (ed.), *Different Rainbows*. London: Gay Men's Press, 137–56.

Appadurai, Arjun. 1996. 'Disjuncture and difference in the global cultural economy', in *Modernity at Large: Cultural Dimensions of Globalization*. Minneapolis: University of Minnesota Press, 27–47.

Baral, S., *et al.* 2007. 'Elevated risk for HIV infection among men who have sex with men in low- and middle-income countries 2002–2006: a systematic review', *PLoS Medicine* 4(12).

Bleys, Rudi. 1995. *The Geography of Perversion: Male-to-Male Sexual Behavior outside the West and the Ethnographic Imagination, 1750–1918*. New York: New York University Press.

Boellstorff, Tom. 2011. 'But do not identify as gay: a proleptic genealogy of the MSM category', *Cultural Anthropology* 26(2): 287–312.

Bullough, Vern. 1976. *Sex, Society, and History*. New York: Science History Publications.

Cant, Bob. 1997. 'Introduction', in Bob Cant (ed.), *Invented Identities? Lesbians and Gays Talk about Migration*. London: Cassell, 1–17.

Chin, J. and J. Mann. 1988. 'The global patterns and prevalence of AIDS and HIV infection', *AIDS* 2(Suppl. 1): S247–52.

Cole, Jennifer and Lynn M. Thomas. 2009. *Love in Africa*. Chicago: University of Chicago Press.

Cooper, Barbara. 1997. *Marriage in Maradi: Gender and Culture in a Hausa Society in Niger, 1900–89*. Oxford: James Currey.

Cox, M. 2002. 'The long-haul out of the closet: the journey from smalltown to boystown', in Stephen Clift, Michael Luongo and Carry Callister (eds), *Gay Tourism: Culture, Identity and Sex*. London: Continuum, 151–73.

Donham, Donald. 1998. 'Freeing South Africa: the "modernization" of male–male sexuality in Soweto', *Cultural Anthropology* 13(1): 3–21.

Drucker, Peter. 2000. 'Introduction: remapping sexualities', in P. Drucker (ed.), *Different Rainbows*. London: Gay Men's Press, 9–41.

Epprecht, Marc. 2012. 'Sexual minorities, human rights and public health strategies in Africa', *African Affairs* 111(443): 223–43.

Esiet, U.E. 2001. 'Nigeria – HIV/AIDS', in R.T. Francoeur (ed.), *The International Encyclopedia of Sexuality*, vols I–IV. New York: Continuum.

Executive Board, American Anthropological Association. 1947. 'Statement on human rights', *American Anthropologist* 49(4): 539–43.

Federal Ministry of Health. 2010. *Nigeria Integrated Biological and Behavioural Surveillance Survey*. http://www.popcouncil.org/pdfs/2011HIV_IBBSS2010.pdf.

Foucault, Michel. 1990 [1978]. *The History of Sexuality: Volume 1, An Introduction*. New York: Vintage Books.

Gaudio, Rudolf. 2009. *Allah Made Us: Sexual Outlaws in an Islamic African City*. Malden, MA: Wiley-Blackwell.

Hallah, Tashikalmah, Francis Okeke and Abbas Jimoh. 2009. 'Homosexuals storm National Assembly', *Daily Trust* (Nigeria), 12 March, p. 1.

Halperin, David M. 2012. *How to Be Gay*. Cambridge, MA: Belknap Press of Harvard University Press.

Hannerz, Ulf. 1992. 'The global ecumene as a network of networks', in Adam Kuper (ed.), *Conceptualizing Society*. London: Routledge.

Herdt, Gilbert and Andrew Boxer. 1992. 'Introduction: culture, history, and life course of gay men', in G. Herdt (ed.), *Gay Culture in America: Essays from the Field*. Boston: Beacon Press, 1–28.

Johnson, Mark. 1998. 'Global desirings and translocal loves: transgendering and same-sex sexualities in the southern Philippines', *American Ethnologist* 25(4): 695–711.

Khan, Badruddin. 1992. 'Not-so-gay life in Karachi: a view of a Pakistani living in Toronto', in Arno Schmitt and Jehoeda Sofer (eds), *Sexuality and Eroticism among Males in Moslem Societies*. New York: Haworth Press, 93–104.

Kugle, Scott Siraj al-Haqq. 2003. 'Sexuality, diversity, and ethics in the agenda of progressive Muslims', in Omid Safi (ed.), *Progressive Muslims: On Justice, Gender, and Pluralism*. Oxford: Oneworld.

Kulick, Don and Margaret Wilson (eds) 1995. *Taboo: Sex, Identity, and Erotic Subjectivity in Anthropological Fieldwork.* London: Routledge.

Lewin, Ellen and William Leap (eds) 1996. *Out in the Field: Reflections of Lesbian and Gay Anthropologists.* Urbana: University of Illinois Press.

Markowitz, Fran and Michael Ashkenazi (eds) 1999. *Sex, Sexuality, and the Anthropologist.* Urbana: University of Illinois Press.

McLean, H. and L. Ngcobo. 1995. 'Abangibhamayo bathi ngimnandi (those who fuck me say I'm tasty): gay sexuality in reef townships', in Mark Gevisser and Edwin Cameron (eds), *Defiant Desire.* New York: Routledge, 158–85.

Merrigan, Mike, Aderemi Azeez, Bamgboye Afolabi, Otto Nzapfurundi Chabikuli, Obinna Onyekwena, George Eluwa, Bolatito Aiyenigba, Issa Kawu, Kayode Ogungbemi and Christoph Hamelmann. 2011. 'HIV prevalence and risk behaviours among men having sex with men in Nigeria', *Sexually Transmitted Infections* 87: 65–70.

Murray, Stephen. 1995. 'Discourse creationism', *Journal of Sex Research* 32: 263–5.

Murray Stephen and Will Roscoe. 1997. *Islamic Homosexualities: Culture, History, and Literature.* New York: New York University Press.

Myers, Steven and Helene Cooper. 2011. 'U.S. to aid gay rights abroad, Obama and Clinton say', *New York Times*, 6 December. http://www.nytimes.com/2011/12/07/world/united-states-to-use-aid-to-promote-gay-rights-abroad.html?pagewanted=all.

Nasidi, Abdulsalami and Tekena Harry. 2006. 'The epidemiology of HIV/AIDS in Nigeria', in Olusoji Adeyi, Phyllis J. Kanki, Oluwole Odutolu and John A. Idoko (eds), *AIDS in Nigeria: A Nation on the Threshold.* Cambridge, MA: Harvard University Press.

Odets, Walt. 1995. *In the Shadow of the Epidemic: Being HIV-Negative in the Age of AIDS.* Durham, NC: Duke University Press.

Padilla, Mark, Jennifer Hirsch, Robert Sember, Miguel Munoz-Laboy and Richard Parker (eds) 2007. *Love and Globalization: Transformations of Intimacy in the Contemporary World.* Nashville: Vanderbilt University Press.

Pew Research Center. 2007. *The Pew Global Attitudes Project.* http://pewglobal.org/files/pdf/258.pdf.

Pincheon, Bill. 2000. 'An ethnography of silences: race, (homo)sexualities, and a discourse of Africa', *African Studies Review* 43(3): 39–58.

Reid, Graham and Liz Walker. 2005. 'Sex and secrecy: a focus on African sexuality', *Culture, Health and Sexuality* 7(3): 185–94.

Said, Edward. 1978. *Orientalism.* New York: Vintage Books.

Schmitt, Arno. 1992. 'Different approaches to male–male sexuality/eroticism from Morocco to Usbekistan', in Arno Schmitt and Jehoeda Sofer (eds), *Sexuality and Eroticism among Males in Moslem Societies.* New York: Haworth Press, 1–24.

Smith, Adrian D., *et al.* 2009. 'Men who have sex with men and HIV/AIDS in sub-Saharan Africa', *Lancet* 374: 416–22.

Stoler, Ann. 1995. *Race and the Education of Desire: Foucault's History of Sexuality and the Colonial Order of Things.* Durham, NC: Duke University Press.

Suganuma, Katsuhiko. 2007. 'Associative identity politics: unmasking the multi-layered formation of queer male selves in 1990s Japan', *Inter-Asia Cultural Studies* 8(4): 485–502.

Taussig, Michael. 1999. *Defacement: Public Secrecy and the Labor of the Negative.* Palo Alto, CA: Stanford University Press.

Urban, Greg. 2001. *Metaculture: How Culture Moves through the World*. Minneapolis: University of Minnesota Press.

Wright, Timothy. 2005. 'Gay organizations, NGOs, and the globalization of sexual identity: the case of Bolivia', in Jennifer Robertson (ed.), *Same-Sex Cultures and Sexualities: An Anthropological Reader*. Malden, MA: Blackwell Publishing, 279–94.

Young, Rebecca M. and Ilan H. Meyer. 2005. 'The trouble with "MSM" and "WSW": erasure of the sexual minority person in public health discourse', *American Journal of Public Health* 95(7): 1144–9.

Zanghellini, Aleardo. 2010. 'Neither homophobic nor (hetero) sexually pure: contextualizing Islam's objections to same-sex sexuality', in Samar Habib (ed.), *Islam and Homosexuality*, vol. 2. Santa Barbara: ABC-CLIO, 269–96.

16

Epilogue

The Strings, Strains and Strides of Transnational Competencies and Complex Ambiguities

RIJK VAN DIJK

WHILE ONE OF THE SUCCESS STORIES of globalisation has been the establishment of the nation-state as the model *par excellence* for the geo-political and socio-economic ordering of people and place, which Lissa Malkki (1992) once called the rise of the 'national order of things', this order brought with it a myriad of ways in which a national dominion over territories and identities could be undercut, negotiated, dissolved or questioned. Loosely called the field of the 'transnational', the chapters in this book have explored the ways in which nation-states, also in Africa, cannot be considered iron cages with full control over their territory, people and policies. As Glick Schiller (2005) argues, transnational social fields have become part of the modern reality of the nation-state in all corners of the globe.

Even in the African context where the fragility of the nation-state and the limited success of its modes of operation have been captured by such terms as 'failed state' (Rotberg 2003) or 'fragile state' (Osaghae 2007), a patchwork of singular nation-states cannot be denied. Perhaps more than anywhere else, the strong force of transnational powers capable of crosscutting and undercutting nation-states' borders and boundaries can be felt. As the chapters in this volume show, religious and therapeutic/medical formations are crosscutting and undercutting national boundaries in Africa, and are shaping and are part of communities and institutional frameworks that transcend ideas of nation-state dominion. Disease is a transnational phenomenon as such (with the spread of HIV/AIDS as a prototypical example) and so is the medical regime that is curtailing and controlling it (Dilger *et al.* 2012). In this epilogue, I venture to highlight a number of themes that have emerged from the chapters in this volume and that are setting a new research agenda on why the interlinkage between the religious response to HIV/AIDS and the medical regime requires this transnational lens.

While globalisation is shaping economic, cultural and political processes through the expansion of markets, media, migration, exchange and communication, the rise of transnationalism relates to the formation of specific and direct connections that governments, institutions, social groups and individuals can establish across nation-states with induced distinctions in terms of identity, belonging, policies and interests. Whereas the process of globalisation is diffuse, dispersed, generic and based on broad patterns of influence, exchange and information, the analysis of transnationalism requires a much more profound exploration of how linkages work; who and what is being connected; and what the connecting across borders signifies for a particular setting or social formation. If we follow Basch *et al.*'s (1994: 7) definition of transnationalism as 'processes by which immigrants forge and sustain multi-stranded social relations that link together their societies of origin and settlement', we can note that the idea of a link across a border or a cultural, social or economic divide is crucial in the study of transnational processes. The difference between the study of globalisation and the study of transnationalism is thus located in distinguishing the level of entanglements that individuals, groups or institutions are engaging with and the way these entanglements set the terms and conditions under which links operate. The transnational perspective immediately sets a research agenda for the politics of connectivity (across borders of a political, economic or cultural nature) and the manner in which power is distributed in the face of all sorts of global processes (de Bruijn and van Dijk 2012). If we maintain the analytical distinction between transnationalism and globalisation, we can see that while each of these chapters deals with the global disease that AIDS is and the globalised (medical and religious) responses, they underscore the need to understand the nature and impact of the transnational linkages that are vital in the fight against it. The chapters all revolve around the experience of the transnational appearing as a source of ambiguous potential because these linkages transgress (socio-cultural, political) formations that are otherwise ideologically perceived as bounded and autonomous entities.

While this boundedness of the nation-state may not function particularly well, the experience of the transnational is one often fraught with sentiments ranging from fear to fascination, and from anxiety to hope and aspiration. One type of sentiment is what seems to be an anxiety related to the fear of the transgressive power of transnational connections. While individuals, institutions or governments may see the opportunities and potential benefits that a transnational connection can bring, these chapters interestingly describe a fear that is commonly typical of the national political establishment, national elites and national institutions. This is a fear best described as apprehension surrounding a loss of control that engaging with transnational actors (often donors) from elsewhere may bring, while the transnational connection can bring new resources. There is simultaneously a fear of embedded (unequal) hierarchies and expectations that can involve disempowerment and confrontations with structures emerging from elsewhere but effectively capable of having an impact on domestic affairs, policies and public debates. This is a fear of modern times and, in the case of Africa, of a relatively new experience (see Ferguson 1999).

Whereas the (political) elite are usually described as the class exhibiting what Bayart (2000) has called 'extraversion', i.e. an eagerness to engage with international contacts and resources, there is often an ambiguity among these elites about the nature and content of this connectivity. There is a gamut of transnational organisations capable of effectuating a boundary-crossing power that undercuts and crosscuts the dominion of the nation-state in ideological, moral and human-rights terms. These organisations include Amnesty International and Greenpeace but, in the context of this book, a variety of international AIDS agencies, women's groups and LGBT pressure groups too. Here it is usually the national (political) elites that express a kind of transnational anxiety, precisely because transnational effectiveness is based on the establishment of concrete linkages across boundaries and between individuals, organisations, institutions, modes of expression and resources in the pursuit of ideological-cum-structural changes. Especially in cases of protest, resistance and advocacy work, the transnational demonstrates the limitations of a nation-state's governmentality. The nation-state's hegemony is never complete, never total, never fully comprehensive, as James Scott (1985) demonstrated in a number of his works.

Transnational sentiment

The paradox here is that while nation-states, governments and political elites may be fearful of what transnational connections can do and may signify for the power of individuals, groups and communities in a nation-state, the experience of the transnational is marked by strong sentiments of the opposite. In fact, marginalised or disenfranchised groups can be anxious to engage in such transnational relations that may come to support their case or struggle. Local religious congregations and communities can be seen to be highly interested too in developing such linkages. In these situations their transnational anxieties may have more to do with the danger of losing a particular life-line that a transnational connection represents in terms of survival, access to resources and assistance, international recognition of one's plight and so forth. Transnational relations can thus involve critical and progressive engagement with the powers of the establishment and can be significant in fighting indifference towards their plight. This is indicated in the chapter by Ajibade who, as a (religiously inspired) activist herself, positions her work between Africa and the UK such that it becomes a vehicle for local organisations to reach platforms where their concerns may be expressed and, above all, heard. She is a representative of a London-based Anglican church but, through her local community work, has come to realise how important transnational relations have become for many of the people she is in contact with and has turned herself into a transnational activist with contacts in Africa as well.

What we learn from the contributions in this volume is that transnational sentiments are always pivotal and positional. They are pivotal because they revolve around the question of the relative transnational positioning of nation-states, (institutional) power holders/stakeholders and other (sometimes marginalised) groups in society that represent a particular interest. All of these revolve around transnational relations as producing sentiments of enthusiasm as well as fear. What is fearful for one may be eagerly pursued by the other group or body. They are positional in the sense of enhancing or reducing positions of power, authority and control. After all, the established powers in a nation-state can develop transnational connections that transcend the boundaries of the nation-state they aim to control.

Transnational connections, however, may not necessarily always be perceived as beneficial by other groups in society. In fact, they can easily develop transnational anxieties as well because such groups can become fearful of the connections that a nation-state may establish with powers elsewhere that are beyond the dominion of the state's territory. For example, the Ugandan government's connections with the US-initiated PEPFAR funding scheme, through which millions of US dollars flooded into the country for AIDS campaigns, developed into a formidable transnational relationship enhancing the power of the state, while its conservative moral and political influence was both welcomed and at the same time feared. One element of fear was that PEPFAR's moral agenda of encouraging abstinence and being faithful was a type of public campaigning, downplaying the availability of and access to condoms, since condoms were perceived in many Christian circles as antithetical to a disciplined sexuality. This created a fear of increased infection rates. Another anxiety of this transnational connection was the danger of hetero-normativity and the further marginalisation of sexual minorities in the country, especially in the gay community. On this point, the authors of Chapter 1 clearly state how religious moralities that travel along the transnational connection have tainted the public image of the religious groups involved in PEPFAR-sponsored campaigns by stating that it may represent:

> a linkage that we find deeply problematic since it seems to corroborate stereotyped ideas of what religion is doing in the context of AIDS and sexuality, while ignoring counter-movements among both Christian and Muslim communities and organisations aiming to move away from that conservatism and find new ways of approaching the moral dilemmas posed by HIV/AIDS.
>
> (Beckmann *et al.*, Chapter 1, pp. 3–4)

The explicit connections between players and agents that are thus fostered by transnational contacts have the potential for becoming more of a superimposition than an experience of the global, which can be more easily ignored. This is because the transnational connection provides for greater impact and regulation in the way it shapes and provides the conditions under which an interest, policy or resource becomes noticeable in terms of its local ramifications.

Emotions in the religious transnational connection

By discussing the strings attached to the transnational, this volume clearly demonstrates that the religious factor can deepen the experience and the sentiments attached to transnational connectivity. In a sense, the religious transnational connection of local congregations with larger outside religious actors places sentiments in more extreme positions. On the one hand, these sentiments may stress enthusiasm, hope and consolation regarding what the outside connection may bring, while on the other hand there are deep concerns, fears and anxieties about how connections may disrupt and disturb the local balance of power, moral agendas or religious interests. Ehrisman (Chapter 13) adds a deeply historical connotation to this perspective of the ambiguities of these sentiments by looking at how British missionaries among the Baganda emphasised a strict heteronormative moral landscape in which anxieties about same-sex relations were attributed to the 'perverse' influence of Arabs across the border from the missionary dominion. Ehrisman writes about these transnational sentiments *avant la lettre*:

> I argue that British missionaries proselytising in Buganda between 1875 and 1910 reconciled their metropolitan preconceptions about African sexuality as well as their own utopian visions for the region and its people with the same-sex relations they witnessed or heard about, by implicating 'decadent' Arabs as the importers of 'unnatural vice'. British missionaries somewhat opportunistically utilised and exacerbated anxieties about male–male sex to garner support from the colonial government during a time when a violent clash between religious sects (Catholics, Protestants and Muslims) compromised the Protestant missionary project.
>
> (Ehrisman, Chapter 13, p. 273)

This historical record shows that, in many cases, the transnational connection is starting to change the position and social (moral) location that a religious body occupies in the social fabric of the nation-state in Africa. In the cases of Zambia, Zimbabwe and Uganda, for example, the important and transnational connections that are part of the success of the popular Pentecostal churches in these countries have not only resulted in a different positioning of these religious groups *vis-à-vis* the former mainline missionary churches, but have also impacted on their upward socio-political mobility in the way they have become much closer to the political elite in these countries. Müller (Chapter 14) indicates how the missionary record of anxieties surrounding same-sex relations was not only continued with the arrival of the new transnational Pentecostal churches but was intensified when these churches clearly related to state policies in the field of HIV/AIDS:

> Uganda's widely extolled HIV/AIDS strategy and its internationally abhorred homophobic legislation are inextricably related, and [. . .] both can be traced back to transnational religious and conservative movements, most notably evangelical organisations in the United States and Uganda.
>
> (Müller, Chapter 14, p. 290)

From the perspective of the nation-state, the Abrahamic traditions of Christianity and Islam are marked by a long history and experience of crosscutting and undercutting cultural, political, social and economic boundaries and establishing links that connect individuals, communities and institutions across great distances and divides. Tocco (Chapter 15) alerts us to the fact that in this domain of religious transnationalism of Abrahamic traditions, pursuing transnational relations cannot and should not be equated with the adoption of Western identities, modes of organisation and an appreciation of various forms of sexual relationships:

> Scholarship on homosexuality and globalisation has focused overwhelmingly on how Western identities, discourses, and cultural productions affect non-Western people. Yet to the extent that homosexuality is 'othered' by Northern Nigerians, it is *Larabawa* (Arabs) who are more commonly professed to be its progenitors than *Turawa* (Europeans/Whites). That this is the case is unsurprising: Islam and other longstanding trade and cultural connections have meant that Middle Eastern influences are much more pronounced in Northern Nigeria than Western influences.
>
> (Tocco, Chapter 15, p. 322)

Yet Tocco indicates that, despite longstanding and developed transnational connections, Nigeria's LGBT groups receive limited financial and strategic support from organisations in the Islamic world and from organisations such as the International Gay and Lesbian Human Rights Commission, FBOs and other religious bodies in the West.

Even when an Africanisation of these Abrahamic traditions started to take place and led to a rise in the so-called Africa-initiated (or instituted) churches (AICs) or localised forms of Islam, these new churches and movements also began to spread across (post-)colonial boundaries, sweeping through wide areas of southern and West Africa. Churches like Maranke or the Masowe Apostles that originated in South Africa in the 1920s were not only the product of long-distance labour migration to the mines from present-day Malawi, Zambia and Zimbabwe, but began spreading to these regions and establishing branches there. In a sense, these religions are transnational and transcultural *par excellence* and their loyalty to any nation-state project concerning the creating of dominion over a particular territory and people has been only partial. While they may maintain their headquarters in South Africa where the church is organised, such religious transnational connections remain largely unscrutinised and beyond the control of nation-states in terms of resources, personnel, ideas/ideologies and moral agendas. Religious transnationalism has a long history in Africa and suggests a degree of fascination with what links may bring to the religious body and its sources of inspiration.

Within the religious context, transnationalism can still be fraught with ambiguities since the religious field allows for extensive contacts beyond nation-state borders in a myriad of ways, something the younger, Pentecostal, religious movements in and from Africa specialise in. The ways in which they use modern modes of communication, travel and media with ease have been well documented and this offers a thick tapestry of highly influential connections (van Dijk 2001, 2002, 2004; Englund 2003; Maxwell 2007). These connections are intricate in the sense that they are capable of reaching into the micro levels of everyday relations of ordinary members in their daily routines and concerns. Especially in the religious field, the transnational connection can be said to have arrived on members' doorsteps and this exposes them to links with fellow believers in other parts of the world in direct forms of exchange.

The exchange of moral views and agendas that may have a direct bearing on everyday decisions has become very immediate, much in the way some of the chapters in this volume demonstrate the choices related to HIV/AIDS treatment and care. Religion, in other words, seems to be able to bring the transnational connection, impact and influence closer to the individual than other types of transnational organisations can, basically because it generates so much sentiment. In Pentecostal meetings, messages are pre-eminently enveloped in emotional styles, in weeping, sobbing, electrifying moments of ecstasy and an outpouring of manifestations of the Holy Spirit. The moral messages never come without emotion, and visits by international leaders and other contacts are often displayed as moments of spiritual fervour. While medical practice and religion may not differ much in how they situate themselves in the intimate life spheres of members and/or patients, religious bodies *a priori* sentimentalise whatever message they may bring, including those relating to a transnatioanl connection or source. Mediating messages concerning HIV/AIDS and mediating (moral) concerns about safe-sex practices, abstinence, antiretroviral medicine (ARVs) or condom use are becoming more emotionally charged since sentiments surrounding these matters are seen to relate to much deeper existential truths than just the plight of the individual sufferer. They are often rephrased as directly impinging on the order of society or on any divine plan for the redemption of a community. The sentiments these concerns produce cannot easily be ignored and they make dialogue between religious adherents and biomedical practitioners difficult. The contributions in this volume not only highlight the existing sentiments of religion and its dealings with HIV/AIDS but also how transnational connections may deepen or fuel these emotions, as Müller has demonstrated for the case of homosexuality in Uganda.

Transnational competence

Given the dynamic of fear and fascination, anxiety and enthusiasm of transnational relations, this volume draws attention to the socially felt need for what I perceive as a 'transnational competence'. In many situations, and especially in the field of AIDS, experience has demonstrated that no engagement with transnational relations and connections can be pursued without specific skills and competences. While the notion of transnational competence comes close to what Bourdieu called 'cultural competence', there is a level of know-how involved that is not cultural but has to do with the technicalities of the pursuit, exploration and use of transnational connections. This know-how of procedures, policies and lines of communication is not evenly spread but positions individuals, groups, communities and institutions differently in this field. At the level of individuals, groups, institutions and even governments in the West that are exploring and setting up transnational links in Africa, there is a constant quest for knowledge, expertise, relevant contacts and for knowing what works. As Bartelink and Meinema (Chapter 8) demonstrate for the Netherlands, Dutch FBOs became interested in articulating partnerships with FBOs in the South in the late 1990s. This was partly inspired by the context of secularisation in the Netherlands and by the fact that the role of religion in development cooperation provided additional support. Svensson (Chapter 11) also shows how, in the context of the development of the South African NGO Positive Muslims, development agencies such as Oxfam Novib, USAID and UNAIDS contributed funds to the formulation of the organisation's 'theology of compassion'. This is a set of ideas and insights that helped shape interaction with AIDS policies, treatment and awareness campaigns in the context of Islam. The dynamics and politics surrounding claims of competence are usually formidable as access to resources is frequently directly dependent on the manner and extent to which transnational know-how can be demonstrated.

The contributions in this volume highlight how extremely important it is for individuals, groups and institutions in Africa to have transnational connections and foster specific transnational know-how. The creation of these competences pertains to many levels and dynamics, and it is knowledge about the transnational social field that is important in order to know who the players are, what the contacts and links are and require, and how to present oneself and demonstrate one's capacities, needs and weaknesses. Some of the chapters in this volume demonstrate how local individuals, groups and organisations forge skills in how to negotiate, mediate and accommodate the policies, messages, strictures and requirements of their transnational linkages so as to produce them in a way that is locally acceptable. In his study of the Positive Muslims, Svensson shows how an intellectualist approach to AIDS in the context of Islam was developed that fostered the ambition to accommodate authentic Islam with concepts and values associated with modernity. This has led to a high level of acceptance internationally whereby both condom use and sex education can be promoted within the Positive Muslims' agenda of a 'theology of compassion'. It is a 'way in which a shared "pool of resources" – the Qur'an, early Islam and established ethical principles – is applied in contemporary Muslim politics' (Svensson, Chapter 11, p. 229).

Transnational skills and competences can be viewed as being similar to those commonly attributed to brokers. The anthropology of brokerage (Mosse and Lewis 2006) does indeed show how Janus-faced local brokers usually need to be so as to skilfully position themselves *vis-à-vis* their local communities and the external partner to whom they are linked. On this dynamic, the authors in Chapter 1 point to the room for manoeuvre that needs to be created in view of the force by which transnational connections make their presence in the local situation felt:

> on the one hand, one can observe the presence of powerful transnational forces directing the development of HIV prevention programmes through the injection of large amounts of money and the design of universal, blueprint approaches to HIV interventions implemented across the globe; on the other hand, ethnographic research evidences the presence of a certain room for manoeuvre at the local level, where the universal, often oversimplifying messages contained in international policies are re-elaborated and negotiated to fit with local contexts.
>
> (Beckmann *et al.*, Chapter 1, p. 9)

Transnationalism does not exist without such brokerage. That said, the question is clearly what this means for the religious factor in a context of AIDS. The chapters show that this engagement of religion with the field of AIDS, involving international partners and contacts with governments and governmental policies, creates a special kind of brokerage that requires moral skills and competences in the first place. Obbo (Chapter 2) explains how, under the weight of the impact of PEPFAR funding in Uganda that emphasised an agenda of abstinence and being faithful but discouraged the promotion of condom use, 'Project designers became skilled in self-censoring their experiential grassroots knowledge in favour of condom marginalisation' (Obbo, Chapter 2, p. 39).

In addition to the obvious brokering of transnational relations as relating to access to (external) resources, ideas and personnel, these skills of transnational connectivity require what I would like to call 'moral brokering', especially in the religious domain. This is a notion of the mediation between different sets of moral values and ideas and of mediating the acceptance or rejection of certain moral agendas and programmes between different groups or institutional partners. FBOs, churches or other religious bodies in the West may, for example, have more liberal moral notions about sexuality than their partners in Africa, a situation that often requires them to engage in careful moral brokerage to avoid a total disconnect occurring in the partnership. In the field of HIV/AIDS, moral brokerage has been part of programmes aimed at behavioural change where, for example, the problem of how to convince the public domain of this form of morality where it is not common has become a serious matter of skills and competences for the religious groups concerned. As Sadgrove (Chapter 5) indicates by exploring the life of Pentecostal students on their campus in Kampala, this moral brokerage can be difficult and may lead to tensions since what people proclaim publicly about their (moral and sexual) conduct may be very different from what is happening in the more intimate domains of their lives. Sadgrove claims that a better understanding is required of 'how the management of such tensions relies on and produces moral strategies of concealment, and how such moral strategies and ethical systems are antagonised by and antagonise many of the transnational morality discourses that abound within Kampala' (Chapter 5, p. 108). In a sense, each of these students has learnt how to broker different antagonistic moral sets of values, something that living in a situation of AIDS and their involvement in a particular form of Christianity appear to require them to do. This volume sets a future research agenda of understanding about the transnational features of such skills and competences, and how, with religious involvement with disease and behavioural change, this know-how is directed towards the formation of effective moral brokerage.

Mobility and transnational relations

Discussing this level of skill and competence clarifies the transnational connections that are often part of striving towards upward social mobility, in addition to the geographical and political mobility that the term also implies. This expectation is bounded in sentiments of fear and fascination, anxiety and eagerness. Various chapters in this volume demonstrate that the anxiety surrounding the success of establishing transnational connections from the African perspective is often fostered by the prospect of new or better jobs or access to other resources that can provide upward social mobility. There is a class emerging in African societies that has positioned itself in these corners of upward social mobility by being or becoming prototypical AIDS workers, pastoral agents and community workers. While much of their social history still needs to be written, it is clear that the career ladder for many is constructed in a transnational dynamic. This is something that Patterson (Chapter 6), by referring to Bayart (2000), indicates as an 'extraversion' of a particular kind. Mobility is key to this extraversion, i.e. this orientation, not towards internal but external dynamics, partners and prospects. There is a constant 'moving on' that is marking the interlocking of mobility and transnational connections.

Whereas mobility is part and parcel of transnational relations, the question, especially in the African experience, is whether we need to focus on these forms of mobility as something extraordinary. Is mobility *a priori* to be perceived as unsettling to the lives of communities or individuals, as a process that is preferably avoided as it disturbs the common flow of the everyday? Yet the perception of being settled, staying put and being immobile as the natural or normal state of affairs seems counterintuitive and problematises mobility. It does not problematise settledness and being established. In other words, as problematised by de Bruijn *et al.* (2001), what if we de-centre movement and make movement a 'normal state of affairs'? What if we allow for the fact that being involved in mobility does not immediately foster sentiments of uneasiness in African settings but is instead embraced as something that may enrich, and not problematise, everyday existence? Is religious mobility, as it is being witnessed in the transnational movement in Africa, similar? Is it being embraced and not avoided?

The portability of religion and AIDS moralisation

Csordas (2009) has been exploring what he calls the (trans-)portability of religion, religious practices, ideologies and institutions in the current context of globalisation, arguing that successful religions foster portability. Their easy insertion into new cultural, political and economic contexts is often based on explicit attempts to render religious practice, ideology and institutions fit for adaptation into different national contexts. Pentecostals again excel here in explicitly fostering, managing and designing the portability of many of their practices, such as those related to healing and divine revelation, and practices relating to sharing and spreading of ideological messages and moral dictums. Pentecostals are renowned for the ease with which they introduce their ritual practices in different cultural contexts and in different socio-economic milieux, and seem to be able to make them relevant to the people concerned wherever they intend to establish their churches. Csordas (2009: 5) in this sense draws attention to what he calls the 'plasticity' of religious messages and practices, which means that Pentecostals entertain ideas of how to mould and shape these practices such that they become relevant to the context in which the faith is spreading either locally or internationally. The moralisation of AIDS has become part of this portability since religious practices and engagements (such as those of counselling, fellowship and deliverance) allow for easy adoption into any nation-state irrespective of the state's health policies, institutions and the like. Nation-states cannot therefore be conceived of as being containers of a 'national culture' or a 'national identity' and many religious formations in Africa are demonstrating and producing such plasticity to allow their messages to move and travel far and wide by not maintaining an 'iron-cage' notion of the nation-state either.

The chapters in this book recognise the portability of practice and ideology. It is an important contested reality and care must be taken not to perceive these forms of mobility as an extraordinary and/or unsettling condition. As has been argued elsewhere (de Bruijn *et al.* 2001), for many African societies, the mobility of people, objects and ideas is not an extraordinary condition but a profound daily reality. In a sense, what is much more a condition requiring exploration is what Appadurai (1995) called 'the production of locality', the idea of being settled and staying put. From this perspective, the transnational portabilities that religion and medical regimes may produce so forcefully should not be over-emphasised or made to appear as extraordinary phenomena that African societies need to adjust to. Instead, the opposite may be true, namely that the extent to which something or somebody resists mobility, exchanges extraversion for intraversion or resists engagement with the transnational may be in need of careful study. The non-transnational can *not* be taken for granted.

The contributions by Niehaus and Bochow (Chapters 9 and 12) speak profoundly to this experience. For Niehaus, the transportability of ideas and practices from elsewhere is hampered, if not obstructed, by a local emphasis on silence, total discretion and non-communication regarding intimate and sensitive matters, while much of the organisational engagement with AIDS expects speech and communication. This is a (local) form of anti-portability and intraversion that many of the transnational organisations involved in AIDS care and treatment run up against, and a form of anti-portability that is confrontational to the religious field involved. Silence does not foster upward social mobility since this would require AIDS workers to speak and communicate in order to do their jobs of testing, providing care and treatment effectively, something they now find difficult. The production of locality can thus develop into a serious force by making transnational brokerage impossible, by making the formation of a class of AIDS workers impossible since their role will not be acceptable, and by increasing resistance to the transmission of certain new ideas and moralities.

In Bochow's chapter, the de-centring of mobility is at stake since while the elite women she is dealing with seem cosmopolitan in orientation, they hold on securely to their upwardly mobile position, also with regard to the ways in which Pentecostalism and medical practice are relevant for them. They seem little interested in creating greater upward social mobility for others, or in turning the negotiation of infertility into a force for other women to engage in to achieve a better position in society. Again, as is the case in the chapter by Niehaus, infertility is a matter of silence (and shame) and stands diametrically opposed to the kind of extraversion that Patterson (Chapter 6) and Bayart (2000) attribute to the engagement with transnational organisations, their personnel, ideas and policies.

The transnational perspective of this book is fostering yet another future research agenda, one that focuses on how far the 'production of locality' is actually the result of transnational success. Can the ambiguities of transnational engagements be so extensive that certain communities, individuals or groups opt for a new kind of 'settledness', of 'splendid isolation' and an emphasis on locality that would otherwise not have existed. If the local cannot be taken for granted but requires explanation, and if containment (of local practices and ideas) becomes an effect of transnational portabilities of religious and medical practices, then what are the limitations of the transnational perspective? The answers that I suggest this volume offers fall into three groups that can best be captured by the words 'strings', 'strains' and 'strides'.

Conclusion: the strings, strains and strides of transnational connections

At the level of strings, this volume warns against a celebratory perception of transnationalism and points to the danger of a naïve appreciation of transnational engagement to and from Africa. Important strings can be attached, such as the insertion through transnational linkages of highly conservative public and moral agendas that may go against the interests of marginalised groups in society. An analysis of transnational mobilities, especially in the context of religion and AIDS, that does not pay due attention to the strings attached runs the risk of violating realities on the ground and of uncritically endorsing policies that were formulated under the weight of transnational interests.

Another important limitation of the transnational perspective can be overlooking or not recognising the strains that transnational connections can create for the local, for the workers, brokers and communities involved to live up to the expectations of external partners, donors and policies. The transnational perspective must acknowledge that extraversion is not always perceived as a plus, irrespective of the fact that transnational connections have become so much a part of the reality of people's everyday lives. Careful (social-science) analysis is required to determine how debilitating religious and medical transnational connections can become, how much input and effort such engagement may require, and how new inequalities and conflicts may result from these linkages in a local domain.

At the same time, we must acknowledge that transnational connections have allowed local people, organisations and institutions to take big steps forward in using religious linkages in the fight against AIDS and in changing notions of sexuality. This progress is sometimes hidden in the nooks and crannies of everyday life so that it is only visible from a bird's-eye transnational perspective. The limitation of this perspective can be that the transnational appears to dictate the kind of lens used to measure or describe what a particular transnational linkage has meant in the social fabric of the people concerned. Especially in sensitive fields such as AIDS and sexuality, the strides that have been accomplished in terms of improving conditions can require a lens that is not determined by the transnational connection itself. The contributions in this volume clarify how these strides can appear in unexpected places. Rasmussen (Chapter 7), for example, demonstrates how local staff learn to reshape, with masterful skill, the ethics of the Roman Catholic AIDS organisation and thereby make the transnational connection relevant in entirely new and ethical ways. Running against the official Roman Catholic apprehension of promoting condom use, and searching to embrace a global health perspective concerning ethical issues, local staff have created their own rationale when counselling clients. As Rasmussen states:

> I do not want to suggest that the counsellors are merely foot soldiers of a global health intervention. They themselves identify with and seem motivated by a wish to see their clients stay healthy and alive and to prevent new HIV infections [. . .]
>
> In fact, as mentioned earlier, abstinence was sometimes given as an option and so was the practice of reducing the frequency of sex (this was presented as a method to minimise the risk of re-infection), but mostly [. . .] the counsellors recommended condom use.
>
> (Chapter 7, pp. 147, 149)

In conclusion, the perspective on the strings, strains and strides of transnational connections that this book provides opens up a line of investigation that has, to date, lacked research into religious engagement with HIV/AIDS in Africa. This is a line of investigation that is lending shape to a future research agenda and one to which each of the chapters in this volume makes an important contribution.

References

Appadurai, A. 1995. 'The production of locality', in R. Fardon (ed.), *Counterworks: Managing the Diversity of Knowledge.* London: Routledge.

Basch, L., N. Glick Schiller and C. Blanc-Szanton. 1994. *Nations Unbound: Transnational Projects, Postcolonial Predicaments and Deterritorialized Nation-States*. New York: Gordon & Breach.

Bayart, J.-F. 2000. 'Africa in the world: a history of extraversion', *African Affairs* 99(395): 217–67.

Csordas, T.J. 2009. 'Modalities of transnational transcendence', in T.J. Csordas (ed.), *Transnational Transcendence: Essays on Religion and Globalization*. Berkeley: University of California Press.

De Bruijn, M. and R. van Dijk (eds) 2012. *The Social Life of Connectivity in Africa.* Basingstoke: Palgrave Macmillan.

De Bruijn, M., R. Van Dijk and D. Foeken (eds) 2001. *Mobile Africa: Changing Patterns of Movement in Africa and Beyond.* Leiden: Brill.

Dilger, H., A. Kane and S. Langwick (eds) 2012. *Medicine, Mobility, and Power in Global Africa.* Bloomington: Indiana University Press.

Englund, H. 2003. 'Christian independency and global membership: Pentecostal extraversions in Malawi', *Journal of Religion in Africa* 33(1): 83–111.

Ferguson, J. 1999. *Expectations of Modernity: Myths and Meanings of Urban Life on the Zambian Copperbelt.* Berkeley: University of California Press.

Glick Schiller, N. 2005. 'Transnational social fields and imperialism: bringing a theory of power to transnational studies', *Anthropological Theory* 5(4): 439–61.

Malkki, L. 1992. 'National geographic: rooting of peoples and the territorialization of national identity among scholars and refugees', *Cultural Anthropology* 7(1): 24–44.

Maxwell, D. 2007. *African Gifts of the Spirit: Pentecostalism and the Rise of a Zimbabwean Transnational Religious Movement.* Athens, OH: Ohio University Press.

Mosse, D. and D. Lewis. 2006. 'Theoretical approaches to brokerage and translation in development', in D. Lewis and D. Mosse (eds), *Development Brokers and Translators: The Ethnography of Aid and Agencies*. Bloomfield, CT: Kumarian Press.

Osaghae, E.E. 2007. 'Fragile states', *Development in Practice* 17(4/5): 691–9.

Rotberg, R. 2003. *State Failure and State Weakness in a Time of Terror*. Washington, DC: Brookings Institute Press.

Scott, J.C. 1985. *Weapons of the Weak: Everyday Forms of Peasant Resistance*. New Haven, CT: Yale University Press.

Van Dijk, R. 2001. 'Time and transcultural technologies of the self in the Ghanaian Pentecostal diaspora', in A. Corten and R. Marshall-Fratani (eds), *Between Babel and Pentecost: Transnational Pentecostalism in Africa and Latin America*. London/ Bloomington: Hurst Publishers/Indiana University Press.

Van Dijk, R. 2002. 'Religion, reciprocity and restructuring family responsibility in the Ghanaian Pentecostal diaspora', in D. Bryceson and U. Vuorella (eds), *The Transnational Family: New European Frontiers and Global Networks*. Oxford: Berg.

Van Dijk, R. 2004. 'Ghanaian identities in the transnational domain', in W.M.J. van Binsbergen and R.A. van Dijk (eds), *Situating Globality: African Agency in the Appropriation of Global Culture*. African Dynamics Series 3. Leiden: Brill.

Index